CAN YOU CATCH A
COLD?

Untold History &
Human Experiments

DANIEL ROYTAS
Foreword by Dr Samantha Bailey

Disclaimer

The information contained within this book is for general information and education purposes only. It is not a substitute for professional advice. Before taking any actions based upon such information, consult with a suitably qualified professional. The use of or reliance on any information contained within this book is solely at your own risk.

Acknowledgements

Dr J.A. – Thank you for truly understanding what this book is all about—I don't think I could have found a better editor-in-chief. Your ability to take an ordinary piece of writing and transform it into something great is unparalleled. I am forever grateful for the time, care, and attention you have invested in this undertaking. Without your honesty, persistence, and patience this work would not be half of what it has become.

Dr Sam Bailey – Despite facing considerable adversity over the last four years, you continue charging forward. Your tireless and unwavering efforts have inspired and motivated me to do the same. Thank you for being a beacon of hope for humanity. My excitement was palpable when you agreed to write the foreword. Your words will undoubtedly leave a lasting impression on those who read them. I am honoured to have been able to work with you on this project.

Dr Mark Bailey – I was thrilled when you offered to edit this book. Words cannot express how indebted I am for the sheer amount of time and effort you spent meticulously reviewing and critiquing my manuscript. Your encouragement and support is nothing short of a blessing. You have not only helped shape this book but my life as an independent researcher.

Roman Bystrianyk – Never in my wildest dreams did I think I'd be collaborating with an accomplished author like yourself. Thank you for giving me the idea to write this book, as well as reviewing and editing it. I am truly humbled by how generous you have been with your time to help a fledgeling author. Without your superb guidance, genius mind, and literary prowess, this piece of work would not have been possible.

P.H. – Your expertise as a virologist and microbiologist has been instrumental in ensuring the information presented herein is accurate, informative, and engaging. Thank you for taking the time to thoroughly review and critique my work. Your dedication towards making this book a reality is appreciated more than you know.

Dr Jordan Grant – Few people in this world have an intricate comprehension of logic, reasoning, epistemology, and the scientific method quite like you. There are even fewer who can teach these concepts in a way that can be easily understood. I consider it a privilege to have learned so much from you. Thank you for reviewing this book and for continuing to challenge the status quo.

Emrys Goldsworthy – Having you as someone to confide in, bounce ideas off, and seek guidance from has been pivotal in the development of this text. Never let go of your willingness to question long-held beliefs and your desire to challenge clinicians about theirs. Your support and friendship means the world to me.

B.R. – I have decided to save the best till last. For all of the long days and nights you spent by my side formatting, proofreading, and cheering me on—thank you. This journey would have been infinitely more difficult and considerably less enjoyable without your moral support, unconditional love, and friendship. Thank you for believing in me.

Table of Contents

Foreword

By Dr Samantha Bailey

Can you catch a cold? When I was a doctor in the 'mainstream' system, I would have dismissed this question as folly. Why ask such a question when every doctor knows that contagion (the transmission of disease by 'germs') had been proven by medical science long ago? However, like almost all of these doctors, there was something I neglected to do: look at the claimed evidence for myself. When I opened that door, a dramatic cascade of events unfolded, starting with being fired from a network television role and then being blocked from my clinical work as a doctor. There were even gag-orders and ongoing prosecution attempts by the so-called authorities as I communicated my new-found discoveries to the world. Challenging the medical establishment can be risky, but from my point of view, I have never looked back.

So, when I was approached to write a foreword for this book, I was delighted to be aligned with another fully independent researcher and dissident. My husband, Mark, and I have known Daniel Roytas for a couple of years, but it has always felt like we were old friends. Our journeys were similar to Daniel's, and in retrospect, it was natural that our paths would be brought together. We all received years of formal university education in the natural sciences and eagerly absorbed the material. Like most students, we assumed that the theories we were being taught were nothing less than rock-solid scientific facts. In fact, when I was at medical school and then a practising doctor, I did not know that questioning contagion or the concept of 'pathogens' was even a thing.

That worldview came crashing down in early 2020 with the onset of the COVID-19 era. Many of us instantly felt that something was wrong with the narrative being promulgated and it triggered a drive to start scratching beneath the surface. The initial step was letting go of everything we thought we knew, whether it be the concept of contagion, disease, infection, 'germs' and even the very existence of particles known as 'viruses'. It was the first time we examined the source documents and foundational scientific publications for ourselves and what we found was truly astounding. For me personally, one of the greatest shocks was the consistent experimental failures to demonstrate the transmission of influenza between individuals. The 500-page textbook of influenza in our collection conveniently omitted such facts and the authors simply asserted that it is a contagious entity through epidemiological data and other indirect 'evidence'.

It is important to state at the outset that the occurrence of people getting sick in clusters is not being denied by the author. As is pointed out in this outstanding book you are reading, conditions such as scurvy and pellagra were once thought to be contagious diseases because groups of people would experience the same symptoms at the same time. Only later was it 'discovered' that these conditions were the result of nutritional problems. (I put 'discovered' in quotation marks because sometimes when one searches historical records it is evident that the causes had been described long before.) People are also affected by others in numerous ways and this book documents fascinating 'outbreaks' of illness due to psychological factors alone, a phenomenon that is all too often ignored.

As for the special 'Common Cold Unit' (CCU) that operated over many decades until 1989, we can only conclude that the experimental results were not exactly what was expected by the germ and virus enthusiasts. Perhaps this is the reason why the history of the unit remains unknown to the vast majority of health professionals. As Daniel observed, although the CCU is reported to have discovered, 'more than 100 common cold viruses', there was a fatal flaw in every single one of them—a lack of adequate controls and insufficient methodologies to demonstrate an independent variable. In effect, a complete failure to provide any evidence that the infectious particles they were reportedly finding even existed! The question of what causes colds and flu (and by inference, other 'infectious' diseases) is one of the most important of the current era.

The claim, or more importantly the belief, that they are caused by germs has resulted in widespread lockdowns, severe infringements on human rights, and the mass deployment of both old and new pharmaceuticals.

If the germ hypothesis is incorrect, then it is clear that there is no possible excuse for this kind of oppressive behaviour which has forced the world into psychological and economic hardship. Without a doubt, the fear of contagion and being made sick by others has been used to drive the self-destructive behaviour we have witnessed during the COVID-19 era. Additionally, the collapse in such beliefs would mean the collapse of vaccines, 'anti-viral' drugs, and a large section of the medico-pharmaceutical industry, not to mention numerous so-called public health institutions. With so much at stake, we cannot expect the vested interests to let this debate happen on a level playing field. That is why books like this are taking the information directly to the public so they can see the state of the science for themselves.

This book is a vital contribution in its field. While there are dozens of interviews, podcasts and forums discussing the common cold and the concept of contagion, there are few formally written treatises dealing with the subject in such a complete and extensively referenced manner. Daniel is a natural teacher and he does not tell you what to conclude. Instead, he invites the reader to look into the facts for themselves. He has done the hard work finding and analysing all the relevant studies and they are summarised in a concise and easy-to-understand manner. Everything is carefully cited so there is no doubt about the facts in this revealing and enjoyable read. Following his extensive research over the past few years, it is clear that Daniel himself is genuinely astounded that the 'science' that has been espoused by the most famous institutions in the world is decidedly tenuous. I hope that, like me, you find some life-changing information in these pages which brings about a better understanding of health and wellbeing for you and your loved ones.

Dr Samantha Bailey
Medical Doctor, Content Creator, and Health Educator
Her books include Virus Mania, Terrain Therapy & The Final Pandemic
www.drsambailey.com

Preface

By Daniel Roytas

Almost 20 years ago, I attended a lecture on immunology as part of my undergraduate degree in naturopathic medicine. This class was just like any other until the teacher brought up an unfamiliar concept that was not mentioned anywhere in the prescribed textbook—the *terrain theory*. They professed there is an understanding, held by practitioners of natural medicine, that germs are not the *cause* of disease, but are in fact, the *consequence* of it. This assertion seemed rather preposterous because it contradicted my belief that the germ theory had been proven long ago by men like Louis Pasteur, Robert Koch, and Joseph Lister. I gave no further thought to this fantastical idea and continued my studies in blissful ignorance.

In the years that followed, I opened a clinical practice, obtained various post-graduate qualifications, and worked as a lecturer and senior lecturer of naturopathic and nutritional medicine at educational institutions around Australia. For the next decade, I taught university and college undergraduate students about the prevention and management of infectious diseases with nutritional, herbal, and lifestyle interventions. Then, in early 2020, I heard several doctors and scientists making claims similar to the ones my immunology lecturer had made all those years prior—that *germs don't cause disease.* Although their words resonated with me, I wanted to appraise the literature myself, to see if there was any validity to these newfound revelations.

I began systematically searching through the medical and historical literature for experiments demonstrating human-to-human disease transmission. My investigation also extended to experiments that proved germs are capable of infecting a healthy host and causing illness. Within 18 months, I had amassed a repository of hundreds of scientific journal articles. To my astonishment, not a single one contained a scientific experiment verifying either of these phenomena (i.e. infection or contagion). This lack of evidence came as quite a surprise, considering infection and contagion are touted as irrefutable facts. It wasn't long before people started becoming aware of the work I was doing. As fate would have it, one of those people was Roman Bystrianyk, co-author of *Dissolving Illusions: Disease, Vaccines, and the Forgotten History*. In late 2022, he suggested that I compile the results of the papers I had accumulated into a book. At that time, I was already working on another book dismantling common misconceptions plaguing the field of nutrition. However, given the state of worldly affairs, I realised this new undertaking was far more important and deserving of my time.

No sooner had Roman made this suggestion, than the work on *Can You Catch A Cold?* began. My initial aim was to tabulate the results of the studies I had accrued into a booklet. However, I noticed that in several experiments, healthy participants became sick after direct contact with sick people or being inoculated with their bodily fluids. Given the lack of evidence demonstrating these ill effects were caused by a pathogen (i.e. a bacteria or virus), I decided to dig deeper to see if other plausible explanations existed. It was at this point I realised a booklet wasn't going to do this topic justice. As it turns out, many brilliant scientists and doctors have proposed all kinds of ideas over the last century about why we seem to catch colds and flu. The problem is that very few people know about these alternative explanations because they have been overshadowed by the prevailing theory on germs—*until now*. This book not only highlights failed contagion experiments, but brings these forgotten ideas to the forefront of a debate that has never been more deserving of humanity's attention—*the terrain versus germ theory*.

Approach this book with an open heart and an open mind. May it help you unlock a new realm of possibilities.

Daniel Roytas
Author & Educator

Part 1

Untold History

Chapter 1

Introduction

C an you catch a cold? If you asked this question to everyday people, chances are the vast majority would answer something along the lines of, *"Of course you can,"* whilst giving you a strange look for asking something so obvious. But what if you ignored their puzzled glare and probed further, asking how they knew this to be true? No doubt, they would offer up personal tales as proof, recounting times they had caught a cold or flu themselves. Maybe it was from snotty-nosed kids who brought a cold home from school, or from an inconsiderate co-worker who spread their flu around the office. Others might offer more elaborate explanations of how sick people infect healthy people with disease-causing germs. Although these kinds of answers seem reasonable on the surface, they are limited in obvious ways. These anecdotes certainly do not prove you can catch a cold or flu, nor do they adequately account for how it happens. It seems—as is the case in many walks of life—that people hold beliefs they cannot justify with supporting evidence *or* explain in sufficient detail. Why, then, are they so strongly convinced they can catch a cold?

Well, from an early age, we are taught to believe in the concept of contagion—that a cold or flu can be *caught* from another person. Those in positions of authority like parents, teachers, doctors, scientists, and government officials all reinforce the same story to us: when people are sick, they spread disease-causing germs to others. Accordingly, we are warned to keep a safe distance from anyone who has symptoms, in the hope we can evade their germs and avoid *catching their disease*. We go out into the world equipped with this understanding, before eventually coming into close contact with a sick person. A few days later, we fall ill with the same symptoms. This experience confirms the story we were told and solidifies our beliefs about germs and contagion. We are sufficiently convinced by this model of reality that we spend the rest of our lives in fear of an invisible enemy and wary of our fellow man. We become so invested in this worldview that few of us ever think to give it a second thought, let alone question it. Anyone who does is likely labelled conspiratorial and heretical, which adds even more social pressure to conform to the tale of contagion.

With such societal weight and cultural momentum behind this story, one would assume good evidence and explanations for contagion exist, even if the average person cannot provide them. But, as we will come to learn throughout this book, the available scientific support is lacking or contradictory, and the current explanatory models are inconsistent or incomplete. More generally, it is deeply problematic how little people—even qualified health professionals—know about this topic, despite being utterly convinced of it and willing to structure their entire lives around it. So, to remedy these issues, let's imagine an alternate reality for a moment. One where we have all the necessary information to form our own understanding, rather than blindly accepting what the authorities profess. This world is better on two fronts. First, we have a more complete and accurate knowledge of the truth. Second, we are more empowered and self-determined because we can make up our own minds, instead of having them made for us. It would put us in the best position to appraise the dominant paradigm. At the same time, however, this alternative world also contains an uncomfortable possibility—one of *disillusion*. Whilst we may discover that the enduring and widespread story of germs and contagion is invalid, it would allow us to find a better explanation to account for why people *seem* to catch a cold. Though this might be shocking, the uncertainty would only be temporary and, ultimately, for the best. The role of this book is to bring about this new reality by giving you the information you need to dismantle the current one.

The World's Dirtiest Man

In orienting you to the issues that plague germ theory and contagion, consider Amou Haji, a 94-year-old Iranian who held the title of "World's Dirtiest Man". For 67 years, Haji *never* set foot in a bathroom and avoided soap and water because he was worried it would make him sick. Haji was so averse to bathing, he once jumped from a moving vehicle when concerned townsfolk tried to take him to a local river for a bath. Not only that, but Haji lived in absolute squalor. His residence was a run-down shack located on the outskirts of the city of Dejgah, Iran. It was dusty, rusty, exposed to the elements, and crawling with wildlife. He survived on a diet of fresh roadkill, consisting mainly of uncooked (and tragically tenderised) porcupine, which he collected from the roadside. Every day, Haji smoked animal dung from a pipe and sourced water from muddy puddles, which he drank out of an old oil can. Not only was Haji dirty on the outside, but much of this dirt also found its way inside him, too.[1-3]

Science would have us believe this lack of personal hygiene, poor diet, and questionable lifestyle habits would weaken Haji's immune system, making his body the perfect breeding ground for the deadly germs he would undoubtedly ingest and inhale. This belief, however, was disproven after scientists ran a battery of tests on Haji several years before he died. Not only did the scientists fail to find any pathogens, but they discovered—much to everyone's surprise—that he was in a decidedly good state of health. Given these findings, it was a rather cruel and ironic twist when Haji died in late 2022, one month after local villagers forced him to take a shower.

Following Amou Haji's death, the title of "World's Dirtiest Man" was bestowed upon Kailash Singh, an Indian man from the city of Varanasi. Singh, now aged 77, has not showered for almost 50 years 'out of love for his country'. Every evening, Singh opts for a 'fire bath' instead, which involves standing on one leg, lighting a bonfire, smoking marijuana, and praying to Lord Shiva.[1-3] Again, these unconventional hygiene practices (if you can even call them that) are a far cry from what mainstream medicine advocates to maintain a healthy and disease-free existence. Yet, Singh, like his predecessor Haji, has managed to escape the clutches of infectious germs and disease.

So how is it that men like Haji and Singh can live a lifestyle contrary to the best health advice and, against all odds, remain in a good state of health well into old age? How are their immune systems strong enough to protect them against germs when they do nothing to support their immunity (and, indeed, actively undermine it)? Strong immunity is supposedly attained by eating healthy food, washing frequently, exercising, having access to proper housing and plumbing, limiting exposure to unsanitary conditions, and abstaining from substances like cigarettes and alcohol. Given this, how is it possible that Haji, Singh, and others like them can live in filth, drink contaminated water, and share a bed with some of the most infectious organisms, yet waltz through life largely unaffected? There are two broad possibilities: (1) they are both *freaks* of nature whose constitutions defy our current understanding of germs, or (2) they are *normal* humans, and our current understanding of germs desperately needs updating.

Long-Standing Questions

Critics have argued fervently for the latter possibility since the late 19th century by challenging contagion and germ research. One exceptional example is Dr John E. Walker, who published a paper titled *"The Etiology of Colds"* in a leading medical journal in 1932.[4] At the time, several researchers had conducted experiments apparently demonstrating human-to-human transmission of influenza and the common cold.[5-10] Their experimental methods were simple, in principle. They obtained respiratory mucus from a person suffering a cold or flu. They then filtered the mucus to remove any particulate matter or bacteria. Finally, they instilled this filtered mucus (known as a *filtrate*) into the nose, throat, eyes, or mouth of healthy volunteers. In some instances, the researchers injected the filtrate intramuscularly (into the muscle), subcutaneously (under the skin), or intravenously (directly into the bloodstream). When healthy recipients developed flu-like symptoms, the researchers concluded a contagious virus was responsible.[4]

In response to this research and its claims, many doctors, like John Walker, were sceptical. As Dr Walker stated in his critique of the emerging field of virology, *"such assertions are full of pitfalls"*. He was particularly critical of human experiments claiming to have demonstrated contagion because they failed to define what a cold was, or what constituted successful transmission of the disease. Also, he noted *none* of the studies used proper controls, which is problematic for several reasons. First, inoculating even inert substances into the nasal passages is known to cause cold and flu-like symptoms by irritating the mucous membranes. Second, the symptoms produced by inoculated filtrate could also reflect various inflammatory or allergic-type responses, so they were not necessarily proof of a viral infection. Third, the power of suggestion is large enough for participants receiving a saline placebo to develop a cold merely because they believe they have been inoculated with a filtrate. Finally, there are many other substances contained in the mucus secretions of sick people, any number of which could produce cold and flu-like symptoms. It is for these reasons, among others, that Dr Walker considered the results of human contagion studies allegedly demonstrating person-to-person transmission of the common cold to be unreliable.[4] Most of the shortcomings he highlighted have not been addressed since they were published over a century ago, which is why they continue to be raised by doctors and scientists.[11-14]

Indeed, Walker was far from the only one to question the lack of evidence for contagious germs. Many others have publicly challenged the official story over the last century.[15-23] Like Walker, they highlighted the absence of human experiments that delineate person-to-person transmission of respiratory illnesses.[24,25] As you will find out in later chapters, this is not for lack of trying. Dozens of unsuccessful attempts have been made trying to transmit the common cold and influenza from the sick to the well—more than 200 of which will be covered in this book. Even modern epidemiological data are inconsistent with the theory of an infectious particle spreading between people.[17,25,26] For example, despite decades of intense research, epidemiologists cannot reliably predict the timing and severity of cold and flu outbreaks using virus-based models.

More recently, these sorts of gaps and inconsistencies prompted several well-credentialed, highly experienced, and widely respected members of the academic and medical communities to systematically appraise the scholarly literature on germs. They wanted to get to the bottom of this issue, so they reviewed the available evidence (as of the early 2020s) supporting the claim that the cold and flu are caused by respiratory viruses and that these viruses are passed from sick people to healthy people. What they uncovered would shake the field of infectious disease to its core.[11,12,14,27,28]

Their findings can be summarised into *three* main points;

1. **Viruses do not cause disease.** There is an *absence* of direct evidence demonstrating a cause-and-effect relationship between viruses and infectious diseases.

2. **Viruses are not contagious.** Few, if any, published scientific studies have unambiguously established sick-to-well transmission (i.e. contagion) of *any* infectious disease.

3. **Viruses may not even exist.** No published scientific studies have ever truly isolated a *pure* sample of a virus and then documented its characteristics.

Taken together, these points undermine the current understanding of germs and contagion. They argue we simply do not have enough high-quality scientific evidence to support a model wherein contagious pathogens cause disease. In their book *"The Final Pandemic"*, Dr Samantha Bailey and Dr Mark Bailey drive these points home in an exemplary critique of the germ theory.[29]

Unsurprisingly, word spread quickly about these bold assertions. The novel and somewhat controversial perspectives shared by these doctors and scientists captured the attention of millions of people worldwide. Meanwhile, the claims polarised the scientific and medical community, generating significant debate. Although several institutions were quick to dismiss the claims outright,[30-32] they nevertheless piqued the interest of many other doctors,[33] scientists,[13] statisticians,[34] and independent journalists.[35-37] These professionals were all left wondering, *"Where is the evidence germs cause disease?"* This same line of questioning has now been levied for almost 150 years. Yet, for reasons unknown, mainstream institutions have largely ignored the constructive criticisms, opposing views, and results of scientific experiments contradicting germ theory and contagion.[38-47] As it stands, we still do not have good answers to these long-standing questions.

New Understandings

At first, it might seem preposterous for anyone, especially medical doctors, microbiologists, epidemiologists, and virologists, to ever challenge the currently accepted theory about the cause of the cold and flu. You could be forgiven for dismissing this line of inquiry as uneducated, narrow-minded, or downright delusional. But historically, there have been plenty of things we have been wrong about, like the safety of cigarettes,[48] asbestos,[49] thalidomide,[50] and lead.[51] What about when we wrongly believed depression was caused by a serotonin imbalance,[52] that cholesterol and saturated fat caused heart disease,[53,54] or that sodium was solely responsible for the hypertensive effects of table salt?[55] In the not-so-distant past, doctors thought lobotomies were the cure for schizophrenia and other mental maladies,[56] that mercury could treat syphilis,[57] and that bloodletting was an appropriate intervention for the common cold.[58] Of course, it is now unfathomable to think these interventions were once considered 'settled science' and common practice in the field of medicine. Imagine if those who opposed these ideas were dismissed as 'science deniers', publicly ridiculed, beaten into intellectual submission, and forced into silence. We might still be blindly following these archaic ideas today, and many more people would have been injured, killed, or forced to suffer needlessly. If no one dared to challenge the consensus, we would never have been able to advance our understanding and progress forward as a society.

Rightfully so, challenges to science continue to happen on many fronts. For instance, some scientists argue cellular structures like the Golgi apparatus, endoplasmic reticulum, unit membrane, nuclear pores, and membrane receptors are simply artefacts that result from preparing tissue samples for electron microscopy.[59-65] If what these scientists say is true, it would disrupt the entire field of microbiology and virology as we know it. Without these cellular structures, it would be impossible for viruses, microorganisms, and white blood cells to work the way they are claimed to. In this way, the current scientific understanding is always contested and updated, as it should be. Given this, what else will we look back on years from now and wonder how we got it so wrong? Even Thomas Rivers, the man who created *River's Postulates* (a set of rules that, if satisfied, would establish a cause-and-effect relationship between viruses and infectious disease), admitted his postulates will one day become *obsolete*.[66] The only way such a thing could ever happen is if people dare to ask questions, criticise theories, and propose new ones.

Revising our understanding of widely accepted concepts is a natural and necessary part of the scientific process. It happens all the time, like when new research emerged against the safety of cigarettes, thalidomide, and lead additives. Guess what happened when science challenged these long-standing beliefs and practices? Despite initial resistance, people eventually accepted it and moved on once the truth came to light. We made the necessary changes and proceeded with our lives in a better direction. In this way, humanity is incredibly adaptive and resilient. Likewise, if we are wrong about germs, who's to say people won't simply shrug their shoulders and carry on with a new and improved understanding as if nothing had ever changed? It is possible, but we are getting ahead of ourselves. Before society can course-correct, we first need to lay out all the pieces of the puzzle and see how they may (or may not) fit together. This book will accomplish this by addressing *three* aims.

Aim #1: Joining the Dots

Remember playing connect-the-dots as a child? Drawing the pictures was relatively straightforward. No guesswork was involved because each little black dot peppered across the page was individually numbered. All you had to do was draw lines between the dots in sequential order and, before long, you would produce a clear and recognisable image on the page before you. Now, this process is straightforward precisely because you are given enough *detail* (i.e. dots) and *guidance* (i.e. numbers) to arrive at a solution. But, without either one of these, it would be much harder (if not impossible) to complete the puzzle. In other words, you cannot see the 'bigger picture' without some minimum number of data points and enough information about how they relate to one another. So, if you turned to a page that contained just four dots, it might seem reasonable to connect them into a square. However, it's entirely possible the correct answer was a circle—or something far more complex—yet you simply didn't have enough detail and guidance at your disposal to deduce this.

Now, when it comes to infectious diseases like the cold and flu, people assume science has identified all of the dots, numbered them, and connected them in the proper order. But, as discussed earlier, these same people aren't aware of the available evidence (dots), nor can they provide a satisfactory explanation (numbers), so they're unknowingly and incorrectly drawing whatever picture they want. Even if they did have access to the research, the science is limited in both *perspective* (i.e. it presents a one-sided view) and in *method* (i.e. it is noisy and confounded). Given this state of affairs, the first aim of this book is to set the record straight by laying out a raft of overlooked evidence and alternative explanations so you, the reader, can arrive at an informed understanding of how people get sick. For this reason, the book is extensively cited, drawing on over 1,000 citations. Every effort has been made to obtain information from sources such as academic journals, scientific textbooks, and official news articles. A virologist and microbiologist, several medical doctors, and a psychologist were also engaged to review this book to ensure the accuracy of the information being put forward. Across the chapters, you will accrue enough 'dots' and 'numbers' to be able to join them together and form your own bigger picture.

Critically, on this last point, the book will not tell you what to think. It does not claim germs do not exist, nor does it claim that germs cannot infect a healthy person and cause disease. Neither does it make any medical claims (and, therefore, no person should take any of the information presented within these pages as medical advice or use it to inform decisions they make about their health). Instead of telling you *what* to think, it is simply getting you *to think*, and giving you the materials to do so. The book strives to be as impartial as possible, erring on the side of neutrality by presenting a balanced, well-rounded overview of a topic that has never been more relevant. Please take the information presented herein as a resource and starting point to draw your own conclusions from.

Aim #2: Asking Hard Questions

In the same spirit, the title of this book is deliberately posed as a question (i.e. 'Can you catch a cold?'), rather than a statement (i.e. 'You can't catch a cold'). Though the latter is provocative and has far more potential to gain attention, it is making an outright claim, which is a perilous task that requires new research to substantiate it. On the other hand, asking a question is not only simpler but more effective in the long run. It invites curiosity and promotes dialogue, rather than creating adversaries. It also implies a broader point about the degree of uncertainty surrounding contagion. As such, this book does not claim either side of the argument (i.e. terrain vs germ theory) is right or wrong because, for all we know, *both* sides of the debate could be incorrect. If we align ourselves too closely with one paradigm, we might overlook some far more important concepts. After all, the human body is incredibly complex, so we must constantly update our understanding of its functions and how it interacts with the outside world. There is so much we still do not know, so getting too attached to any one idea might impact our ability to see things clearly.

With all of this in mind, it is critical to practice humility and accept that we might be wrong about long-standing and commonly held beliefs, like what causes a case of the sniffles. Can anyone say with 100% certainty the currently accepted theory about contagion is true and correct? Certainly not. Therefore, scientists and the public must keep the channels of discussion open so a lively and intellectual discourse can take place *without* fear of reprisal or judgment. If something else is responsible for causing these seasonal ailments, surely the world would want to know about it. But the only way to make new discoveries and confirm or invalidate our current understanding is to think outside the box, ask questions, and engage in discussions—precisely what this book seeks to promote.

Accordingly, the second aim of this book is to encourage you to ask difficult questions more generally in your life. There are many instances where we acquire basic knowledge from our parents, school, institutions, or popular media and then carry this forward with us—completely unchanged—until we die (or are fortunate enough to be disillusioned). These imperfect 'models of reality' become entrenched and rigid across the population. This is not to say all commonly held views are wrong, but that we should be cautious in holding ideas so confidently just because they are familiar and approved. Modern society places a great deal of trust in authorities to provide true and accurate information. But what if these sources of truth are corrupted or misguided? What if they have ulterior motives or vested interests? What if they are simply wrong? We should follow the data into the unknown, rather than attack people or silence ideas in the hopes of clinging to false certainty. Reading this book will inspire healthy scepticism and invite you to interrogate any idea considered too sacred or comfortable.

Aim #3: Opening up to Possibility

While people hold ideas—such as contagion—with such certainty, it is also well known that the potential of the mind and body are far greater than we currently comprehend. Throughout history, men and women have achieved truly incredible and seemingly superhuman feats by harnessing the power contained within.[67-69] For instance, the world record for deadlifting is 524 kilograms. While this lift is mind-boggling in itself, there are also documented cases of mothers lifting cars weighing more than 1,500 kg off their children who were involved in an accident.[70] How are such extraordinary displays of strength possible? Well, that's the mystery. We do not yet know. But there is a profound mind-body connection we have only scratched the surface of (and must remain open to). What's more, this isn't only reserved for other-worldly strength—it can affect everyday functions. Several studies have shown that just imagining lifting weights can yield results that are comparable to performing actual exercise.[71,72] Similarly, although it is believed humans can only go without oxygen for a matter of minutes, free divers can hold their breath underwater for around 25 minutes, while reaching depths of 250 metres.[73,74]

The untapped power of the body and mind also relates to illness and wellness. A group of young men allergic to Japanese lacquer or 'wax trees' (which produces an effect similar to poison ivy) were touched on one arm with the leaves of a harmless plant but were told it was the wax tree. On the other arm, they were touched with the leaves of the wax tree but were told it was the harmless plant. Of the 13 participants, just two (13%) had an adverse skin reaction to the wax tree, whereas every single one developed contact dermatitis to the harmless plant. People have also been able to harness the power of their minds to protect themselves against harm after being injected with endotoxins (i.e. the fragments of bacterial cell walls) intravenously. They counteracted the harmful effects by learning how to activate their autonomic nervous system and influence their immune response. These are physiological systems that were once considered impossible to control voluntarily.[67] Countless others afflicted with chronic health conditions have been able to reverse their disease with a range of mind-body, consciousness, meditative, and relaxation-based techniques—an indication that the power of the mind is far greater than we give it credit for.[69,75-78]

Concerning contagion more specifically, many controlled human experiments have documented volunteers developing a cold or flu through *expectation* after being inoculated with sterile saline solution.[10,79,80] In the same way, placebo-controlled studies have shown the duration and severity of the common cold are significantly reduced when people are given a placebo pill they believe is a medicine designed to treat the cold.[81] More generally, there is evidence published in the medical literature demonstrating the ability of people to induce the symptoms of respiratory illnesses, and also rapidly recover from them, using nothing more than mind power alone.[10] In sum, humans can both create and eliminate sickness *psychologically*.

These mind-body phenomena raise a host of intriguing possibilities. If people can make the seemingly impossible become possible, what other feats are we capable of when it comes to germs and contagion? If the mind can cause a cold or flu, might we compromise our health by being so single-mindedly hung up on contagious viruses? Similarly, if we can learn to use our mind to voluntarily activate our immune, and autonomic nervous system, might the effect of germs take a backseat in the story of illness anyway? That is, if their negative effects can be thwarted with mental power alone, it makes no sense to live in fear of germs. Conversely, if it is the case that germs *do not* cause disease—yet we merely *believe* they do—how might this needlessly contribute to disease burden? Perhaps, instead of focusing our time and attention mindlessly wedded to an idea, our efforts are better devoted to harnessing mental might and directing it more constructively towards better health.

The sentiment behind these sorts of ideas, and the third aim of this book, is to open your mind to new possibilities. These factoids alone should encourage anyone to approach this book (and life) much more receptively. We certainly do not know everything. What's more, the things we think we know might also be wrong, or only reveal part of the picture, especially when it comes to what we are capable of. Nothing is ever 'proven', and the science is never 'settled'. As such, we need to think beyond our rigid assumptions and be willing to suspend pre-conceived ideas, particularly on topics affecting all of us. Instead, it is crucial to consider what else could be and evaluate these possibilities with open-mindedness.

Structure of the Book

To achieve these three aims of *informed sense-making*, *humble inquiry*, and *open possibility*, this book will take you on a comprehensive tour of twenty chapters. This is a lot of content, no doubt. But tackling such a vast topic is no simple feat and to do it justice requires diligence. For this reason, and to assist you as a reader in parsing through the breadth of information written on these pages, this book is divided into *three* sections.

Section one clarifies *foundational and historical misconceptions*, equipping you with the necessary principles and context required to grasp the rest of the book. Specifically, after setting the scene here in the introduction, Chapter 2 gives a historical account of many diseases we mistook as contagious. Chapter 3 extends this history by exploring how the world worked before the advent of germs. Then, Chapter 4 recounts the rivalry between two seminal thinkers, Louis Pasteur and Antoine Béchamp. Chapter 5 documents the fracture in the medical and scientific community split by Pasteur's *germ theory* and Béchamp's *terrain theory*. Chapter 6 dives into spontaneous generation—the lynchpin in the debate between contagionists and anti-contagionists. After this tale of two theories, you will then see how germ theory, despite winning the battle, is inadequate because it fails to meet the criteria of Koch's postulates (Chapter 7) and fails to adhere to the scientific method (Chapter 8). Chapter 9 uncovers the issues surrounding virus isolation and the failings of various analytical techniques such as plaque assays and electron microscopy.

Once equipped with this foundational knowledge and history, section two will guide you through *the untold scientific literature*, bringing to light data from hundreds of human experiments. Broadly, it covers the many instances where academic and government institutions attempted to prove germ theory, yet produced contradictory or inconsistent findings. You will gain insights into what happened during the Russian Flu (Chapter 10) and the human contagion experiments that followed (Chapter 11). The peculiarities of the Spanish Flu will be discussed in Chapter 12, and experiments attempting to prove its contagiousness will be presented in Chapter 13. You will then learn about conclusions drawn from studies on the common cold (Chapter 14) and a range of anomalous instances involving sailors and explorers that challenge the underlying premise of germ theory (Chapter 15).

After highlighting issues with germ theory and its empirical support, section three attempts to *expand your horizons* with some alternative explanations of what might be going on when people get sick. You will come to appreciate the power of expectation in the form of placebo and nocebo (Chapter 16). You will realise how mind viruses can spread via social contagion and explore the concept of mass psychogenic illness (Chapter 17). The relationship between meteorological phenomena and the symptoms we normally associate with colds and flu will be established in Chapter 18, and Chapter 19 will make the case for why colds and flu may actually be our *friend*, rather than foe. To conclude, the book brings these ideas together and highlights the personal and societal implications (Chapter 20).

Critically, the book also contains a substantial reference section for you to check sources and follow up with your own research. This is further supplemented by an extensive appendix that summarises the results of more than 200 human contagion and challenge studies. After reading the book, and digesting this information, you may very well be left asking, "Can you catch a cold?"

Chapter 2

Confusing Contagion

G roups of people routinely fall ill at the same time. A famous example of this occurred in 1977 onboard an Alaskan jetliner. The plane was forced to ground on the tarmac for almost five hours when an engine failed during take-off. One of the passengers on board reportedly had influenza. Within 72 hours, 38 of the 54 passengers (~70%) also developed an influenza-like illness characterised by one or more of the following symptoms: cough, fever, headache, sore throat, and myalgia.[1] Epidemiological evidence like this seems to suggest sick-to-well transmission occurred.[2,3] But simply observing a group of people becoming sick with the same symptoms does not, in and of itself, constitute proof that a pathogenic microbe passed between them. Experts and laypeople frequently point to these kinds of events as proof that influenza spreads from person-to-person. However, the data are correlational and, therefore, do not demonstrate cause-and-effect.[4]

It is incorrect to claim a disease is contagious because one person gets sick, and then other people in proximity also become sick shortly afterwards. This supposes that because X preceded Y, then X must have caused Y.[4] Sure, this is one possible explanation, but there is also a chance it is wrong because we cannot rule out alternatives. The key problem is this logic *assumes* rather than demonstrates sick-to-well transmission. In reality, all we can deduce is that people on the plane were exposed to some common causal or contributing factor. There are a multitude of possible environmental conditions that might explain why passengers developed flu-like symptoms on board the stranded aircraft. For instance, the ventilation system was inoperative while the flight was grounded, and the doors were kept closed for at least two hours.[1] This means passengers could have been inhaling all kinds of impurities suspended in the communal, re-circulating air. Regardless, making firm conclusions about what caused the symptoms based on this kind of epidemiological data is inherently problematic. The causal or contributing factor *cannot* be determined by observation alone. Instead, it can only be confirmed by a series of controlled scientific experiments.

As this book will reiterate at various points, there is no convincing evidence published anywhere in the scientific literature demonstrating sick-to-well transmission of a respiratory illness under strictly controlled conditions. In fact, when researchers have performed these experiments, their attempts have almost always ended in complete failure. Despite this, epidemiological observations continue to treat pathogenic microbes as the only possible explanation for the apparent spread of disease amongst a group of people. By relying on such a flawed research design, is it possible to confuse contagion for some other process? Well, there are certainly many examples of this phenomenon occurring throughout history, such as scurvy, pellagra, and mercury exposure. In each case, it appeared as though groups of people were making each other sick when they were actually suffering from a nutritional deficiency or poisoning. This is not to say colds and flu are necessarily caused by deficiencies or poisons. Rather, these examples simply highlight how easy it is for non-contagious diseases to be incorrectly classified and treated as though they are contagious. As you will learn in this chapter, viewing the world single-mindedly through the lens of contagion not only causes confusion but can result in harm.

Confused About Scurvy

Just a few hundred years ago, scurvy was believed to be a communicable illness. After several months of navigating the high seas, sailors often fell ill with the same symptoms, one after the other. Their gums would begin to bleed, their teeth would fall out, and red and blue lesions would appear on their skin. Within weeks of the first case breaking out, the entire crew would succumb to the disease. Naval doctors considered scurvy's pattern of spread to be proof of its contagiousness.[5] This false belief proved extremely costly as more than two million sailors died from scurvy between 1500 and 1800.[6] Had countless decades not been wasted perpetuating this incorrect line of thinking, the true cause may have been realised much sooner.

A typical English sailor's diet in the 1500s consisted of a small portion of butter and cheese, a pound of bread or biscuits, dried beef, pork, or fish, and one gallon of beer. Fresh food was available, but because sailors had to pay for it out of their own pocket, few could justify the additional expense for what was considered a non-essential luxury.[7] People did not yet fully appreciate the importance of consuming fresh, whole food at this point in history—an oversight that proved to be an Achilles heel for naval forces across the world for at least three centuries.

By the 1700s, scurvy had become the greatest enemy to naval forces worldwide, yet no one knew how to defeat it. Scottish surgeon to the Royal Navy, James Lind, exemplified how serious the problem was in his mid-1700s treatise on scurvy. Lind said, *"Armies have been supposed to lose more of their men by sickness, than by the sword. But this observation has been verified in our fleets and squadrons; where the scurvy alone, during the last war, proved a more destructive enemy, and cut off more valuable lives, than the united efforts of the French and Spanish arms".*[8] Aware of the magnitude of this threat, Lind took it upon himself to discover the cause where so many before him had failed.

To investigate the issue, Lind adopted a logical and systematic approach, which turned out to be the first controlled trial in clinical medicine.[9] During a 1747 voyage, 80 men aboard Lind's ship contracted scurvy. Twelve of these men were quarantined and fed the same diet for a short period. Soon thereafter, Lind divided the men into six groups of two and then fed each group a different diet. He observed that sailors who received fresh oranges and lemons recovered from their affliction in under a week, whilst the health of those who were denied these foods continued to deteriorate.[8] Though Lind concluded scurvy was *not* a contagious disease, he failed to recognise the true importance of his discovery. Instead of concluding scurvy was a deficiency of fresh fruits and vegetables, Lind believed these foods merely protected against what he believed was the true cause: *dampness*.[10]

While this discovery dispelled sailors' fears of contracting the dreaded disease from their fellow shipmates, Lind did not recommend that sailors consume fresh fruit or vegetables because they were perishable and prohibitively expensive. Instead, Lind advocated for a juice concentrate called 'rob'. Unbeknownst to him, rob's complicated preparation method negated its 'anti-scorbutic' (i.e. anti-scurvy) properties, rendering it useless.[11] Although sailors drank rob daily, they still developed scurvy. Tragically, it would take another 40 years until fresh lemon and lime juice were included as a standard provision aboard British Naval vessels.[6,9,12] Just before the turn of the century, in 1795, the navy mandated that three-quarters of a fluid ounce (22 mL) of fresh lime juice be included as part of the daily rations for all British sailors.[13] With a simple squeeze of citron, scurvy's three-hundred-year curse was lifted.

Despite Lind's research findings, the idea that scurvy was a contagious disease persisted well into the early 1900s. Some doctors, like Hugo Bofinger, argued scurvy was transmitted between people by a virus or bacteria. Bofinger was head of the Natives' Sick Station and Laboratory Field Hospital XII on Shark Island, positioned off the coast of Namibia. The island was used as a prisoner-of-war camp for native Africans who rebelled against the German empire during the Herero and Namaqua genocide, which occurred between 1904 and 1908. Bofinger argued the unhygienic nature of the camp was a breeding ground for pathogens that caused diseases like scurvy. Attempting to prove his hypothesis, Bofinger conducted various human experiments where he injected prisoners with arsenic, opium, and various other noxious substances. Unsurprisingly, his attempts were met with complete and utter failure.[14–16] The final nail in the coffin for scurvy's contagiousness occurred in 1928 when the Hungarian biochemist Albert Szent-Györgyi is said to have isolated vitamin C, the substance claimed to be deficient in scorbutics.[6]

Confused About Pellagra

Pellagra is now considered to be a nutritional deficiency of niacin (vitamin B3). However, less than 100 years ago, it was thought to be contagious because people living in the same towns, prisons, hospitals, or orphanages began falling ill with identical symptoms around the same time as one another.[17–19] The pathology of pellagra was defined by four D's: dermatitis, diarrhea, dementia, and death.[20] The symptoms were cyclical in nature and they typically presented in the springtime.[17] These factors gave the illusion that the disease was spreading from person to person.[21–23] Meanwhile, the relative absence of pellagra amongst prison guards, doctors, and nurses led some to wonder if they had developed immunity against the pellagra pathogen, whereas others took this as evidence against pellagra's contagiousness.[18,19] These conflicting views caused significant confusion amongst physicians, leading them to refer to the disease as *"The greatest riddle of the medical profession"*.[24]

People were so fearful of catching pellagra that a wave of 'pellagra-phobia' swept across the United States in the early 1900s.[25,26] Many hospitals refused to admit pellagrins, and it was not uncommon for nursing staff to refuse treatment for those admitted with the affliction. Some nurses even went on strike after being instructed to treat pellagra patients for fear of being infected themselves.[27] Quarantine measures were implemented by hospital staff in the hope of reducing transmission of the disease, but all to no avail. Elementary schools barred children from school grounds if any of their family members were ill, while hotel patrons threatened to leave en masse if guests displaying even the mildest pellagra symptoms were not promptly vacated from the premises.[28–30]

As the cause of the disease was unknown, doctors began treating patients with a range of different toxic substances, including arsenic and mercury. Dr Roy Robinson believed pellagra was caused by a parasite, so he lathered his patients' skin with bichloride of mercury. Within three weeks of commencing treatment, the dermatitis in 13 of his patients had *"practically disappeared"*. He then gave the drug internally for two weeks, and the patients' diarrhea also vanished.[31] Similarly, the physician L. P. Tenney reported exceptional outcomes from treating pellagrins with arsenic-based drugs. Tenney prescribed this toxic heavy metal to his patients, in his own words, *"Indefinitely, or until symptoms cleared up; then I continued its use once a week for some two or three months longer. The idea is to keep the patient saturated with arsenic, and it's surprising how much they can stand"*. Tenney also insisted his patients consume plenty of eggs and milk, but he overlooked their curative effect in favour of the arsenicals.[32] Strangely, arsenic held 'chief place' in the treatment of pellagra until the 1930s.[33] Both of these radical treatments, determined to kill a non-existent germ, undoubtedly took their toll on patients.[34]

At the turn of the 20th century, pellagra was thought to be one of three things: a nutritional deficiency disease, an intoxication disease, or an infectious disease. In 1911, the Illinois Pellagra Commission concluded the disease was caused by a living micro-organism of unknown nature.[35]

The following year, the Thompson-McFadden Commission was tasked with further investigating the cause. Two years after its commencement, the Commission concluded pellagra was not a nutritional disease but an infectious, contagious, gastrointestinal disease.[36] Not content with this conclusion, the surgeon general turned to an infectious disease 'specialist', Dr Joseph Goldberger, for a second opinion.[17]

Goldberger continued where the Thompson-McFadden commission left off. To determine whether pellagra was contagious, Goldberger held 'filth parties' where volunteers would eat pills made from the skin, faeces, nasal secretions, blood, saliva, and urine obtained from pellagrins.[17] When these experiments failed, he injected 16 healthy volunteers with blood and nasopharyngeal secretions taken from pellagrins. In no instance did any of the volunteers develop pellagra, nor did they become sick with any disease.[37] Goldberger didn't stop there, though. He then injected himself and his wife with the bodily fluids of pellagrins, yet they both remained completely well. These findings demonstrated pellagra was not contagious and must have been caused by some other factor.[17] It seems ironic that this handful of experiments is considered proof against pellagra's contagiousness when the results of dozens of similar experiments failing to transmit the cold and flu are dismissed as *specious*. It is also rather curious that recipients remained well considering the array of undesirable, germ-ridden, human byproducts entering their bodies.

Based on this work, Goldberger reasoned pellagra was either a nutritional deficiency disease or a toxicity disease. To test his hypotheses, he conducted several experiments in prisons, orphanages, and insane asylums, where he fed participants a range of different diets. In one of the more notable experiments, the Governor of Mississippi recruited a group of inmates from a prison farm to assist Goldberger. To entice the men to participate, the Governor offered them a full pardon upon successful completion of the experiment. The inmates were called 'The Pellagra Squad' and were fed a meagre diet consisting of corn grits, pork fat, molasses, collard greens, and sweet potatoes for six months. At the end of the experiment, six of the eleven inmates (54.5%) developed pellagra.[17,38]

Goldberger considered the results of his experiments proof that a 'poverty diet' of the three Ms (i.e. corn meal, meat, and molasses) was the cause of pellagra. He also believed this could explain the seasonality of the disease.

During the winter months, when the most impoverished people ran out of money, they would consume the cheapest food they could find, which tended to be corn meal, meat, and molasses. These dietary choices persisted into the springtime, resulting in a chronic deficiency of what Goldberger referred to as 'pellagra preventive factor',[35] which later became known as niacin (vitamin B3).[17,38] People living in the same households became sick at the same time, not because something was being transmitted between them, but because their niacin reserves were becoming depleted at the same time. This also explained why medical staff and prison guards remained well despite their close contact with pellagrins. It wasn't that they were immune to the (non-existent) pellagra germ; their diets were just superior.

The final proof that pellagra was a nutritional deficiency disease came about in 1927 following the Mississippi River Flood. Goldberger instructed authorities to feed brewer's yeast to the 50,000 survivors. A considerable number of survivors suffering from pellagra, were cured in a matter of weeks after ingesting the yeast. These results led Goldberger to conclude that pellagra is a disease caused by a deficiency of niacin.[17,39]

Now, it is important to mention that pellagra (and scurvy) were not the only deficiency diseases once thought to be contagious. Although not discussed here, beriberi, an alleged deficiency in thiamine (vitamin B1), and rickets, an alleged deficiency in vitamin D, were also considered contagious or infectious.[40] In fact, Robert Koch, one of the pioneers of the germ theory, convinced Japanese scientists investigating beriberi in the early 1900s that it was caused by a contagious microorganism. This sent those researchers on a wild goose chase for many years.[41,42] Looking back, it is difficult to grasp how anyone could ever think scurvy, pellagra, rickets, or beriberi were caused by a pathogen, but such was the hysteria caused by viewing the world through the lens of germ theory. At one point in time, this perspective became so dominant that people claimed *all* diseases were caused by pathogenic microbes.[43,44]

Confused About Minamata Disease

Preoccupation with germ theory meant nutritional deficiencies were not the only diseases mistaken for contagious illnesses. In May of 1956, a five-year-old girl was admitted to a local hospital in Minamata, Japan. Minamata was a small fishing village of approximately 50,00 people situated on the coastline of the Yatsushiro Sea. The girl had become acutely ill with unusual neurological symptoms, including convulsions, difficulty walking, and impaired speech. A few days later, her sister and three other people in the town also presented to the hospital with the exact same symptoms.[45,46]

Over the following weeks and months, the number of people in the village falling ill increased rapidly, although it wasn't just townsfolk who were being affected. Large numbers of fish began to swim strangely before dying and being washed ashore. Sea birds were unable to fly and exhibited unusual behaviour. Cats that preyed upon these animals also became unwell, drooling from the mouth and running in circles as if they had gone mad.[47] Was some kind of pathogen being passed between animals and humans? No one knew for sure. However, the outbreak seemed to exhibit all the hallmarks of a contagious disease. After the first case had occurred, an increasing number of people living in the village began falling ill with the same symptoms, one after another. This ignited rumours that some kind of 'strange infectious disease' had broken out.[48] Unconfirmed reports soon began surfacing that the disease was infectious meningitis, sending the community into a wild panic.[49]

The fear of catching the mystery illness was so great, that people from neighbouring towns began ostracising Minamatans, quickly eroding long-established and close-knit community ties.[50] To curb the spread of the epidemic, people's homes were disinfected, and the sick were quarantined.[49] Despite these countermeasures, the disease continued to ravage the local population. Early reports indicated at least 55 people had contracted the disease, and 17 people had died.[45]

After nearly three years, however, the research group finally traced the cause of the disease to a local fertiliser manufacturing company. They had dumped 27 tonnes of methylmercury, a waste product of synthetic fertiliser production, into Minamata Bay.[51] The mercury contaminated local waterways and polluted hundreds of square kilometres of ocean. What was once a beautiful and fertile natural reef became a toxic wasteland, poisoning any human or animal unfortunate to consume its once plentiful bounty.

In February of 1963, a formal announcement was made by the research group investigating the cause of the outbreak. Much to everyone's dismay,

Minamata disease was caused by the consumption of fish and shellfish from Minamata Bay that had been contaminated with methylmercury, *not* an infectious microorganism.[49] Despite officials publicly announcing mercury was the cause, the belief that the disease was transmissible persisted. For many years, victims of the environmental catastrophe were forced to reassure the people they encountered in their daily lives that they were not contagious.[52] In the wake of the disaster, more than 900 people died, and two million suffered chronic health problems.[51]

Confused About Mercury Poisoning

Despite the events that unfolded in Minamata, medical professionals still—to this day—mistakenly diagnose mercury toxicity as an infectious disease. In August of 2018, three siblings, a 15-year-old female, a 13-year-old female, and an 11-year-old male, presented to an emergency department. They were experiencing progressive, non-specific symptoms, including fever, myalgia, skin rashes, and malaise. A barrage of negative tests resulted in the diagnosis of a non-descript 'viral syndrome'. The children were sent home to rest. Three days later, the siblings returned to the emergency department in a much worse condition, with one of the children experiencing neurological impairment. The children were diagnosed with streptococcal pharyngitis (strep throat) and scarlet fever. They were administered a course of antibiotics and discharged.[53]

A few days later, the children were taken to another emergency department for a second opinion. By this time, their symptoms had become significantly worse, and they had developed severe headaches, shortness of breath, numbness and tingling in their hands and feet, and generalised weakness. Instead of jumping to conclusions and blaming a virus or bacteria, the emergency doctors probed further. It was discovered that the children had been playing with a jar of elemental mercury at home, which spilled onto the carpet. Their mother used a vacuum in an attempt to clean up the spill. Unbeknownst to her, this heated and vaporised the mercury, which the children inadvertently inhaled. Curiously, the mother did not develop any symptoms, which made it appear like the illness was an infectious *childhood* disease.

After realising the children had been poisoned with mercury, doctors commenced a course of chelation therapy to remove the mercury from their bodies. Two of the children recovered completely. However, one child suffered from ongoing joint, back, and muscle pain and required a walker. This event was documented in a case study and published in a medical journal in February 2020. The authors concluded that mercury toxicity can mimic an infectious disease.[53] Because the children had been living in the same home and presented with similar symptoms, the doctors at the first hospital incorrectly assumed it must have been a contagious childhood illness spreading between the siblings. Once again, seeing the world through a single-minded lens led to false assumptions, which likely delayed the correct diagnosis and treatment.

Why Does This Matter?

Clearly, it was important to correctly identify the causes of illnesses like scurvy, pellagra, and mercury poisoning. In each case, however, the lens of germ theory interfered with the truth, sending investigators on futile searches and launching the public into a needless panic. In these instances alone, it is difficult to quantify the fallout from applying the wrong explanatory model. Countless resources, time, and lives were lost battling or chasing an enemy that never existed. It is also harrowing to think how many people were ostracised, isolated, treated inhumanely, or denied timely and effective healthcare. This was not because they had a contagious disease, but because people *feared* they did. In this way, the lens through which we view the world is powerful. For better or worse, it colours our every perception and leads us to outcomes consistent with our perspective.

Of course, now we know better—no longer do we see these diseases as contagious. It is easy to look back and realise the error of our ways with diseases like scurvy, pellagra, and Minamata disease. From our current vantage point, it seems barbaric that human beings were branded like lepers, denied care, and locked away like caged animals because they were seen as *unclean* when, in fact, they were *clean* all along. Hindsight is a funny thing, though. We assume we now have all the answers. But what if there are other illnesses, we still consider contagious, that are not? Though we look back proudly at how far we've come, we may be making the same mistakes right now. We charge forward, blinded by pride and naivety, blissfully unaware of the errors we continue to make.

Looking back, it was fortunate, then, that some of the researchers of the past did not fall prey to hubris or conformity. They remained humble, kept their minds open, and acted with courage. If they never thought to challenge the accepted paradigm, what would the world look like today? It's possible we would still consider those diseases contagious and continue to manage them with the same ineffective and inhumane interventions of yesteryear. Imagine injecting heavy metals and being quarantined for pellagra instead of implementing a simple dietary change. Imagine living in fear of contracting scurvy, beriberi, or even rickets from other people. Perhaps we would even try to protect ourselves from these (non-existent) germs using modern methods: vaccinating, hand washing, social distancing, injecting antibiotics, popping antivirals, wearing face masks, and locking down. All the while, people would continue to die needlessly from their lifestyle or environment. These things aren't hard to conceive of because they are how the world operates today for many other diseases like the cold and flu, for example. The only difference is modern researchers believe the model of contagion does accurately explain these ailments. This belief is now so ingrained into the collective psyche that they struggle to entertain the possibility of being wrong. The culture has also shifted such that anyone challenging the accepted paradigm is labelled a crazy conspiracy theorist.

We have become so sure of ourselves, yet this chapter demonstrates how easy it is to get things wrong by observing an effect and *incorrectly* attributing a cause. It also emphasises how important it is to confirm cause-and-effect relationships through rigorous and controlled scientific experiments rather than jumping to conclusions. We have made errors in the past and, if we don't get the causal story straight, we will continue to make them regardless of how advanced we consider ourselves to be. As the mistaken examples highlight, incorrectly diagnosing an illness as contagious produces all kinds of negative consequences. For unwell individuals, it delays access to proper diagnosis and treatment, potentially leading to more severe dysfunction and disability. Collectively, it has far-reaching implications. Indeed, if we confuse the cause of disease with contagion, we cultivate a more fearful and avoidant society, we misallocate resources (e.g. research grants), we prop up false economies (e.g. pharmaceuticals), we cede power to institutions (e.g. governments), and we wear an opportunity cost that ultimately sees more people fall sick and die while we veer down the wrong path.

Chapter 3

A Time Before Germs

The belief that influenza and the common cold can be 'caught' is something that most people accept without question or objection. Yet few realise this line of thinking is relatively new. For hundreds, possibly thousands of years, mankind believed respiratory illnesses were caused by toxins and poisons, meteorological conditions (e.g. exposure to cold-dry weather), celestial activity (e.g. meteors and comets), solar radiation, and various other atmospheric phenomena (e.g. aurora borealis). Only in recent times has the idea of disease-causing germs become the dominant theory.[1]

Testament to this line of thinking, in 1794, Dr Erasmus Darwin (grandfather of Charles Darwin) remarked on the spread of influenza, stating, *"This malady attacks so many at the same time, and spreads gradually over so great an extent of country, that there can be no doubt but that it is disseminated by the atmosphere"*.[2] Darwin's 'environmental' perspective was shared by others around that time, including Dr James Woodforde, who said, *"I am of opinion that it* [influenza] *is not contagious; at least, not primarily so; but that it owes its source to the state of the atmosphere"*.[3] The great epidemiologist, Professor August Hirsch, also expressed doubt about contagion. In 1883, he noted the evidence in favour of influenza being a contagious disease was lacking, and that it would be hard to discover any reason for classifying it as contagious or communicable.[4]

After an influenza epidemic ravaged Great Britain in 1837, a leading medical association wanted to gather as much information about the epidemic as possible to better understand the cause and mode of spread of the illness. The association issued a series of 18 questions to its members, many of whom, were general practitioners or surgeons. One of the questions asked the members if they possessed any proof of influenza being communicated from one person to another. The responses were entirely in the negative—*none* of the doctors had definitive proof of person-to-person transmission. Their answers also indicated it was not uncommon for those who nursed influenza patients to work through the entire epidemic without contracting the disease.[5]

Renowned social reformer and founder of modern nursing, Florence Nightingale, expressed her scepticism about the contagion explanation in a letter to British Surgeon James Pattison Walker. She wrote *"Facts are everything—doctrines are nothing. See what harm the German pathologists have done us. There are no specific diseases. There are specific disease conditions. It is that which is bringing the medical profession to grief, and will, in time, make a great reform—to wit, to make them make the public care for its own health and not rely on doctrines. It is a grand thing for weak minds—the doctrine of contagion".*[6] Even Dr Charles Creighton, the founder of modern epidemiology, was highly critical of the theory that influenza epidemics are caused by the transmission of infectious particles from person-to-person.[7] In 1891, he published his treatise, *"A History of Epidemics in Britain,"* the contents of which would see him denounced by the medical profession. After Creighton conducted a thorough systematic analysis of the literature, he was unable to reconcile himself with the idea that germs caused infectious diseases like influenza. Instead, he contended that meteorological effects and exposure to toxic and poisonous substances offered a far more accurate explanation.[8]

What's in a Name?

Historically, people were so confident in their belief that the cold and flu were not contagious that they literally named these seasonal afflictions after their purported causes. In the 16th century, the common cold was named after the similar symptoms experienced by people following exposure to cold weather.[9,10] The Chinese were even more explicit in their definition, referring to the common cold as 'Gan Mao', which quite literally translates to *a common cold caused by abnormal seasonal changes*, like exposure to cold-damp wind.[11-14]

Influenza was named in much the same way. The term was first coined by John Huxham in 1743, based on the Italian phrase, *"un influenza di freddo"* or *"the influence of the cold"*. However, some suggest it was used as early as 1580, only to become popularised centuries later. The word was widely used to describe the epidemic of 1775,[15,16] and had become commonplace by 1782.[8] Influenza may have also derived from the Italian phrase, *"influenza coeli,"* meaning *"the influence of the stars"*.[17,18] This is likely due to ancient civilisations observing celestial phenomena such as comets, asteroids, and meteorites just prior to influenza epidemics.[19]

The contribution of meteorological and celestial activities stood the test of time, being widely accepted by doctors and scientists up until the early 1900s. In fact, before the adoption of germ theory, the medical orthodoxy acknowledged cold exposure as the cause of the cold and flu.[1,20,21] This is evidenced by the fact that, as of 1910, English dictionaries still defined the common cold as *"an indisposition occasioned by exposure to cold or to a draught of cool air, or to dampness"*. Similar definitions were also published in medical dictionaries, defining the common cold as *"a catarrhal or other disorder, due to exposure to cold and wet"*.[22] The role of cold weather was only challenged in the late 1800s when doctors began asserting bacteria, and not meteorological or celestial phenomena, were responsible. They incorrectly championed the bacterial theory of colds and flu for almost thirty years until scientists started to believe sub-microscopic, diseasing-causing particles known as viruses were the causative agents.[23,24]

In an effort to prove this new theory, scientists conducted many experiments that exposed healthy people to the mucosal secretions of sick people. However, these attempts *failed* time and time again, casting doubt on the fundamental tenets of contagion.[25-27] The results of these experiments led many learned individuals to reconsider whether their forefathers had been right all along about the impact of meteorological effects and toxin exposure, or if the cold and flu might be caused by some other under-appreciated or yet-to-be-discovered mechanism.[1] Just like the doctors of old, modern scientists studying the cold and flu argue the mode of spread is far more consistent with changes in temperature, humidity, celestial activity, and fluctuations in solar radiation than it is with viral spread.[28-30]

Some assert that catching the common cold and influenza 'viruses' have less to do with human interaction, and more to do with the location people are in and the environmental conditions they are exposed to.[31,32] Others have theorised viruses are produced *de novo* (i.e. anew from within the body), or that they have simply been mistaken for cellular debris arising from tissue damage caused by various external aggravating factors.[33–35] Some scientists even postulate that colds are not caught, but instead arise from an ongoing battle between the immune system and normal internal flora, which contains 'viruses' residing inside the respiratory tract. Only when the battle tips in favour of the 'viruses', does a person develop symptoms.[36] While it is not yet clear which (if any) of these alternative models is correct, the same is true for the current model which is plagued with issues.

Sir Christoper Howard Andrewes, the man credited with the discovery of the influenza A virus, was also perplexed by epidemiological peculiarities. He published a journal article in 1942 asking, *"Where is the virus between epidemics?"* Andrewes noted that, in Britain, influenza was only prevalent every other year in January, February, and March. He wondered how it was possible the influenza virus could disappear for 21 out of 24 months. To this point he remarked that it was hard to imagine an influenza virus keeps spreading from one place to another by means of infection, only to end up back at its point of origin. Even when Andrewes considered the southern hemisphere as part of this equation, he could not make this theory work.[37] Andrewes spent three decades waiting for someone to answer this question. He eventually attempted to answer it again in 1973, proposing several ideas to address this anomaly.[38] Even so, his efforts merely raised more unanswered questions. This uncertainty is typical in the scientific literature, as almost a dozen other influenza conundrums remain unaddressed.[39]

Weather Doctors

For thousands of years, it was believed low temperatures penetrating the body played a central role in respiratory infections.[40] In the 5th century BC, Hippocrates established a connection between meteorological conditions and epidemics. He stated, *"Whoever wishes to investigate medicine properly should proceed thus: In the first place, consider the seasons of the year and what effect each of them produces; then, the winds, the hot and the cold"* and *"If it be thought that these things belong rather to meteorology, it will be remembered that astronomy contributes not a little, but a very great deal to medicine, for with the seasons the digestive organs of men undergo a change"*.[41] Hippocrates formally proposed a theory of 'meteorological causation', which was so widely favoured that it inspired the development of an entire speciality of medicine, known as 'medical meteorology'. Those who studied and practised under this discipline were referred to as 'medical meteorologists' or 'weather doctors'.[42,43]

Weather doctors reported that influenza did not behave like a contagious illness, but was instead consistent with changing meteorological conditions.[44] More specifically, it was thought changes in barometric pressure, temperature, atmospheric electrical influence, wind, ozone, and actinic effects triggered influenza outbreaks.[45] They believed the secrets of cold and flu epidemics could be unlocked by understanding how subtle fluctuations of these meteorological phenomena impacted the human body.[44,46] Even though the concept of contagion was proposed by the Persian physician, Ibn Sina, in the Canon of Medicine in the year 1025 (some 1,500 years after Hippocrates), the idea that influenza was caused by meteorological conditions prevailed over that of contagion for centuries. In the years and decades that followed, the idea of contagion progressively waned. By the mid-1800s the doctrine had all but collapsed and was considered nothing more than a remnant of childish ideas.[47,48]

There was no shortage of weather doctors who carried Hippocrates' legacy forward throughout the ages. The renowned English physician, Dr Thomas Sydenham, who was known as the 'English Hippocrates' and the 'Prince of English Physicians', was convinced of an atmospheric cause.[49] Sydenham had become interested in understanding why people exhibited identical symptoms simultaneously to epidemic diseases like influenza. After much deliberation, Sydenham and his colleague, Robert Boyle, theorised that 'effluvium' released from under the Earth contaminated the atmosphere and interacted with perceptible physical qualities such as moisture, dryness, heat, and cold, which induced various atmospheric changes. Sydenham argued these changes disrupted one of the four 'reciprocal humors' of the body, which were also moist, dry, hot, and cold. This disruption, in turn, caused conditions like influenza.[49-51]

Later, physician and polymath, John Arbuthnot, published *"An Essay Concerning the Effects of Air on the Human Body"* in 1733. In this work, Arbuthnot described the effects of different seasons on people and proposed that specific atmospheric characteristics of each season could induce different disease states.[52] That same year, Benjamin Franklin tried to quash such ideas, proposing that contagion, not meteorological effects, caused influenza and the common cold.[53] It seems, however, that public perception was not swayed by Franklin's testimony because the belief that weather conditions caused colds and flu persisted for at least another 150 years.[1,10] This is shown in the results of a survey of over 2,000 people conducted in 1925, where only half of the respondents considered the common cold to be contagious.[54] This is not to say that the work of men like Benjamin Franklin went unnoticed. His words undoubtedly planted the seed in the minds of some physicians that contagion caused influenza, even though by that time, the field of medicine had already begun to abandon the idea.[48,55]

Throughout the 1700s, anti-contagionism gained wide acceptance, with just a handful of medical men desperately clinging to the doctrine of contagion. By the early 1800s, a mere ten per cent of the medical profession in the United Kingdom held onto the belief that influenza was contagious, while the other 90 per cent remained completely unconvinced. This is evidenced by the work of Dr Thomas Beddoes, a prominent physician, scientific writer, and public figure, who conducted an extensive inquiry during the epidemic of 1800 to better understand the nature of influenza. The overwhelming majority of the 170 physicians surveyed reported that influenza was not contagious, largely because healthy people failed to contract the disease despite living, working, and socialising with the 'infected'.[56-62] At this point, Dr Beddoes called for the idea that influenza was contagious to be relinquished entirely. He stated, *"After thorough investigation of the opinions adduced, respecting the disease entitled influenza; when a majority amounting to nine-tenths of the medical world are agreed with respect to its non-contagious nature, all controversy should now cease, as it is certain that the proof, though not positive, is sufficiently presumptive".*[58]

The sentiment towards contagion was reciprocated by physicians in the United States, owing to the numerous inconsistencies with the theory. At the turn of the 19th century, American revolutionary Benjamin

Rush recanted his position on contagion and argued for cleanliness over quarantine.[48] He asserted that quarantine laws were worse than useless, declaring, *"Thousands of lives have been sacrificed, by that faith in their efficacy, which has led to the neglect of domestic cleanliness".*[63] Rush, a professor of medicine inspired his students, like Charles Caldwell, to also adopt an anti-contagionist stance. In 1803, Caldwell was appointed to the Board of Health in Philadelphia and made his position on the matter well-known.[64] The work of men like Caldwell and Rush had such an impact, that by 1820, less than half a dozen physicians in the entire city practised under the failing doctrine.[48]

In 1825, Charles Larkin expressed his perspective on 'contagion' in a prominent medical journal. He declared, *"This dogma which in my judgement has no foundation in fact, but is based on misapprehension and inaccurate observation, is revered by those who cannot say anything else in its defence than that it was believed by their fathers and grandfathers".* Like other weather doctors, Larkin pointed towards environmental factors as causal, or at the very least, a significant contributing factor of epidemic outbreaks.[65] Around the same time, Dr Alexander Jones proposed that influenza could not possibly be contagious because the pace at which it spread across North America and the West Indies was faster than it could spread from person-to-person. He concluded this fact alone was sufficient to dispel the idea that influenza was propagated from one person to another by means of contagion.[66]

Shedding light on this mystery, Dr George Ross noted how drastic changes in weather conditions preceded the influenza epidemics of 1832, 1837, and 1842. In every instance, the weather was dry and frosty for several days prior to the epidemic. When the weather abruptly changed and became damp and foggy, influenza became widespread shortly thereafter. Ross believed that air saturated with moisture impairs the normal functions of the respiratory tract and other mucous membranes, causing a disturbance in the body that results in influenza.[67] In line with this thinking, English chemist and physician, William Prout, published his *"Bridgewater Treatise"* in 1836. In it, Prout described the first-ever empirical observations linking atmospheric pressure to disease. He claimed the weight of the air increased positively during the first outbreak of cholera in England. Prout also posited the amount of particulate matter dispersed into the air following a volcanic eruption, or through a crevice in the Earth after an earthquake, was sufficient to contaminate the atmosphere and cause diseases like influenza over a vast area.[68,69]

During the same period, Dr Robert Tytler, a surgeon in the Bengal Infantry, thought it strange Hippocrates never thought to mention contagion. In his 1834 lecture, *"Refutation of the Doctrine of Contagion,"* he remarked, *"If contagion were a truth, how comes it that the venerable founder of the healing art* [Hippocrates] *should have omitted such a conspicuous fact in those splendid aphorisms, each of which seems to contain the concentrated wisdom of ages?"* Tytler dissented further, asserting, *"If gentlemen, contagion be an error, as I contend it is, here is a dreadful and most mischievous error, indeed permitted to pervade the whole of our science".* He continued, *"But contemplating as I do, the baneful doctrine of contagion, as a most dreadful and destructive delusion, which tends to the establishment of the horrible quarantine laws, and leads to the violation of every duty of humanity...It is the science itself which requires to be reformed, and this beneficial alteration can alone be affected by the members of the profession themselves".*[70]

Given these sorts of strong views, as well as the long history of meteorological accounts, The Royal Society of Medicine set up a statistical committee in 1845. Their task was to investigate the relationship between the weather and epidemic diseases (like influenza) with the sole focus of identifying the causal factors. The committee collected data across 11 European countries for periods of four to seven years. In total, their dataset encompassed over four million cases. Although it was difficult to establish any firm cause-and-effect relationships, one particularly interesting finding resulted from the investigation. One of the committee members, Frederik Bremer, tested the hypothesis that easterly winds carried bad air ('miasmas'), which is why epidemics spread from east to west. Contrary to his expectations, but interesting nonetheless, Bremer found that epidemics always spread east to west, irrespective of which direction the prevailing winds blew.[71,72] English member of parliament Henry Labouchere referred to this fact in 1890, stating that pandemics always spread from east to west, never from west to east.[73] Other historical and epidemiological data does indeed show most major epidemics spread from east to west.[25,74-76] This broad environmental trend is *incompatible* with contagion. Specifically, if influenza spreads from person-to-person, why would it follow a preferred direction of travel across large distances?

Contagious epidemics should have an epicentre and spread outwards in all directions following human social behaviour.

Lending further support to the environmental account, Dr John Charles Atkinson published a book titled *"Change of Air: Fallacies Regarding It"* in 1848, and a journal article in 1850 detailing how changes in temperature, humidity, and atmospheric pressure were inextricably linked to influenza outbreaks. Atkinson found significant differences in atmospheric conditions over relatively short distances (i.e. a matter of metres), which might explain why some people and not others become unwell, particularly when they are close to one another. He noted that people living on one side of a road or stream developed influenza, yet those living on the other side remained completely unaffected. Like Ross, Atkinson also found epidemics seemed to be triggered when conditions changed from cold, frosty, and dry, to damp and humid.[77,78]

The Dutch physician, Dr Christian Fibiger, also firmly believed that meteorological conditions caused influenza epidemics. Fibiger ran his own weather station and took measurements up to nine times per day. By 1860, he had recorded more than 50,000 atmospheric observations. He was able to statistically analyse whether any relationship existed between weather events and epidemic disease. This work formed the basis of Fibiger's doctoral dissertation titled *"On the Influence of Climate on the Genesis of Disease"*. He concluded that meteorological changes, particularly hot or cold temperatures, were the primary cause of diseases like influenza, casting further doubt on the theory of contagion.[72,79]

A Change in the Weather

The accumulating meteorological accounts were dealt a major blow when the first part of Louis Pasteur's *germ theory* was published in 1861. This perspective was seen to undermine the validity of the work weather doctors had undertaken to that point. Supporters of contagion argued influenza epidemics occurred independently of meteorological changes, and that person-to-person transmission could explain the spread of the disease.[80] Despite the medical elite opposing and dismissing medical meteorology, many weather doctors remained undeterred in their pursuits. They adamantly resisted, and maintained germ theory was not required to explain the cause and spread of influenza.[72] They also challenged the notion that germs could account for influenza appearing and simultaneously affecting (within a single day) large numbers of people over vast distances, despite the majority of them having no direct contact with each other. Given these sorts of inconsistencies, many physicians found it difficult to concede influenza was contagious.[16,81]

For example, in 1885, Dr Frederick Campbell wrote, *"If we reject germ theories, the relation between atmospheric changes and disorders of the human body is even more easily comprehended. The organic chemical processes in plants which depend entirely upon soil and climate for their development, have their analogies in the human system which are also influenced by meteorological changes".* He argued that any physician who points towards a microbe as the cause of influenza without understanding the role of environmental changes is only doing half his duty.[43] A few years later, in 1899, Dr George Poore gave a lecture at a prominent medical college in London where he argued that properly studying the diseases of mankind requires us not to simply focus on man, but also on what goes on in nature, *outside* of the human body. Poore believed nature is where the field of medicine must look if they are to solve the problem of infectious diseases, particularly when it comes to epidemics.[82]

Despite their resistance, the work of medical meteorologists was largely overshadowed by the advent of viruses at the beginning of the 20th century. However, germ theory never fully dispelled the meteorological accounts and the intuitive appeal of their ancient wisdom. Indeed, to this day, a considerable proportion of the world's population still believes colds and flu are caused by weather conditions, not germs.[83–86] The data, as well as the questions it raised about the pace, scope, timing, and direction of spread, remain unaddressed. There are still many open threads from this era, even if most scientists and doctors moved on.

The Story of Dr Ashbel Smith

In the years before Louis Pasteur published his germ theory, there were signs that the medical profession was going to abandon the concept of contagion for an environmental model of infectious disease causation. The final push towards shifting the consensus was championed by the work of people like Dr Ashbel Smith, the first Surgeon General of Texas. Shortly after his appointment, an epidemic of yellow fever broke out in 1839 on the island of Galveston. Smith decided to travel to the island to see if he could assist the 2,500 or so inhabitants who were in dire need of help. The town was divided into two sections, with the main part positioned barely above the water level. As a result, the ground was muddy, and a considerable amount of human filth had accumulated on top of the waterlogged soil behind the buildings. The other part of town sat on dry ground, owing to the fact it was positioned slightly above sea level and located further inland. According to Smith, this second area was neat, comfortable, and clean. It was also largely free from serious diseases, unlike the damp, filth-laden main streets.[87,88]

At this point in American history, the medical profession was convinced yellow fever was a highly contagious illness (not a mosquito-borne one like it is today).[89-92] The belief that it was contagious stemmed from nothing more than observations: large numbers of people in the same location falling ill with identical symptoms, one after another.[89] Some medical practitioners proclaimed yellow fever was so infectious that a bag filled with earth taken from a disease-ridden area could be transported to another disease-free location and infect the inhabitants who lived there.[93] Dr Smith was sceptical about such unfounded claims. He was a man of science who believed that experimental evidence, not hearsay, should inform medical opinion about the nature of illnesses like yellow fever.[87,88]

If yellow fever was contagious, Dr Smith reasoned that exposure to the bodily fluids of those with the disease should be able to recreate it. During his post-mortem examinations, Smith would immerse his hands in the black vomit and other bodily fluids of the dead. When he failed to contract the illness after holding his hands close to his face and inhaling the fetid matter, he decided a more extreme approach was required. Smith collected fresh samples of black vomit ejected from the ill, which he then consumed. Despite doing this on several separate occasions, Smith never contracted yellow fever. He also observed that when ill people were relocated from the infected areas of the main city into the outer areas free of the disease, no person-to-person transmission occurred.[87,88]

These negative results led Dr Smith to conclude yellow fever was not contagious but rather the result of exposure to noxious gasses emanating into the air from piles of garbage and stagnant pools of contaminated water.[87,88] Smith contended that understanding the nature of yellow fever was of great importance due to the fact that *"a belief in the contagiousness of this disease would deprive the sick of the most necessary attentions"* and because *"non-contagion destroys many of the horrors of an epidemic".*[87] In other words, he understood that, as long as yellow fever was incorrectly classified as contagious, (a) steps to prevent outbreaks would be ineffective, (b) people would be denied access to the correct treatment, and (c) the ill would continue to be subjected to inhumane and ineffective practices like quarantine.

By discovering yellow fever was not contagious, Smith implemented targeted strategies like personal hygiene, sanitation, good nutrition, herbal medicine, and bed rest.[94] He found that these simple measures usually resulted in the rapid recovery of those affected. Unfortunately, owing to social and political factors, and what Smith described as the *"absurd denial of a few who feared their pecuniary interests would be damaged,"* his anti-contagionist views were dismissed in favour of medications, and the cruel and ineffective use of quarantine.[87,88] Consequently, many preventable deaths ensued as the outbreak ravaged the city. As there was no cemetery on the island, the people of Galveston buried the bodies of the deceased in mass shallow graves near the shoreline of the gulf.[94] These unsanitary practices likely contributed greatly to nine other yellow fever epidemics that intermittently plagued the island over the next thirty years.[88]

Smith's work garnered the attention of fellow weather doctors and anti-contagionists. His conclusions, along with the work of others, prompted the medical profession to question the nature of *all* so-called contagious fevers.[95,96] Physicians wondered, if they had been wrong about the aetiology of yellow fever, what other diseases they had also been wrong about. The dissent towards contagion by the medical profession continued to gain traction over the next few decades, as evidenced by the proceedings of a meeting at the New York Academy of Medicine in 1858. During this meeting, Professor Smith read an elaborate paper that contained the testimony of the most eminent and trusted physicians from the United Kingdom, Europe, and America. The contents of this paper were the culmination of fifty years of evidence demonstrating yellow fever was not communicable.[97]

Upon the conclusion of Professor Smith's presentation, Dr John W. Francis, president of the academy, made an earnest address to those in attendance, *"We only wish that the equally baseless superstition of contagion in other epidemic and infectious diseases were as fully repudiated as in yellow fever. For as American physicians were the first to explode this heresy of contagion in this fever, and compel all the medical world to abandon it; so should they be foremost in driving out of the profession the dogma of contagion in any fever but small-pox"*. Francis continued, *"The time is not distant when our profession shall see eye to eye on this subject, and the contagion of any other fever* [than smallpox] *will be annihilated, and only remembered as among the relics of ignorance and barbarism".*[97]

By the 1860s, momentum was building in the medical profession to free itself from the idea of contagion entirely. Physicians were washing their hands of the idea in droves and the word 'contagion' seldom appeared in journals of sanitary medicine before this time, unless to be branded as dangerous heresy.[98] The outspoken minority of physicians in favour of contagion seemed like they were on the back foot until 1861 when they were thrown a lifeline. Just three years after the meeting at the New York Academy of Medicine that denounced the doctrine of contagion, Louis Pasteur released his germ theory to the world, breathing new life into the woefully deflated concept. Contrary to popular belief, this new theory was met with considerable opposition. Many doctors and scientists publicly contested Pasteurs assertions and 'germ theory' seldom appeared in any dictionary, encyclopedia, or medical textbook, particularly in the United States until 1878—almost two decades *after* its inception.[99]

Germ theory, despite its prevalence today, has not been the dominant model for long. Instead, for most of human history, environmental accounts of illness prevailed. The tradition of medical meteorology documented a fascinating relationship between environmental events and illness. Weather doctors were unconvinced by the contagion model, noting how it was unable to account for the *pace* (i.e. near simultaneous), *scope* (i.e. across entire countries and continents), *timing* (i.e. coinciding with atmospheric phenomena) and *direction* (i.e. from east to west) of sickness spread. There are also other remarkable examples, such as Dr Ashbel Smith, who found contagion to be hopelessly inadequate in accounting for yellow fever outbreaks. Once again, others' preoccupation with germs interfered with the truth and promoted unnecessary suffering. Despite its days being numbered, it was only after the 1861 release of germ theory that consensus began to shift in its favour, albeit reluctantly. There is, however, much more to this shift than meets the eye, notwithstanding the unanswered questions left hanging by weather doctors about the environmental impact on human health.

Chapter 4

Béchamp Versus Pasteur

The last chapter alluded to an ongoing tension between meteorological and germ-based accounts of illness. Before proceeding, it's imperative to dive into both perspectives in more detail to clarify the context behind them and establish the claims each makes. Theories are only as strong as the foundations they are built upon. Just like a building, weak or faulty foundations compromise the entire structure—despite outward appearances. To understand the relative strengths (and weaknesses) of each perspective, it is necessary to return to their beginnings and ascertain the fundamental principles upon which each is based. This history will provide a basis for evaluating their merits and making a judgement about whether they are fit for purpose.

The debate between Pierre Jacques Antoine Béchamp and Louis Pasteur has spanned more than one and a half centuries. It is arguably one of the longest-running and well-known debates in modern history. Both put forward such compelling arguments for their respective positions that supporters for either side have been steadfast in their conviction the other is wrong. Béchamp's essential premise was that exposure to environmental conditions determined the health of an organism, whereas Pasteur proposed microscopic pathogens floating through the air were the cause of disease. Which perspective is right? This chapter (along with the information presented in the following chapters) will allow you to answer this question yourself.

Béchamp Versus Pasteur

In 1854, Antoine Béchamp, a physician, pharmacist, and Chevalier of the Legion of Honour (France's highest order of merit) began conducting experiments to determine what caused sugar to ferment and form alcohol. The consensus at the time was that fermentation occurred spontaneously (i.e. without the presence of microorganisms). Whilst it was noted that the growth of mould coincided with the fermentative process, their importance in catalysing this process was unknown. Furthermore, the origin of the moulds had not been discovered, although many scientists pointed towards a phenomenon known as spontaneous generation. Also defined as 'Heterogenesis', spontaneous generation occurs when living organisms develop from non-living matter. Essentially, it is the belief that germs could arise *de novo,* completely anew without 'parents'. This contrasts with 'Homogenesis' or 'Generation from Parents', which states that different species of bacteria can only arise from a parent bacterium of the same species.[1,2] However, Béchamp was not initially convinced of spontaneous generation. Through a series of experiments, he discovered that tightly stoppered flasks containing a solution of sugar and water began to ferment rapidly, but only *after* mould (yeast) appeared. Accordingly, he noticed moulds would not grow, and fermentation failed to take place when he added various chemicals to the solution.[3]

Béchamp continued to ponder about the origin of these moulds. How did they get into the flask? Were they already present in the solution, or did they arise from some other source? Intent on understanding their origin, Béchamp conducted a second set of experiments in 1857. He found that air was required for mould to grow and start fermenting sugar and concluded fermentation was *not* caused by the spontaneous generation of microbes within the solution itself, but due to something present in the air.[4-7]

While Béchamp had been busy studying fermentation in his laboratory, the French chemist, Louis Pasteur, had also been conducting experiments to determine what caused milk to sour, meat to rot, and grapes to turn into wine. Just like Béchamp, Pasteur observed that mould growth and fermentation occurred only after exposing flasks containing a solution of sugar, water, and albuminoids (proteins) to the air. He also found that when flasks containing beef broth were exposed to the air, microorganisms would appear, and the broth would begin to putrefy.[8,9]

Conversely, when flasks were sealed from the outside atmosphere, microorganisms would not grow, sugar would not ferment into alcohol, and protein failed to putrefy. As a result, Pasteur wondered if mould growth (and the decomposition that followed) might be caused by something in the air, although he was still sympathetic to the idea that the mould may have been generated spontaneously from within the decomposing matter itself. At this point, both Béchamp and Pasteur acknowledged mould was always present during fermentation, though neither man realised mould might have been directly responsible for this process.[8,9]

While Béchamp continued to advance his understanding of the origins of mould and its role in fermentation, Louis Pasteur struggled to do the same. Despite four years of experimental research, Pasteur's understanding had barely progressed since beginning his investigations. He was still convinced the microorganisms involved in fermentation were generated spontaneously. This fact is documented in Pasteur's first work on fermentation, published in 1858, where he claimed mould arose spontaneously in solutions that favoured its growth.[10] Now, it is somewhat peculiar that Pasteur would hold such a position, considering just one year later, he vehemently opposed this very stance whilst embroiled in a heated debate with another French scientist by the name of Félix-Archimède Pouchet. Pouchet was convinced microorganisms arose spontaneously, while Pasteur argued they floated through the air.

In late 1857, Pasteur presented a series of experiments to the French Academy of Science. Due to this work, Pasteur was credited with discovering that moulds caused sugar to ferment into alcohol.[11] Béchamp protested, claiming he had made this discovery before Pasteur, detailing his findings in a memoir submitted for publication in mid-1857—many months *before* Pasteur's submission. For reasons unknown, Béchamp's memoir was only published towards the end of 1858, and because no records were kept about the submission date of the manuscript, his dispute could not be substantiated.[7,12] Though Béchamp later accused Pasteur of plagiarising his work, no action was taken by the Academy due to the lack of corroborating evidence.[13]

In the years after these events had transpired, an American physician and lawyer by the name of Dr Montague Leverson caught wind of the controversy surrounding the purported plagiarism of Béchamp's work and decided to conduct his own investigation. Realising the injustice that had transpired, Leverson travelled to France to speak before the Academy of

Science, but they were not swayed by his testimony. In 1911, Leverson gave a public lecture at a prestigious London hotel titled *"Pasteur, the Plagiarist"*. During this lecture, Leverson is reported to have demanded Pasteur's work be reviewed thoroughly to verify the veracity of his scientific claims and to ascertain whether he had engaged in scientific misconduct.[12] Despite Leverson's best attempts, no such review ever took place.

Though this controversy went unresolved, it was clear Béchamp's understanding of mould and fermentation was superior to Pasteur's in many ways. For example, Pasteur's collaborator Émile Duclaux asked Béchamp, how such a small amount of mould could produce such large amounts of alcohol? Perplexed as to why such an obvious question would need to be asked, Béchamp responded with an analogy: a man of 100 years of age, weighing only 60 kilograms, will have consumed tens of thousands of kilograms of food and produced hundreds of kilograms of urea during his lifetime. Béchamp contended that mould can consume a significant amount of sugar and produce alcohol in much the same way. Béchamp also discovered that mould produced an enzyme he called 'zymase', which catalysed the fermentation reaction, a concept unfamiliar to Pasteur.[14] Although Pasteur argued 'albuminoids' were required for the fermentation of sugar to take place, Béchamp proved they were not required, and that fermentation was possible with a solution comprised of nothing more than sugar and water.[12] In these ways, and more, Pasteur's understanding of mould and fermentation seemed to lag behind Béchamp's. It is strange, then, that Pasteur was seen as the world's leading expert on this topic, given Béchamp needed to educate him on such elementary concepts.

Pasteur's Path

Both Béchamp and Pasteur originally proposed germs in the air ultimately caused fermentation. As time went by, however, Béchamp wondered if there might be another plausible explanation. Meanwhile, Pasteur remained firm in his belief about airborne germs. In 1859, Pasteur conducted a series of experiments that solidified his position on the matter. One such study involved passing 1,500 litres of air through a glass tube that had a gun-cotton filter inside it. Pasteur then removed the guncotton, dissolved it in ether and collected the resulting sediment. He then repeatedly washed the sediment and placed it inside a small amount of distilled water, which evaporated over 24 hours. Following this, Pasteur placed the dry sediment on a glass slide smeared with a solution of potash, on top of which he placed a glass cover slip. When Pasteur looked at the slide under a microscope, using about 180x magnification, he saw thousands of little microorganisms. Given Pasteur's repeated efforts to wash and sterilise the specimen, these results led him to conclude that the germs must have come from the air.[2] In some cases, Pasteur also took the gun-cotton and placed it into sterile solutions which resulted in the growth of microorganisms, a result which he asserted confirmed the existence of airborne germs.[15] In 1861, Pasteur drew on these experiments to publish what would become the first part of his germ theory, which states germs do not spontaneously generate, but instead derive from the air.[8]

But how did Pasteur know the germs he detected in a gun-cotton filter came from the air without ever directly observing them floating there? With this question in mind, many scientists set out to reproduce Pasteur's experiments but were unable to demonstrate the presence of airborne germs. In attempting to replicate Pasteur's methods, researchers hung cotton wool out in the open for weeks on end. Yet, when they examined it microscopically, they were unable to observe any germs. Similarly, in other studies, researchers examined fresh snow, rain, and dust, but found germs were absent in these samples too. The negative results ultimately led sceptics to conclude germs were not widely present in the air in the manner Pasteur had claimed.[16,17]

The challenges continued when other scientists calculated the amount of airborne nitrogen required to demonstrate the presence of germs. They concluded germs could not possibly exist in the air because there wasn't enough nitrogen to support them.[18] Others criticised Pasteur's work on methodological grounds. For example, Professor John Bennet Hughes pointed out several experimental design flaws, such as a lack of adequate control measures. Without including these in his studies, Pasteur's results could be confounded by other factors.[2] More generally, others have highlighted the ways in which direct evidence for the existence of germs in the atmosphere is curiously lacking.[19]

An Inspired Germ Theory

Regardless of its flaws, Pasteur proudly presented the second part of his germ theory to the world in 1878, which posited airborne germs cause infectious diseases.[20] This came after Pasteur observed the microbial spoilage of food. He theorised the same airborne germs that spoiled food could also explain why people get sick. Germs would infect a completely healthy person, replicate inside them, and turn healthy tissue into diseased tissue. Critically, Pasteur argued all of this with scant direct scientific evidence that germs existed in the air or caused disease.[12,21,22] How then did he arrive at this conclusion?

Although Pasteur was heralded as the progenitor of germ theory, the idea that invisible germs could cause disease was not original. In 1546—more than 300 years prior—Italian physician, Girolamo Fracastaro, believed contagious diseases were caused by 'minute bodies' or 'seeds of contagion'. He defined these units as chemical substances that could be transmitted through the air.[23] A little over 100 years later, in 1658, a medical practitioner by the name of Athanasius Kircher is said to have observed 'tiny worms' invisible to the naked eye, present in vinegar, milk, and the blood of those with febrile illnesses. Kircher thought epidemic diseases were the result of these 'tiny worms' floating through the air and entering the body.[24] In 1677, following the discovery of spermatozoa by the Dutch microscopist, Antoine van Leeuwenhoek, people believed 'real animals' lived inside them. It was assumed Kircher's 'tiny worms' must also be animals and, as such, were illustrated as having crooked bills and sharp claws. People thought these creatures could be killed during epidemics by blowing horns and firing cannons into the air. Such fantastical ideas were indistinguishable from superstition, hence theories of disease involving germs stayed dormant for some time.[25]

Later, in 1762, a similar theory was proposed by Austrian physician, Marcus Plenciz.[26] Like Fracastaro two centuries prior, Plenciz contended that contagious diseases were also caused by 'seeds' and that every disease was seeded by its own specific causative agent.[27] Again, in 1813, the idea that air contained disease-causing entities was suggested by Charles Astier.[28] Once more, three decades later, a French physician named Jean

Hameau, proposed a theory not dissimilar to Pasteur's: that infectious diseases were the consequence of exposure to airborne germs.[29]

It is rather curious, given how many similar ideas were put forth by scholars and physicians across history (even as late as 1847), that Louis Pasteur was proclaimed the father of germ theory. In spite of those who came before him, Pasteur received all the credit and enjoyed considerable recognition for his theory on disease-causing germs. Others who proposed essentially the same idea have since been forgotten, relegated to the annals of history. Meanwhile, Pasteur's work on germs was widely embraced. Esteemed scientists, like Robert Koch and Joseph Lister, expanded upon and legitimised the theory, further propelling it into the mainstream. In contrast to germ theory's widespread adoption, it is also peculiar how this same idea repeatedly failed to gain traction and support with multiple attempts over 350 years. Perhaps there was something unique about Pasteur's approach that separated him from the rest.

The Other Side of Pasteur

Before Pasteur died, he explicitly instructed his family to keep his laboratory notebooks a secret. Pasteur made it abundantly clear no one was to ever have access to them. Pasteur's wishes were honoured until 1964, when his grandson, Dr Pasteur Vallery-Radot, donated more than 140 laboratory notebooks to the national archive in France. Following Vallery-Radot's death in 1971, historians, academics, and members of the public were finally able to put Pasteur's work under the microscope, so to speak. Scholars studied the notebooks for many years and published books and reports detailing their findings on the life and work of Pasteur.[22,30-32]

As a person, Pasteur was reported to have been unfair, arrogant, dogmatic, greedy, misogynistic, and ruthless. During his time educating teachers and professors as administrator and director of scientific studies at École Normale Supérieure, over 70 students *un-enrolled* themselves from the institution, owing to Pasteur's authoritarian attitude, inflexibility, and numerous conflicts with the students. This resulted in the Minister of Education intervening, which ultimately led to Pasteur's resignation.[33] Though his character does not necessarily speak to the quality of his experimental work, it has also been claimed that on more than one occasion, Pasteur engaged in scientific misconduct. He massaged and manipulated his own data, failed to adhere to the scientific method, acted unethically, deliberately published false and misleading information about a number of his discoveries, and modified the results of his experiments before publishing them to align with his preconceived ideas. More than once, Pasteur was also reported to have checked the results of other scientists' work prior to publication, before proceeding to publish them as his own.[22,33,34] Ironically, it was argued (sometimes by the same people who accused Pasteur) that these 'minor discrepancies' and oversights should not detract from or diminish his considerable accomplishments and contributions to science.[35–38]

Béchamp's Little Bodies

In contrast to Louis Pasteur, Antoine Béchamp shifted his initial position on airborne germs after making a startling discovery. When he crushed up the moulds in his experiments, Béchamp noticed they contained microscopic, indestructible particles, orders of magnitude smaller than a bacterium. He named these particles 'little bodies' or 'microzyma', from the Greek words for 'small ferment'. He also discovered that microzyma were present in inorganic matter like limestone. By adding crushed-up limestone to a pure solution of sugar and water, it fermented rapidly, even in the absence of air. Curiously, though, by adding a pure solution of calcium carbonate (i.e. limestone), no fermentation took place. When Béchamp examined crushed up limestone under a microscope, he found the presence of microzyma. Yet, he did not observe these little bodies in the pure calcium carbonate. Based on this discovery, Béchamp claimed microzyma were 'universal base units' of microscopic life that could take the form of *any* microorganism. He reasoned that just like the internal environment of the body determines which sort of tissue stem cells will differentiate into,[39] the external environment (i.e. the 'terrain') determines which microscopic lifeforms microzyma will differentiate into.[5,12,13]

Many scientists confirmed Béchamp's work on microzymas, including the German microbiologist, Gunther Enderlein, who referred to them as 'Endobionts' or 'Protids';[40] the French biologist, Gaston Naessens, who defined them as 'Somatids';[41] and the Austrian doctor, Wilhelm Reich, who named them 'Bions'.[42,43] It is also possible that Béchamp's work on microzyma was initially inspired by the German polymath,

Gottfried Wilhelm Leibniz. Leibniz published a book in 1714 titled, *"La Monadologia,"* where he theorised that the universe was composed of infinitesimally small, immaterial, indestructible, and soul-like particles called 'monads'.[44] According to Leibniz, monads were sentient and conscious particles, capable of harmonising spontaneously with each other.[45] Frederick Henry Hedge translated this work on monads in 1867 where he elaborated on their function in greater detail—reiterating their indestructible 'soul-like' properties. Each monad was said to have its own unique characteristics and an ability to interact with other monads through a pre-established harmony.[46] In 1873, Dallinger and Drysdale conducted experiments on particles claimed to be monads. They, too, observed them appearing and developing into various microorganisms in sterile solutions that had been boiled to 127°C.[47]

Béchamp also noticed microorganisms were 'pleomorphic', meaning they had complex life cycles and could alter their shape and form dramatically in response to changes in the environment. Pasteur, on the other hand, believed microorganisms were 'monomorphic', meaning they had simple life cycles with no ability to change their form and function.[48] It is possible scientists adopted the monomorphic theory due to the difficulties involved in studying pleomorphic changes of bacteria.[49] However, there may be more insidious reasons why the idea of pleomorphism was stifled.[50]

If bacteria are indeed pleomorphic (and their form and function are determined by the environment), this would mean a simpler and more efficient system exists. Only *one* uniform base unit (i.e. microzyma) is required because it is capable of adapting to whatever environmental conditions are present. Germ theory, on the other hand, requires countless different types of germs to exist ubiquitously, each reliant on the right host to present itself to reproduce. If life was spontaneously generated (from microzyma) and capable of pleomorphism, this would certainly be a death knell for germ theory. Rather than *causing* disease, pathogens could only ever be associated *with* disease because they are a *response to* environmental conditions (i.e. they follow rather than lead). This concept formed the basis of 'terrain theory', which was championed by prominent medical doctors like Claude Bernard. He posited, in line with Béchamp, that germs like bacteria are not the cause of disease, but rather the consequence of an altered environment.[5,12,13,51] As it stands, however, the field of bacteriology generally favours monomorphism (as expressed in germ theory) and dismisses pleomorphism (as expressed in terrain theory), despite the latter also being observed and documented by scientists,[49,52-66] government agencies,[50,67-69] and even the military.[70]

Who Should We Believe?

Presently, Pasteur is regarded as a modern scientific hero. His ideas are the basis of contemporary medicine, virology, and bacteriology. But the documented history reveals Pasteur's story is not so clear cut or polished. Though Pasteur is officially credited with the discovery of mould fermenting sugar into alcohol, Béchamp achieved the same breakthrough first, while also demonstrating a superior understanding of the processes involved. Despite a lack of scientific evidence and the fact that similar ideas were published many times beforehand, Pasteur was credited with, and praised for, his germ theory. Those seeking to corroborate and replicate Pasteur's initial work on germ theory struggled to do so using different methods, challenging the validity of Pasteur's conclusions. To make matters worse, Pasteur allegedly committed various forms of academic misconduct, which calls into question his integrity as a scientist and further undermines the legitimacy of his work.

Though Pasteur and Béchamp shared similar views, they ended up in very different places. Pasteur started with spontaneous generation and later committed to airborne pathogens as the cause of disease. Béchamp went the opposite route, eventually uncovering pleomorphism in the form of adaptive microscopic base units (i.e. microzyma). His findings were later corroborated and expanded upon to develop 'terrain theory'. Though relatively unknown, this alternative perspective flips germ theory on its head, claiming germs are caused by disease, and not the cause of it. Although Béchamp appeared to come out second best in the fierce rivalry over fermentation, spontaneous generation, pleomorphism, and airborne germs, Pasteur allegedly conceded defeat while on his deathbed in 1895. He is quoted as saying, *"Le terrain est tout, le microbe n'est rien (the terrain is everything, the microbe is nothing)"*.[71-74] However, only those who were present by Pasteur's bedside will ever truly know if he indeed said this. If true, and there is merit to the terrain perspective, this would have far-reaching religious, spiritual, societal, environmental, medical, and scientific implications.

Chapter 5

Terrain Versus Germs

Pasteur's *germs* and Béchamp's *terrain* gathered support in the form of two opposing factions that divided the medical discipline: the 'contagionists' and the 'anti-contagionists'.[1] In a broad sense, the contagionists operated under the premise that germs cause disease, while the anti-contagionists believed disease causes germs (or, at the very least, that a germ-terrain duality existed).[2-6] Looking back from the present-day dominance of germ theory, it is easy to mistake those who challenged its ideas as some small, fringe group stuck in their ways and unwilling to accept the 'new science'. In reality, however, many of the most eminent doctors and scientists from across the world not only opposed germ theory from its inception but adamantly warned against it.[7] In the face of considerable opposition from contagionists, many physicians—particularly those practising in the United States—remained unreceptive to germ theory for decades after its release.[5,6] This may have been due partly to language barriers and partly to inconsistencies inherent to the germ theory itself.[4,8-11]

Physicians on both sides openly and freely debated each other for decades as to who was correct about the nature of disease. However, as germ theory gained wider acceptance, this discourse became stifled, and the fracture between the two sides grew. Over time, the contagionists were increasingly legitimised, while the anti-contagionists were dismissed and labelled 'sanitarian heretics'.[12] Given their views and critiques gradually vanished in the fog of time, this chapter seeks to clear the air. It revisits core anti-contagionist ideas and unpacks each in greater detail. Shining a light onto terrain theory, zymotic theory, and the work of notable 'heretics' offers an alternative perspective against which to contrast the claims made by contagionists, which persist to this day in the form of germ theory.

The Tenets of Contagion

Contagionists generally subscribe to one perspective, 'germ theory'. The central premise is that one specific microorganism causes one specific disease.[13] They assert that disease-causing microorganisms are ubiquitous in the environment, waiting for an opportunity to infect a healthy host and then spread to other unsuspecting victims. According to contagionists, all living creatures are at the mercy of pathogenic microbes, which have one purpose in mind—to invade the body, replicate, and cause disease.[14] Whilst the host's immune system (e.g. innate, adaptive responses), anatomical (e.g. skin, gut mucosa, airway epithelium, etc.), physiological (e.g. temperature, vomiting, diarrhea, etc.), and functional barriers (e.g. mucus, bile, enzymes, etc.) afford a certain degree of protection, microbes can supposedly thwart these defences under the right conditions.[15,16] The interaction between the immune system and microbes is viewed as a warzone, locked in a constant battle for survival.[17]

Contagionists believe germs can be 'kept in check' by the immune system, permitting them to reside within healthy tissue—an enigma known as asymptomatic infection.[18] However, if the immune system were to faulter momentarily, these pathogens would quickly breach the host's defences, resulting in symptomatic disease, and possibly death. They view disease and its associated symptoms as the problem. Consequently, contagionists have pinned humanities hopes of survival on combatting pathogens and suppressing symptoms with vaccines and pharmaceutical drugs like antibiotics, antivirals, antiparasitics, and antifungals.[19-21] Despite this fearful outlook, germ theorists assert that only one in a billion microbial species are pathogenic to humans.[14] Of the ~1,400 alleged pathogens, less than half a dozen have the capability of killing more than 10 per cent of the people they infect.[22,23]

The Tenets of Anti-Contagion

Anti-contagionists, on the other hand, generally subscribed to one of two main perspectives. Namely, 'terrain theory' and the 'zymotic theory'.

The Terrain Theory of Disease

Terrain theory was first conceived by Antoine Béchamp, Claude Bernard, and a collective of other sanitarian physicians in the late 1800s.[24,25] Terrain (i.e. the soil or *milieu intérieur*) refers to bodily fluids (specifically, the blood and extracellular or interstitial fluid) and the physiological processes involved in maintaining these fluids in a steady state.[26] The core premise of terrain theory is that the body's vital mechanisms have one specific objective: to preserve the internal environment.[27] The body exists in a state of dynamic equilibrium that responds to every stimulus with an appropriate counter-stimulus. Walter B. Cannon built upon this early concept and eventually incorporated it under the umbrella term of homeostasis.[28,29]

According to terrain theory, the body is always in an active pursuit of returning to, or maintaining, a state of equilibrium (i.e. homeostasis). From this view, disease and symptoms are not the problem, but an adaptive answer to the problem.[30] On this point, Dr Thomas Sydenham viewed disease as *"nothing more than an effort of nature, who strives with might and main to restore the health of the patient by elimination of the morbific matter"*.[31] Dr William Braithwaite supported this notion stating, *"One great error which has blinded the minds of medical men in observing the true principles or science of medicine is in confounding symptoms with the disease itself"*.[32] These views exemplify the understanding held by anti-contagionists, that disease was, in fact, the body in an active state of returning to homeostasis.[30]

A critical ingredient in achieving homeostasis is Béchamp's microzyma. These universal base units possess the capacity to *pleomorph* or change into any microorganism depending on the environmental conditions.[25,33] So, when the internal environment (i.e. the terrain) becomes disrupted or damaged by a harmful external input (like a toxin, poison, nutritional deficiency, trauma, etc.), these microscopic units migrate to the affected area. Then, the microzyma adapt to specific environmental conditions by changing their form and function (e.g. to metabolise a present toxin). In their morphed state, the relevant microorganisms carry out various processes to help the body restore homeostasis (e.g. by breaking down dead or dying tissue).

However, in the eyes of the terrain theorists, achieving homeostasis was not confined to the body. They appreciated the broader system, noting the inextricable link between the natural environment and the human body. As these are not separate, the state of one influences the other.[5,6,34] This means the health of the soil upon which people live plays a role in disease as much as the internal 'soil' of their body. Therefore, humans can only ever be as healthy as the state of their terrain—in both senses of the word.[35] As an example of this interdependence, an earth that is devoid of minerals will produce crops lacking key nutrients. In turn, those who eat off this land will suffer nutritional deficiencies or disease. It is possible, too, that deficient or sick people are less apt to look after the earth, perpetuating the cycle.

The Zymotic Theory of Disease

The zymotic or 'chemical theory' of disease was first proposed in the 1840s by Justus von Liebig, the father of modern organic chemistry. This theory was also championed by notable figures like William Farr and John Snow.[36,37] Although zymotic theory gained widespread attention in the mid-1800s, it fell out of favour (like most opposing theories) as germ theory rose to prominence towards the end of the 19th century.[11] The central premise of zymotic theory is that infectious diseases like typhoid, tuberculosis, and cholera are caused by a specific toxic chemical or poison known as a 'zyma'.[37] Zymas are waste products produced when saprophytes (i.e. microorganisms that feed on dead and decaying material) ferment and putrefy organic matter. Eventually, the zymotic poisons and toxins that arise from decaying and decomposing matter damage healthy tissue.[37] Some proponents of this theory believed zymas to be contagious, whereas others thought the appearance of contagion was due to common environmental exposure to toxic and poisonous substances.[37–39]

According to the Zymotic theory, zymas originate from *two* sources:

1. **Exogenous sources**: Zymas are produced in the environment when microbes decompose filth, such as raw sewage, animal carcasses, landfill, and other organic matter. As such, it is possible for these external zymas to enter a person's body via ingestion (e.g. spoiled food), inhalation (e.g. toxic air), or transdermal absorption (e.g. swimming in contaminated water). Once zymas

enter the bloodstream, they damage healthy tissue. The dead and dying tissue are then decomposed by saprophytic microorganisms (i.e. germs) native to the host.[40] This process yields metabolic waste products which could be considered endogenous zymas, perpetuating damage to healthy tissue.

2. **Endogenous sources:** Zymas are also produced inside the body when organs (e.g. liver, kidneys, skin, lungs, gastrointestinal tract) struggle to eliminate metabolic waste products such as urea, ammonia, and hydrogen from the body. This might be catalysed by the presence of toxins and poisons that interfere with various enzymatic detoxification pathways, or the lack of essential nutritional co-factors that facilitate them. As metabolic waste accumulates in the blood, it damages the internal tissues of the body.[41] Consequently, the dead and dying tissue is decomposed by saprophytic microorganisms native to the host. This bacterial decomposition releases zymas into circulation, which can further damage other tissues in the body.[37,39]

Regardless of their source, the zymotic process could reproduce itself indefinitely for as long as zymas remained within the body.[11,42,43] In order for the body to return to homeostasis, anti-contagionists focused on removing *morbific* matter from the body, via the use of treatments that augmented the body's natural pathways of elimination (i.e. urination, sweating, defecation, hepatic and renal detoxification pathways, etc.)

From the perspective of zymotic theory, infectious and contagious diseases were thought to be caused by nothing more than poisons, toxins, unsanitary conditions, and poor nutrition. Critically, it argues germs do not attack healthy tissue, but only break down dead and dying tissue.[34,44] This premise was supported by Ferdinand Cohn (the founder of modern bacteriology) and John Burdon-Sanderson's discovery that bacteria acquire their food source (i.e. nitrogen) by decomposing dead and dying tissue, not healthy vitalised tissue. In other words, the decomposition of tissue *precedes* bacterial growth.[34] Other animal experiments have shown diseases like typhoid fever can be induced by exposure to endogenously produced waste products, lending further credence to zymotic theory.[45]

Integrating the Theories

According to these two theories, disease results from altered internal physiological activity occurring when an organism (a) is exposed to harmful external inputs, and (b) lacks essential health-promoting inputs required to maintain normal metabolic and tissue functions. Both paradigms are very similar in the way they view germs—not as the cause but as the *consequence* of disease. Specifically, when tissue within the body dies or becomes de-vitalised (e.g. due to a lack of nourishment or poisoning), bacteria migrate to the area to decompose it, ultimately removing the poison from the tissue. This fermentative process liquifies the compromised tissue and turns it into pus so the body can eliminate it. In turn, the body also generates new tissue to replace what was lost.[6,46-50] From a contagionist's perspective, this would be seen as an infection, whereas anti-contagionists viewed this as the body's waste removal and recycling process.[3,30,32,47,51]

In the eyes of anti-contagionists, germs are incapable of causing disease in healthy tissue. Not only are 'disease-causing-germs' found in healthy individuals, but the introduction of germs into healthy hosts is *inconsequential*. If germs could cause disease in healthy tissue, it would lead to the rapid extinction of humanity because the so-called immune system would be useless against the ever-present onslaught of pathogens living on us and in us. Indeed, in their view, germs are the fundamental elements of life and should be regarded as *friends*, not foes. To them, germs are the enemies of disease because they decompose morbific matter and recycle the by-products for use in other biological processes.

The fundamental principles of the zymotic and germ theory were so alike that they eventually merged. In fact, the relationship between the two theories was so similar that some scientists stated the word 'virus' could quite easily be substituted for 'poison'.[11] Interestingly, the word 'virus', deriving from the Latin meaning toxin or poison,[52] was defined in English dictionaries as *"a poisonous substance produced in the body as the result of some disease"*.[53,54] The definition was only changed to *"a small, non-cellular obligate parasites carrying non-host genetic information"* in the mid-1900s after so-called 'advances' in the field of virology.[53] After the rollout of germ theory, the terms 'zyma' and 'germ' were used interchangeably for some time until the word zyma was eventually phased out.[11,55]

Sanitarian Heretics

In support of these ideas, the anti-contagionists were labelled 'sanitarian heretics'.[12,56] The term heretic is somewhat ironic, given their views were, by and large, quite reasonable. Some modern scholars have looked upon anti-contagionists more favourably, describing them not only as physicians, but as scientists, reformers, and freedom fighters, standing up for human rights and commerce, with the intention of ridding the world from the *'shackles of despotism'*.[57] They believed disease came from raw sewage, garbage, rotting animal carcasses, and unfavourable environmental factors such as poor sanitation and hygiene, squalid housing conditions, poisons, toxins, and poor nutritional status.[57–61] Understandably, they advocated treating diseased patients by improving the internal and external terrain via the use of holistic interventions, including dietary and lifestyle modifications, herbal medicine, personal hygiene, improved sanitary measures, fresh air, sunlight, and bed rest. These sorts of sanitarian approaches had been accepted for well over 2,000 years (in the form of 'miasmatic' theories, which saw toxic air as disease-causing).[62] Despite the reasonable position and long-standing history, anti-contagionists were harshly labelled and pushed aside in favour of the germ theory almost overnight.[8,11,63] Viewpoints seen to directly challenge the tenets of germ theory were dismissed as heretical and then discarded.

This included the views of people like Rudolph Virchow, who is considered one of the most brilliant and influential sanitarian physicians to ever live. He is heralded as the father of modern pathology and the founder of 'social medicine'.[64–66] Just prior to Pasteur's rise to fame, Virchow famously stated, *"If I could live my life over again, I would devote it to proving that germs seek their natural habitat, diseased tissue–rather than being the cause of the diseased tissue"*.[67,68] Virchow believed epidemics were driven by social factors like poverty, poor housing conditions, and malnutrition and that epidemics should be combatted through political, not medical means.[66,67] Echoing this, Sir William J. Collins gave a lecture to the Sanitary Institute in 1902 titled *"The Man Versus the Microbe"*. In it, he declared, *"We cannot see the man for the germs"*. During the speech,

Collins argued that, even if a germ did possess the capacity to cause disease, its effects could be completely nullified when the terrain was healthy. He also recounted many interactions with well-known figures in the medical community, all of whom expressed scepticism about the germ theory.[6]

One sceptic that Collins recalled listening to was Sir William Savory, president of the Royal College of Surgeons, in his 1879 address. Savory argued the focus on germs from a surgical perspective was overstated, and that the antiseptic system had been credited with results that did not belong to it. Collins also told the story of Dr Alfred Carpenter, president of a leading medical association, who delivered a lecture to the Sanitary Institute in 1881. Carpenter stated that although he admired the efforts of Pasteur to stop the spread of alleged infectious diseases, his proposed methods were not the direction humanity should align itself with as it moved into the future.[6]

In 1902, Dr William Howship Dickinson gave a lecture titled *"The Seed and the Soil"* at a London-based hospital, where he proclaimed that medicine had lost its way—paying far too much attention to the microbe and far too little to 'the man'. In Dickinson's opinion, sanitarians had the best interests of humanity at heart, in contrast to contagionists who promulgated questionable theories. He drew an analogy between a seed and a germ, and the soil and the human body. Dickinson argued treating disease should focus on the soil and not the seed, because the activity and growth of the seed is determined by the conditions of the soil it is growing in. Accordingly, he believed in neutralising toxins with anti-toxins to cure disease, instead of killing germs with germicides.[5]

Dr Stephen Mackenzie, senior physician at a leading London-based hospital, formally addressed the Medical Society in 1902, where he raised concerns that the medical profession was giving too much credence to the germ or the 'seed' and too little to the body or the 'soil'. He believed physicians should treat infectious diseases by rendering the conditions of the soil (i.e. the terrain) unfavourable to the growth of 'so-called' pathogenic microbes. That same year, physician and university lecturer, Sir Benjamin Richardson, presented a lecture to the Sanitary Institute where he implored those in attendance not to be led astray by the conceit of trying to prevent one disease with the inoculation of another.[6] Likewise, Professor John Burdon-Sanderson, another prominent sanitarian, also acknowledged how important the terrain was, declaring, *"The influence of the environment upon organisms such as bacteria is so great that it appears as if it were almost paramount".*[34]

Another outspoken advocate of sanitarian medicine, Dr John W. Hodge, drew attention to the fact that the medical profession did not fully support germ theory and that its proponents were misinformed about disease. In a 1905 journal article, Hodge said, *"There is a popular impression among the misinformed that the medical profession is unanimous in its acceptance of the germ theory of disease; that is, the theory that all infectious and most other diseases are due to the entrance of living microorganisms into the bodies of those affected. This impression is grossly erroneous. Many of the most advanced thinkers in the medical profession, both in this country and abroad, are frank in the expression of their convictions that the germ theory has no scientific basis upon which to rest its claims. It is a mere fantasy of fussy microscopists who know little or nothing of the real nature of disease".*[7]

These men, along with countless others, like Sir John Simon (one of the pioneers of disease prevention), Sir Edwin Chadwick, Sir Benjamin Ward Richardson,[6,69] Professor John Hughes Bennet,[70] Professor Tenison Deane,[71] Professor Ashbel Smith,[72] Dr Thomas Southwood Smith,[6] Dr Montague Leverson,[68] Dr F. R Campbell,[34] Dr Carl Strueh,[73] Dr Benedict Lust,[74] Dr Thomas Powell,[69] John. B. Fraser,[75] and an audacious physician by the name of Dr Matthew Joseph Rodermund,[76,77] all openly contested germ theory. Far from a small, fringe group, the full list of professionals all agreed upon the importance of the terrain (i.e. soil) in health and disease.

Rodermund's Experiments

Dr Rodermund, an American ophthalmologist, was a particularly outspoken critic of germ theory. He was so assured in his belief that germs were not the cause of disease, he conducted a rather questionable experiment with smallpox, that would ultimately lead to his imprisonment. On Monday, the 21st of January 1901, Dr Rodermund visited a young female patient with smallpox. Upon entering her room, he asked the girl's mother if she feared contracting the disease. When the mother replied she was not afraid, Dr Rodermund proceeded to burst open several smallpox pustules located on the girl's face and arms to remove the fetid pus from them. He then proceeded to smear his face, hands, beard, and clothes, with the infected fluid. Rodermund was convinced smallpox was not contagious because he had performed this experiment *dozens of times* over the course of 15 years, each time with a *negative* result.[76]

After covering himself in the pus, Rodermund returned home, ate dinner with his family, consulted with patients in his medical practice, and played cards at the local Businessmen's Club. By his own account, Rodermund touched the faces and hands of at least 10 different people that evening. The next day, Dr Rodermund travelled by train to a nearby town, without washing his hands, face, or clothes from the night before, and mingled with those he encountered. Throughout the course of the day, he consulted with a further 27 patients, again touching their faces and hands. For almost 48 hours, Dr Rodermund had been covered in the pus of smallpox which, according to his estimates, he rubbed onto the faces and hands of at least 37 unsuspecting individuals.[76]

When news broke of Dr Rodermund's actions, he was held under police guard in a quarantine facility. He somehow managed to escape this facility the evening of his arrest and travelled to a nearby town to visit an acquaintance. Shortly after meeting with his acquaintance, he was arrested for the second time in 24 hours. After four days in quarantine, he was released when the police could find nothing to charge him with. Despite directly exposing himself and dozens of people to the bodily fluids of a smallpox patient, not a single case of the disease occurred.[77] This is odd considering smallpox is thought to be highly contagious. Dr Rodermund's exploits were so daring, they made headlines across the United States, and his deeds continue to be reported by media outlets to this very day.[78,79]

The Surgeons' Standpoint

At the turn of the 19th century, many outspoken orthodox trained surgeons echoed the sanitarian physicians. To illustrate the role of bacteria in disease, they wrote books, published papers in medical journals, and gave lectures at medical colleges, universities, councils, and other institutions. Their position was that microbes proliferated to a specific area of the body, not to cause disease, but to break down the dead and dying tissue with the sole intention of facilitating waste removal and promoting tissue regeneration.

Dr Lawson Tait, surgeon, and president of two large hospitals in Britain, gave an address in 1887 to medical doctors at the annual Birmingham and Midland County Branch meeting. In his address, Tait argued bacteria did not cause disease, but were merely the agents responsible for decomposing tissue devoid of 'vitality'. He acknowledged there was an enormous difference between living and dead matter, and in the way microorganisms interact with each of these tissues. From the observations he made as a surgeon, Tait concluded bacteria could not possibly attack living, healthy tissue, and the phenomena of decomposition must not be mistaken for that of disease.[51]

Tait's position was informed by several experiments he conducted. One experiment was performed over a three-year period, which involved 100 women who underwent ovariectomy. In 50 women, Tait performed surgeries adhering to strict Listerian principles of anti-sepsis (i.e. the sterilisation of wounds and surgical instruments with carbolic acid). In the other 50, he operated without any such precautions—just the use of general cleanliness and cold water. The women Tait operated on *without* the use of Listerian infection control measures had a significantly lower mortality rate, better post-operative outcomes, a shorter recovery time, and fewer complications.[46] Though these results might seem anomalous, they agreed with other surgeons at the time, like Professor Victor von Bruns,[80] Dr John Lowe,[81] Dr Thomas Keith,[82] and Dr Geo Bantock,[83] who reported that the use of Listerian methods like carbolic acid not only failed to improve post-surgical outcomes but were actually harmful.

Tait also achieved similar results when operating on people with compound fractures. He found suppuration (i.e. pus discharging from a wound) only occurred when following Listerian principles, whereas using pure water to clean his hands, instruments, and surgical wounds resulted in uncomplicated wound healing. Rather than obsess over disinfecting wounds to eradicate every last microorganism, Tait focused on clearing out any dead or dying tissue from the wound. He believed a successful surgery was due to removing the food source of germs, rather than the germs themselves.[84]

Tait gave a rather telling example of the role of germs in an abscess from a surgeon's perspective. He regarded the pus contained within an abscess as partially decomposed dead tissue that had become liquified.

Although the pus was full of bacteria, the healthy living tissue in the immediate vicinity remained free from germs. When the pus was drained from the abscess, the bacteria were starved of their food source and proceeded to evacuate the area, resolving the so-called 'infection'. Despite not removing every single last germ in the affected area, the abscess would heal without complication.[51] If bacteria were indeed the cause of disease, Tait questioned why they did not re-infect the healthy surrounding tissue and create further damage despite being left inside the clean surgical wound.

Three years later, in 1890, Dr Tait published another paper further describing the saprophytic action of bacteria (i.e. the consumption of dead and dying organic matter). He stated that if a piece of dead tissue was introduced into the leg of a man, it would result in the rapid proliferation of germs. These organisms were not there to prey upon healthy tissue and cause infection or disease. Rather, they were simply there to break down the lifeless foreign organic matter. In line with this, Tait noted how no bacteria would grow when a shard of ivory or a lead bullet penetrated tissue. Although foreign material had entered the body, it was inorganic and, therefore, not prone to microbial decomposition. Consequently, no infection occurred because the bacteria could not use the inorganic matter as a food source.[47]

Tait went on to say that dead and devitalised tissue may lie dormant, free from the effect of decomposition, until such time as bacteria come in contact with it. As soon as bacteria are exposed to the compromised tissue, they quickly go to work, doing what they are designed to do: consume de-vitalised tissue. When bacteria perform this saprophytic activity, they yield metabolic waste products, some of which are toxic to the body. It is these waste products that result in symptoms associated with what is commonly thought of as a bacterial infection. Conversely, if bacteria were introduced into tissue that was vitalised and healthy, no decomposition or 'infection' would take place.[47]

Tait was not alone in his beliefs. In 1891, Professor of Clinical Surgery, James William White, published a paper expressing his views on germs concerning surgery. He claimed that if all decomposable matter (i.e. dead and dying tissue) was removed from the site of tissue injury, germs could enter freely into the wound without consequence. He also went on to say that it was impossible to keep germs out of a surgical incision, due to the simple fact they were ubiquitous, existing in the blood, bodily fluids, and tissue. But White reasoned germs could not proliferate as long as they had no 'pabulum' (i.e. food source). As such, he was convinced these microscopic organisms possessed no capability to cause disease in healthy tissue.[48]

Other surgeons convinced their colleagues (who were wedded to germ theory), using a variety of analogies, like the one given by Dr Kadernath Das in 1895. When entomologists want to attract a certain type of insect, they create a specific type of media. If they want to attract a 'gravedigger' beetle, they place dead tissue under a board in the middle of a field. Within two or three days, countless gravedigger's will arrive. Where these insects came from exactly, no man knows. But, without this medium, it would be difficult to attract such an insect. No one thinks this insect caused the dead tissue. Instead, they migrated there after the conditions were favourable and may very well assist in the process of putrefaction and decomposition. No gravedigger's would be found if a vegetable was placed under the board because the conditions would not allow for it. As Das points out, this insect is analogous with a germ. For healthy tissue, they remain absent or inactive, but for diseased tissue, they actively seek it out and assist in breaking it down—a pattern mistaken for pathogenesis. Based on this reasoning, Dr Das also concluded the effects of the bacteria are entirely dependent upon the medium in which they grow.[49]

Following the same train of thought, Dr George Wilson gave an address at the opening of the Section of State Medicine in 1899. In it, he stated pathogenic germs are only found in necrosed (i.e. dead) tissue. Rather than being the cause of the necrosed tissue, Wilson declared germs performed a benign function, changing necrosed tissue into harmless by-products that could then be removed by the body.[50] That same year, Dr Geo Granville Bantock reinforced this view by stating bacteria were not causative of disease, but were scavengers of tissue devoid of its vitality.[85] Dr Robert Ormiston explained how bacteria functioned as scavengers (i.e. saprophytes) rather than pathogens. They merely return the elements of dead or dying tissue back to their original source, thus allowing for the component elements to be recycled or disposed of by the body.[86]

Other doctors like Hugh Cabot, a Professor of Surgery, explained how surgical operations during the First World War cast considerable doubt on germs as the cause of disease, in an address to a major medical association in 1921. He found that when men were admitted to hospital with battle wounds, the key to successful treatment was completely excising the damaged tissue. Cabot considered the presence of germs was neither here nor there—*of no great importance*. He remarked how, in these battlefield cases, bacteria were already present in the wound before the surgery began. Therefore, the wounds were almost never completely free from bacteria, even after surgeons had finished operating and sewn the wound shut. Cabot arrived at the same conclusion as those before him: it was not the removal of germs that prevented infection, but the removal of the *pabulum* (i.e. de-vitalised tissue). To support this, he argued it could be clearly demonstrated that germs grow on dead tissue and clotted blood and not in tissue of a normal condition.[87]

Summing Up

This chapter delved into the forgotten, though once fiercely argued, perspective of the anti-contagionists. This included core ideas like terrain theory, which states that the medium (i.e. soil, terrain, tissue, bodily fluids, etc.) determines the form, and function of microorganisms. It also included zymotic theory, which claims that each specific disease is caused by exposure to a specific toxin or poison. These views were held and supported by many notable sanitarian physicians, like the smallpox-resistant Rodermund, who were convinced *the environment*—not germs—provided a more robust understanding of the aetiology of disease. These ideas, though labelled 'heretical' and shrouded in history, are nonetheless important to revisit. They highlight how germ theorising was not well received and, in fact, vehemently opposed. Also, much like previous chapters, the historical accounts of sanitarians and surgeons suggest germ theory is inadequate, pointing to documented instances where contagion was unable to explain the course of events. They argue contagionists mistakenly attribute the presence of germs at diseased sites as the cause rather than the consequence and highlight that germs cannot damage healthy vitalised tissue.

Chapter 6

Spontaneous Generation

As the battle raged between Pasteur's germs and Béchamp's terrain, one critical idea held the power to shift the balance: *spontaneous generation*. In short, this idea explains how germs do not infect organisms from the outside air, but rather arise from *within* organic matter in response to disruption (e.g. disease or loss of vitality). If true, spontaneous generation would render germ theory untenable, while simultaneously cementing terrain theory. Given it could single-handedly determine the outcome of the debate, the contagionists saw spontaneous generation as the ultimate obstacle to overcome. In contrast, anti-contagionists saw it as the last bastion of hope to defend. In light of the importance of spontaneous generation, it is necessary to return to this critical juncture in history and lay out arguments for and against it. Though the path society took is clear, it is nevertheless fascinating and helpful to make sense of whether it was the right one.

Back to Redi, Needham & Spallanzani

The theory of spontaneous generation was first proposed by the Greek philosopher and polymath Aristotle in 350 BC.[1] For the next two thousand years or so, people believed life could be born into existence completely anew, without parents (e.g. worms from mud, or rats from filth). Throughout the Renaissance period, the theory became widely accepted by alchemists across Europe.[2] This belief continued until 1668, when the Italian physician Francesco Redi conducted an experiment proving that maggots in rotting meat did not arise from the meat itself, but from the eggs laid in it by flies.[3] The results of Redi's experiment were considered irrefutable proof against spontaneous generation—that life could only come from life. However, just a few years later, in 1675, van Leeuwenhoek's discovery of bacteria and protozoa sparked new interest in the theory once again.[4]

Though people no longer believed organisms like maggots could arise spontaneously from rotting meat, they began to wonder if van Leeuwenhoek's newly discovered, infinitesimally small organisms might be the intermediary between living and non-living matter.[5] Those fortunate enough to have access to a microscope began observing phenomena that suggested spontaneous generation. For example, fresh rainwater, when observed under a microscope, did not contain any life. Yet, after just a few days, it would be swarming with thousands of tiny organisms.[6] Keen-eyed microscopists also began noticing and asking questions about the microorganisms dividing rapidly in fermenting plant material and putrefying animal matter. Were these microorganisms the cause or consequence of decomposition? Did they develop spontaneously from within the plant or animal material, or did they arrive invasively from beyond it?

In 1745, less than 100 years after van Leeuwenhoek's discovery, an English clergyman by the name of John Needham conducted an experiment that was considered by many as irrefutable proof of spontaneous generation. By this time, it was well known that heat killed microorganisms. So, Needham decided to boil chicken broth in a flask, seal it, and then wait to see if anything grew in the sterile broth. To his astonishment, microorganisms did begin to grow, a result he considered proof that life could indeed arise from non-living matter.[7] However, these controversial findings were challenged shortly after by Lazzaro Spallanzani, an Italian biologist. Spallanzani conducted an experiment very similar to Needham's, but instead of sealing the flask after it had been boiled, he sealed it beforehand, preventing contamination with unsterilised air. Nothing grew in the broth and Spallanzani claimed victory over Needham.

Spallanzani concluded that because he sealed his flask first and then boiled it, nothing from the external environment was able to contaminate the broth. He suggested the growth observed in Needham's experiment was not due to spontaneous generation, but the result of substances in the air contaminating the broth before the flask had been sealed.[8] In response, Needham (and others) argued Spallanzani's techniques were so drastic that they damaged the air, the solution, or some other essential component through excessively high temperatures. Therefore, they claimed, it was no longer able to support the spontaneous generation of life.[5]

Pouchet Versus Pasteur

In the mid-1800s, Theodor von Dusch and Heinrich Schröder set out to investigate whether microorganisms could arise from solutions of non-living matter after exposing it to sterilised air. They achieved this by delivering a stream of air through specialised cotton-wool filters into a series of heated glass tubes, which fed into a flask containing a sterile solution. They then hermetically sealed the flask (i.e. so it was airtight) and monitored it for signs of life.[9] Although von Dusch and Schröder's results were negative, a French physician by the name of Félix-Archimède Pouchet claimed he had observed spontaneous generation in a series of experiments employing the same methodology. In 1858, Pouchet submitted his findings in support of spontaneous generation to the French Academy of Science, who were highly sceptical of his claims.[10] Pouchet's experimental results caused quite a stir as they appeared to support the notion of spontaneous generation—bridging the gap between living and non-living matter. If proven to be true, the consequences of Pouchet's findings might well be incalculable, not just for the field of science, but for political, economic, humanitarian, and religious reasons as well.

According to Pouchet, spontaneous generation was more akin to 'spontaneous ovulation'. That is, rather than microorganisms emerging into existence out of thin air, or arising from parent microorganisms, he suggested organic matter contained a plastic force (i.e. *force plastique*) that could be concentrated to form a special organ (i.e. an egg). These 'eggs' would give rise to microscopic organisms when exposed to certain conditions and in the presence of water, air, and heat.[11] Pouchet's theorising was not dissimilar to Antoine Béchamp's, who proposed that all microscopic organisms were derived from 'little bodies' or 'microzyma'.[12]

In March of 1859, several months after Pouchet's original submission, the Academy of Science announced they would be running a contest for participants to submit the results of rigorously conducted scientific experiments proving or disproving the theory of spontaneous generation. While many scientists submitted experiments to the Academy, it was the work of Pouchet and the French chemist Louis Pasteur that took centre stage. Although Pouchet submitted several compelling papers, the Academy ultimately awarded Pasteur the 1862 Prix Alhumbert prize for his elaborate experiments (purportedly) disproving spontaneous generation.[9] Arguably, the Academy sided with Pasteur due to political and religious motives, not necessarily because he had proven his position scientifically.[13,14] The following section outlines several events and experiments to substantiate this indictment.

Newfound Revelations

Despite favouring spontaneous generation in the mid-1850s, Pasteur recanted his position in favour of airborne germs by the end of that decade. It is peculiar how confidently Pasteur argued against spontaneous generation, considering he had been sympathetic to the idea just a few years prior.[15,16] Amassing enough scientific evidence to make fundamental claims about reality generally takes time to accumulate a sufficient body of work. Naturally, then, Pasteur's newfound revelations were met with resistance by many in the scientific community, such as the French chemist Edmond Frémy. Upon hearing Pasteur's new claims, the two men became locked in a heated debate. Pasteur argued sugar solutions only began to ferment after they had become contaminated with the germs floating in the air. Frémy, on the other hand, was convinced otherwise. He insisted microorganisms emerged spontaneously from the solution itself.[17]

Likewise, many other accomplished scientists and doctors were also in disbelief over Pasteur's assertions, including Félix-Archimède Pouchet,[10,11] Professor Nicolar Joly, Charles Musset,[18,19] Victor Meunier,[20–23] Professor John Hughes Bennet,[24] Edward Parfitt,[25] Jeffries Wyman,[26] Professor Dirk Huizinga,[27] Paolo Mantegazza,[28] Albert Wigand,[29] and Professor Henry Bastian.[30–36] They took it upon themselves to conduct scientific experiments to disprove Pasteur's wild assertions. They repeatedly showed that microorganisms did not come from the air but were, in fact, spontaneously generated. Pasteur, shifting his view to airborne germs, caused such a stir that even French newspaper outlets published articles expressing their scepticism. One journalist boldly warned Pasteur's experiments would eventually turn against him.[37]

Pasteur's Experiments

Pasteur claimed that for each type of organic matter to decompose, a specific microorganism would have to arrive on location by floating through the air. This seemed implausible to Pasteur's adversaries who argued too few microorganisms (if any) exist in the atmosphere to facilitate the breakdown of all the different possible types of organic matter. If this were the case, the atmosphere would be so laden with germs that it would appear thick and foggy.[38,39]

Pasteur responded to this objection in 1860, by travelling to a glacier in the French Alps elevated 2,000 meters above sea level. He took with him 20 flasks containing boiled yeast-water and found that after being exposed to the pure glacial air at various altitudes, microorganisms grew in only one of the 20 flasks. Pasteur then went to the foot of the Jura Mountains and opened another 20 flasks, eight of which became contaminated with microorganisms. He then traversed the Jura Mountains to a height of 850 meters and performed the same procedure. This time, five flasks became contaminated.[39] Summarising this work, Pasteur claimed so few flasks became contaminated due to the absence of germs in the atmosphere at high altitudes.[40] He argued the solutions readily inverted at lower elevations due to a greater concentration of atmospheric germs.[39] Although it is generally accepted these experiments proved the presence of airborne germs, critiques by Émilie Duclaux (in 1896),[41] François Dagognet (in 1967),[42] and René Dubos (in 1976),[43] concluded that the scientific validity of these results was in doubt.

Pasteur conducted many other experiments attempting to demonstrate the presence of germs in the atmosphere. In one of his most well-known experiments conducted in 1861, Pasteur showed that beef broth remained sterile after boiling it in a glass flask with a swan-shaped neck. Apparently, the long 'S' shaped neck of the flask trapped dust particles and other contaminants (like microorganisms), while allowing oxygen to come in contact with the boiled, sterile broth. Bacteria only grew after Pasteur either broke the neck off the flask or tipped it downwards (allowing the broth to mix with the trapped dust particles). Pasteur concluded that the microbial growth observed in the broth was caused by airborne germs trapped in the neck of the flask. Pasteur also asserted germs failed to grow in the broth because the heating process had sterilised it. It is this body of work that would form the foundation of Pasteur's germ theory, the first part of which was published in 1861,[44] with the second following in 1878.[45]

Pouchet's Experiments

Pouchet, determined to independently verify whether germs existed in the atmosphere, conducted over 100 experiments employing a range of different methods. One of the first methods involved the use of an aeroscope, a device Pouchet invented himself. This apparatus was comprised of a glass funnel with a wide opening at one end and a narrow opening at the other. Air entered through the wide opening and flowed out of the narrow opening onto a glass slide covered in a thin layer of glycerine. The narrow end of the funnel and the glass slide were enclosed in an airtight chamber connected to an aspirator. Any particulate matter suspended in the air would enter the chamber and become trapped on the glycerine-covered slide. This slide could then be examined under a light microscope.

Pouchet designed the aeroscope in such a way that it was entirely dependent upon the wind. He collected air samples from a range of locations, including mountains, oceans, deserts, and cities. When examining the glass slide to see what the aeroscope captured, Pouchet observed cloth fibres, cotton, wool, silk, combustion byproducts, mineral particles, starch corpuscles, pollen grains, seeds, spores, plant fragments, insects, globules of coal tar, and other non-descript debris. Yet, in almost no instance was a bacterium present.[11,24,46-48]

Pouchet also performed an experiment where he exposed solutions of aconite, flax, meat, China aster, and hay to identical atmospheric conditions. After leaving them to stand, Pouchet later inspected each solution under a microscope, only to find each medium contained a completely different makeup of bacterial life. Pouchet wondered how this was possible given each solution was exposed to the same atmospheric conditions.[49] If germs were really suspended in the air, shouldn't the bacterial profile of each solution be uniform? Pouchet also added dust to some experimental solutions and noticed that the same number of organisms grew compared to flasks that did not have any dust added.[39] The fact that each medium contained vastly different microorganisms points towards the fact that germs don't land on matter arbitrarily. Pouchet argued the medium determined which specific microorganisms were present.

Key Collaborators Join the Fray

After hearing about Pasteur's experiment in the French Alps, Nicolas Joly and Charles Musset collaborated with Pouchet to see if they could reproduce Pasteur's results. Joly, a professor of physiology, and Musset, his student, were working on a thesis on spontaneous generation at the time.[50] The three men travelled together to a glacier in the Spanish Pyrenees, approximately 2,750 meters above sea level. There, they opened four flasks like those used by Pasteur, all of which produced microorganisms.[19] They then travelled down the mountain to a nearby village and opened another four flasks. Once again, microorganisms appeared in all four flasks. The results of this experiment directly opposed those obtained by Pasteur, bringing his claim about atmospheric germs into question.[24,39,51]

This experiment was presented to the Academy of Science but was refuted by Pasteur for several reasons. Pasteur argued that Joly, Musset, and Pouchet's results were invalid because they only had eight flasks, not 20; they shook their flasks before opening them, which Pasteur did not do; and their fingers may have contaminated their samples because they used a short sterile metal file, instead of a long pair of sterile tweezers to remove the material in the flask. The men returned to the Pyrenees several months later, this time with 22 flasks, which were not shaken, and the contents were removed with long, sterile tweezers. In this round of experiments, every flask harboured microorganisms, ending the controversy.[24]

Joly and Musset also conducted experiments examining snow and natural dust deposits for the presence of germs, yet found these substances were often completely devoid of bacterial life. Very infrequently, they would observe the presence of a small number of microorganisms, but nowhere close to the number Pasteur had claimed. They also hung cotton wool six meters above the ground, which they examined for the presence of germs after two weeks. Once again, they were unable to detect any meaningful number of microorganisms. These results, along with those obtained in the Pyrenees, ultimately led them to conclude that germs were not present in the air in the manner Pasteur had claimed.[24]

It wasn't only Joly and Musset who had their doubts. Other scientists calculated the amount of nitrogen in the air and deduced it is insufficient for any meaningful number of germs to be present.[52] Others, like Dr George Child and Professor Lionel Beale, failed to replicate Pasteur's experimental results,[53] as did Dr Jeffries Wyman with the guidance of Professor Asa Gray,[54] and Professor John Hughes Bennet with the assistance of Dr Argyll Robertson.[24] Pasteur and his supporters simply explained away these contrary results as 'contamination' or 'inadequate sterilisation'.[54] They also did not seem to care when highly respected figures like Professor John Hughes Bennet pointed out several methodological issues in Pasteur's experiments, including a lack of adequate control measures that would have the potential to confound his results.[24]

Continuing the Debate: Bastian Versus Tyndall

Less than a decade after the debate between Pouchet and Pasteur came to a head, a similar controversy began. This time, between the English neurologist, Henry Bastian, and Irish physicist, John Tyndall.[55] In 1870, Bastian published a paper describing the observation of spontaneous generation.[35] In the years that followed, Bastian published several other papers detailing a series of controlled experiments he claimed were proof of spontaneous generation. In these experiments, Bastian sterilised solutions in hermetically sealed glass flasks by heating them to very high temperatures. After being left to sit for an extended period, he viewed the sterile solutions under a microscope only to find they were not sterile at all. To Bastian's surprise, these solutions (which should have been sterile) were teeming with a range of microorganisms.[33,34,36,56]

Upon hearing about Bastian's achievements, scientists from across the world began trying to replicate his experiments. Although some were unsuccessful in their attempts,[57,58] many others were able to replicate his results.[25,57,59] To ensure his methodology was sound, Bastian even performed experiments under the close supervision of bacteriology and chemistry professors from several respected scientific institutions.[57] His findings in support of spontaneous generation caused such a stir that questions were raised as to whether atmospheric germs actually existed in the manner Pasteur so vehemently asserted.[52] Many others before Pasteur had worked tirelessly to find germs in the air, but to no avail.[24,60] Even Pasteur himself had difficulty obtaining direct evidence germs existed in the atmosphere.[61]

In response to Bastian's findings, John Tyndall was motivated to conduct his own experiments, for which he developed a method of detecting the presence of microorganisms using a beam of light. When a torch is shone in the darkness, tiny particles can be seen shimmering in the light—some of which are claimed to be germs.[24] This is the same principle that Tyndall used to inform his light-beam experiments. He started by adding a solution containing animal matter to a flask and then sealing it. Tyndall then boiled the flask at a high temperature. When he shone a beam of light through the flask containing the sterile solution, it was completely devoid of suspended luminous particles. When he exposed the solution to purified air, he produced the same negative result (i.e. no germs). However, when he exposed the solution to normal air, the material began to putrefy, and the solution became turbid. Accordingly, when he shone the beam of light through this turbid solution, Tyndall could see countless luminescent particles floating within it. As such, he claimed this indicated the presence of germs and was further proof they existed in the air, rather than being generated spontaneously.[55,62] This conclusion was called into question in 1951 when Nelson and Pickett published two papers. They inoculated sterile broth with red blood cells that had been broken apart (lysed), and then incubated it at 37°C. Like in Tyndall's experiments, the solution became turbid, which suggested the presence of bacteria. Yet, upon closer examination, Nelson and Pickett could neither observe nor isolate bacteria from the solution.[63,64] These results are at odds with Tyndall's indicating the presence of bacteria are not required for a solution to become turbid.

The debate between Bastian and Tyndall came to a head in 1876. Bastian published the results of an elaborate controlled experiment he believed proved spontaneous generation beyond all reasonable doubt. This experiment involved filling a small flask with a solution of sterile potassium salt and then hermetically sealing it in such a way that no outside air could contaminate it. Bastian then placed the small flask inside a much bigger flask containing sterile urine, which was also hermetically sealed. The larger flask containing the small flask was then boiled at 100°C for 15 minutes to sterilise the contents once more. After the sealed flasks had been boiled, Bastian was able to break the smaller sealed flask contained within the larger flask by giving the larger flask a swift shake. The sterile potassium solution leaked out of the smaller flask and mixed with the sterile urine contained within the sealed larger flask. Within 12 hours, the potassium-urine solution began swarming with bacteria. As both the potassium and urine solutions were sterile and remained hermetically sealed from the outside air throughout the entire experiment, Bastian considered the growth of bacteria irrefutable proof that spontaneous generation was indeed possible.[32]

Bastian's detractors dismissed his experimental results by claiming the bacteria were simply the remnants of dead microorganisms left over after the solution had been boiled. Louis Pasteur even involved himself in the debate when, later that same year, Bastian presented his results to the Academy of Science.[31] Pasteur strongly criticised Bastian's methodology, claiming bacteria grew in the sterile urine solution because it was either not boiled for long enough, or because the temperature achieved during boiling was too low to achieve complete sterilisation. Though these seem like fair criticisms, it is important to note that in some of Bastian's experiments, he boiled solutions at 150°C for up to four hours.[52] In defence, Bastian asked Pasteur to demonstrate how bacteria can survive the boiling process employed in his experiments.[30] However, Pasteur flatly denied his request.[65] The Academy intervened and requested Bastian replicate his experiments using a modified methodology they had devised. Bastian was not agreeable to the Academy's stipulations and withdrew from the public debate in 1881.[66]

In the years that followed, however, Pasteur proceeded to conduct several experiments attempting to disprove Bastian's initial findings. Meanwhile, Bastian continued his research on spontaneous generation while working as a professor of medicine at a well-known London university.[67] In 1912, Bastian once more obtained experimental results he regarded as conclusive evidence proving spontaneous generation. He submitted his results to the Royal Society, of which he was a Fellow, but they refused to publish his findings.[2] Undeterred, Bastian published his results one year later,[68] only to receive a less than welcoming response. Critics dismissed his observations as nothing more than artefacts and Bastian's experiments never received the attention they deserved before his death in 1915.[67]

Burdon-Sanderson's Unknown Substance

Though Bastian's work failed to gain traction, experiments by people like John Burdon-Sanderson also challenged the existence of airborne germs.[69] Burdon-Sanderson was a professor of medicine at one of the most prestigious universities in England, where he gave several lectures questioning the nature of infectious disease.[70,71] Despite conducting experiments that suggested spontaneous generation,[72] Burdon-Sanderson officially remained impartial to the idea as he did not want to become embroiled in the controversy.[73] His cautious nature regarding germ theory and spontaneous generation makes it difficult to know his true position on these matters.

Nevertheless, Burdon-Sanderson's experiments are worth discussing because they yielded some very telling results. In one experiment, he took the fluids from the muscle of an animal with sepsis (a so-called bacterial infection of the blood), which he then precipitated with alcohol and filtered. This solution was free of bacteria, but when Burdon-Sanderson injected it into healthy animals, the solution induced a fever. He then took the septic fluid and filtered it, under pressure, through a paper filter or a porcelain filter. When he observed the solution filtered through the paper, it contained many minute particles even though it was free from bacteria. This filtered solution was also capable of producing a fever when injected into a healthy animal. When he observed the solution filtered through a porcelain filter, however, it did not contain any bacteria or particles, nor was it capable of inducing a fever when injected. Burdon-Sanderson let the paper-filtered solution sit for an hour and upon re-examination, noticed it was teeming with bacteria. When he did the same thing with the porcelain-filtered solution, even after 24 hours, it remained completely sterile. This led Burdon-Sanderson to conclude that, not only did the porcelain filter remove the substance responsible for producing a fever, but it also removed some unknown substance essential for bacterial growth.[74,75]

Burdon-Sanderson also conducted other experiments where he intravenously injected animals with a sterile chemical irritant like liquor ammonia. Within 24 hours, 'swarms of germs' were found in the pathological fluids, indicating the bacteria arose from inside the blood in response to the injected irritant.[74] These results were replicated by Bert,

Panum, Coze, Bergman, Schmiedeberg, Vulpain, Clementi and many others, all of whom produced septicaemia in animals by injecting sterile solutions.[76] These results are at odds with the widely accepted belief that sepsis is caused by the introduction of germs into the bloodstream.

Germs in Sterile Air

On the 17th of January 1868, Professor of Medicine, John Hughes Bennet delivered a lecture to the Royal College of Surgeons titled *"On the Atmospheric Germ Theory and Origin of Infusoria"*.[24] In this presentation, Bennet detailed a series of six controlled experiments he conducted with the assistance of Dr Argyll Robertson and Dr William Rutherford. The experiments were performed with the intention of proving or disproving spontaneous generation.

In their first experiment, the researchers passed air through a series of glass tubes, which fed into a collection flask at the other end. The flow of air passed through (1) a glass bulb containing boiling decoctions of liquorice root and hay, (2) a U-shaped glass tube that contained liquid potassium, (3) a 'Liebig' bulb containing sulphuric acid, (4) a hollow glass tube containing gun cotton, and (5) a final U-shaped glass tube containing sulphuric acid. After being sterilised by these stages, the air entered a collection chamber that had been hermetically sealed. Crucially, all instruments and glass tubes were also sterilised thoroughly beforehand to avoid contamination. Then, after a period of four to nine months, organisms began growing in the hermetically sealed flask. For comparison, the researchers captured unsterilised air in collection flasks. Organisms began growing in these 'control' flasks within a few days. The three researchers replicated the experiment a year later, along with several others, all of which yielded essentially identical results.[24] Taken together, Bennet, Robertson, and Rutherford's findings indicate that microorganisms can arise from within sterile solutions in the absence of air, pointing towards spontaneous generation.

These remarkable results caught the attention of Louis Pasteur. He argued their findings were invalid because the bent tubes had acted as a reservoir for germs. So, Bennet modified the apparatus and repeated a series of adapted experiments disproving Pasteur's refutation. In turn, Pasteur argued the temperature at which the infusions were boiled (i.e. 100°C) was insufficient to destroy all of the microorganisms. Pasteur said that a temperature of 130°C must be used to achieve complete sterilisation. In response, Bennet pointed to similar experiments undertaken by Felix Pouchet, where organisms grew even after being exposed to temperatures between 150 - 200°C. However, Pasteur was not receptive to this explanation. Regardless, Bennet concluded spontaneous generation was possible, and that fermentation and putrefaction did not depend on atmospheric microorganisms, much to the displeasure of Pasteur.[24]

A Straw to Break the Germ's Back?

Several decades later, an Austrian physician by the name of Wilhelm Reich began reviewing the literature on germ theory and spontaneous generation. Reich argued the conclusions drawn by Pasteur did not prove the existence of airborne germs, and that the dust in his flasks contained infinitesimally small 'bions'—the lifeless precursors that give rise to microorganisms. To prove this point, Reich conducted a series of controlled experiments, which he published in 1938. Reich added sterilised dust particles to a series of flasks containing either sterilised or unsterilised broth. Curiously, organisms grew more abundantly in the sterilised preparations compared to the unsterilised ones.[14,77–79]

One of Reich's collaborators, Professor Roger Du Teil, conducted similar experiments and yielded comparable results. Reich also allowed Norwegian scientists, Leiv Kreyberg and Theodor Thjøtta, to examine his preparations under a microscope. Whilst Kreyberg and Thjøtta confirmed Reich's starting solutions were sterile, the bacteria that grew in them were ordinary staphylococci. They explained away the growth of these bacteria in sterile solutions by suggesting they had somehow become contaminated by germs in the air.[79] If this was indeed the case, the Norwegian's would also need to account for why only *one* form of bacteria grew, given countless different types of bacteria are supposedly omnipresent in the air.

Beyond Reich's alternative explanation, there are other potential interpretations of Pasteur's results. For example, it could be that, rather than 'sterilising' the broth, the heat simply changed the properties of the broth in such a way that it was no longer conducive for the spontaneous growth of microorganisms.

Final Thoughts on Spontaneous Generation

For a theory thought to be disproven, it is curious so many scientists produced results supporting spontaneous generation (or at least contrary to germ theory). This trend continued throughout the 20th century, with many other published instances of 'particles' displaying characteristics and behaviours remarkably similar to microorganisms arising from sterile conditions.[80–87] In fact, between 1907 and 1957, there were more than three dozen experiments published in the scientific literature, documenting *organised structures* appearing in *sterile media*.[88,89] There is clearly more to this story than meets the eye. But, whenever researchers report findings in favour of spontaneous generation, others promptly dismiss these as nothing more than artefacts or methodological errors.[90,91] Over the last century, there have also been several calls for scientists to carefully reconsider and re-examine the evidence for spontaneous generation.[2,92,93] However, all such requests have been ignored.

While mainstream science has moved on from spontaneous generation, many peculiarities and open threads remain. The contagionists held up Pasteur's experiments as infallible proof against spontaneous generation, yet he never directly witnessed a single germ floating through the air—nor did anyone else.[60,94] Pasteur simply observed an effect and assumed the cause, an approach that flies in the face of the scientific method. Furthermore, despite Pasteur's experiments being seen as dealing the 'fatal blow' to spontaneous generation,[95,96] they did not necessarily disprove this theory—something he, himself, confessed.[78] Indeed, Pasteur admitted his results could be used to support *either* side of the argument.[89,97] Consequently, many historians, scientists, and philosophers from across the world have continued to ask whether spontaneous generation was ever sufficiently disproven, and call for the experimental work of people like Béchamp, Pouchet, Jolly and Musset, Bastian, Burdon-Sanderson, and Reich to be reconsidered.[14,38,92,98–101] Although not common knowledge, Pasteur was still open to the idea of spontaneous generation long after he supposedly disproved it.[97] In the face of these peculiarities and open threads, the reluctance of many to take this alternative theory seriously stemmed from an 'unstated belief' in germs.[89] This view ultimately took us down the path we still find ourselves on. But was it the right one?

Chapter 7

Botched Postulates

U pon its release, germ theory stood on shaky ground and physicians were reluctant to accept it for a range of reasons. Superficial issues certainly stood in its way, such as the language barrier between French and English. However, these paled in comparison to more substantial issues. The chief complaint among the medical community was the absence of scientific experiments demonstrating microorganisms caused disease.[1,2] Without sufficient evidence, many notable physicians, including Professor Horatio Wood and Professor Austin Flint, withdrew their support for germ theory despite being initially receptive to the idea. Widespread acceptance did not follow until the 1880s, when the German physician and bacteriologist, Robert Koch, published his work on tuberculosis.[1]

In 1882, Koch claimed he had proven tuberculosis was an infectious and contagious disease caused by the bacterium *Mycobacterium tuberculosis*. This bacterium was found in animals with tuberculosis, which led Koch to believe it must be the causative agent. After isolating *M. tuberculosis* from sick patients, Koch proceeded to inject pure cultures of it into the abdominal cavities of guinea pigs. The animals became unwell soon after being injected. Importantly, however, they developed completely different symptoms to those animals who had acquired the disease naturally. Koch continued his experiments, seemingly oblivious to the inconsistencies between naturally acquired and experimentally induced tuberculosis. He obtained *M. tuberculosis* from the sick guinea pigs and injected pure cultures of it under the skin, into the abdominal cavities, into the eyes, or directly into the bloodstream of healthy guinea pigs. Unsurprisingly, the animals became unwell soon after that. Again, Koch concluded the bacterium was the causal agent, even though none of the animals developed symptoms resembling naturally acquired tuberculosis.[3]

To make matters worse, Koch never used proper controls, nor did he infect animals via natural routes of exposure. Tuberculosis is supposedly acquired in nature by inhaling the *M. tuberculosis* bacterium. But Koch made no attempts to infect animals in this way, so how could he conclude the symptoms were actually tuberculosis and not just a consequence of being injected (in unusual places) with large quantities of bacteria swimming in growth media? Koch had no control groups to compare his experimental findings with, so the answer to this question is unclear. Now, even if Koch did successfully recreate the disease in animals, it is not appropriate to extrapolate this result directly to humans. Generalising the results of animal studies is invalid without further data.[4]

Taking a step back, it's quite a mystery how Koch justified the broader claim that a specific bacteria caused tuberculosis in people. His experiments reproduced a different illness, using a non-normal mode of transmission, in a species other than humans, with no controls. Somehow, in the face of such oversights and assumptions, Koch's chain of evidence convinced others that *M. tuberculosis* caused tuberculosis. Even more remarkable is the methodologies he employed in his experiments went on to dramatically shape the fields of bacteriology and virology because they formed the basis of what became *Koch's postulates*.

Koch's Postulates

Koch's postulates are a set of criteria scientists and physicians must satisfy to prove whether a microorganism causes an infectious disease.[5,6] It is important to note that, while these postulates were originally designed for bacteria, they also apply to viruses.[7,8]

The postulates are as follows:[9]

1. The microorganism must be found in diseased but not healthy hosts.

2. The microorganism must be isolated from the diseased host and grown in a pure culture.

3. Inoculating a healthy individual with the cultured microorganism must recreate the disease.

4. The microorganism must then be re-isolated from the newly infected host and matched to the original microorganism.

Although Koch was officially credited with formulating these postulates, many critics wondered if they were even his.[10] Some suggest Koch used the work of his colleagues as a 'blueprint' to create the postulates.[10,11] Others claim Koch was merely the 'assumed inventor', though he never drafted, nor conceived of any postulates himself.[12] It is said that Koch's postulates originally stemmed from the work of three men: Koch's teacher and German physician, Jacob Henle, as well as two fellow German bacteriologists, Edwin Klebs, and Friedrich Löffler.[11]

In 1840, almost forty years before Koch's work on tuberculosis, Henle proposed a framework that must be satisfied to prove a microorganism causes a specific disease. For someone to empirically demonstrate this phenomenon, Henle stated they would need to (a) isolate the microorganism from the sick host, (b) inoculate a pure sample into a healthy host, and (c) observe the healthy recipient to see if the germ reproduced the same disease.[13,14] Almost three decades later, in 1878, Klebs drafted a procedure on how to ascertain the cause of an infectious disease. He declared that a microorganism would need to be present in the diseased host, isolated, cultivated, and then transmitted into a healthy host to see if the disease could be recreated.[14,15] Klebs was never able to validate his own procedure because he was unable to isolate pure bacteria in cultures. Nevertheless, his work formed the basis of what would become Koch's postulates.[10]

In 1883, Klebs collaborated with Löffler while attempting to discover the cause of diphtheria, which they believed was *Corynebacterium diptheriae*.[16,17] As a part of this work, Löffler too devised a set of three criteria that he claimed must be fulfilled to establish a cause-and-effect relationship between a microorganism and a disease.

Löffler's criteria are as follows:[17]

1. The microorganism in question must be consistently detected in the diseased tissue.

2. The microorganism must be isolated and grown in pure culture.

3. A sample of the bacteria obtained from the pure culture must reproduce the disease.

One year after Löffler produced these criteria, Koch published a paper on tuberculosis where he began to outline his postulates more explicitly. However, it wasn't until 1890 that Koch published them in the format we recognise today.[10] Surprisingly, in this paper, Koch failed to credit Henle, Klebs, Löffler, or any of the other scientists whose work he had utilised in his experiments.[14] Though this does not speak to the validity of Koch's postulates, it is arguably academic plagiarism—a practice generally frowned upon by the scientific community.

Cracks Appear

Koch's postulates became the launch pad for the field of infectious disease. Armed with this new framework, 'germ hunters' began frantically searching for disease-causing pathogens, dozens of which they allegedly discovered within the decades that followed.[18] But while Koch's postulates seemed simple and fool-proof in principle, satisfying them in their entirety was not so straight forward.[11]

According to Koch, all four postulates *must* be fulfilled to prove a specific microorganism causes a disease. It is somewhat ironic, then, that Koch proposed a set of causal criteria he was never able to satisfy. This is true even in Koch's original paper on tuberculosis. The disease that resulted when he inoculated healthy animals with *M. tuberculosis* was different from that of animals who acquired the disease naturally.[3] As the bacterium did not replicate the disease, one could argue Koch never truly fulfilled his third postulate. Shortly after his work on tuberculosis, Koch conducted similar work with *Vibrio cholerae*, the bacterium claimed to be the cause of cholera.[19] This time, he was unable to fulfill the first postulate because he found *V. cholerae* in completely healthy hosts.[9] Now, tuberculosis and cholera were not simply exceptions to the rule. The bacteria claimed to cause typhoid fever, diphtheria, leprosy, and relapsing fever all failed to satisfy more than one of the postulates. The germs claimed to cause these diseases were not only present in both healthy and sick people, but they also failed to recreate the disease when exposed to healthy hosts.[4,14] In light of these failures, Koch himself admitted he could not fulfil his own postulates shortly after developing them.

Likewise, no sooner had Koch developed his postulates, than other scientists and doctors reported experiencing problems. They too were unable to strictly satisfy all the postulates. So-called pathogenic microorganisms were found in completely healthy people (violating postulate #1). Many alleged human pathogens could not be grown in culture (violating postulate #2).[14] Healthy hosts failed to fall ill when directly exposed to bacteria alleged to cause disease, and the same disease could not be replicated following exposure to various types of germs (violating postulate #3).[4,20] Consequently, germ hunters struggled to provide convincing evidence for the causal role of germs in disease.

Whenever one scholar published a paper suggesting they had found a microorganism in diseased tissue (and assumed it was the cause), another was just as quick to find the same microorganism in healthy tissue, annihilating the possibility that the germ was the causative factor.[21] This conundrum occurred time and again. So, in an attempt to reconcile these contradictions, Koch and the germ hunters were forced to alter and expand the original postulates so they could conclude a particular germ was indeed pathogenic.[14,22] But, after witnessing the fallibility of the concept, many advocates of germ theory turned their back on it in disgust.[21] This disappointment prompted many to consider whether there might instead be validity to the claims made by sanitarian doctors.

Koch's Sceptics

The contradictory findings meant the concept of disease-causing germs was not so simple and fool-proof to verify as Koch had originally proposed. This led many doctors, like John P. Wall, to consider flipping the causal story on its head, asking whether the microorganisms present in diseased tissue were the *cause* or the *consequence* of the disease in question. Like other sanitarians, he figured germs coincided with disease because they scavenged dead, dying, and devitalised tissue.[21] Wall openly expressed his scepticism towards the claims made by Koch stating, *"The germ theory is probably as fallacious as many other theories which have sprung up in medicine, been accepted and flourished for a while, to be finally forgotten or only remembered as curiosities of medical literature"*.[23]

Echoing Wall's sentiment, Dr Montague Leverson exercised little restraint when poking holes in Koch's theories. Leverson authored a paper in 1898 titled, *'An Inquiry into the Logical Basis of the Germ Theory'*. In this paper, Leverson aptly noted how scientists culture bacteria and then inoculate them into healthy hosts was too far removed from what happens in nature. This lack of ecological validity meant it was impossible to make any sense of Koch's experimental results.[24] Leverson and other like-minded physicians also pointed to confounds arising from mixing bacteria (used for inoculation) with culture medium. This contamination meant there was no way to tell whether bacteria, culture medium, or an interaction between the two was responsible for causing symptoms following inoculation.[24-26] Such fundamental oversights—and the inconsistencies that followed—led many to conclude Koch had confused *cause* (disease) with *effect* (germ).[21,26]

Some were so assured in their scepticism, that they were willing to risk their lives by conducting experiments on themselves to subject Koch's claims to the highest level of scrutiny.[27] Take, for example, the German professor of chemistry, Max von Pettenkofer—one of Koch's most outspoken critics. Pettenkofer did not subscribe to the notion that germs alone caused disease. He believed that, when a bacterium acted upon decaying organic matter, it released a toxic waste product which was responsible for the observed symptoms.[28] Therefore, if no decaying matter was present, germs could exist in the host without any untoward effects.

Using this logic, Pettenkofer attempted to disprove Koch outright, by drinking a pure culture of *Vibrio cholerae*, which he obtained from Koch himself. Maybe Pettenkofer was inspired by the likes of Emanuel Klein (the father of microbiology in Britain), François Foy, Scipion Pinel, Emile Veyrat, and Jean-Louis Guyon—all of whom had attempted similar self-experiments without developing the disease.[29,30] In rebuttal, Koch argued stomach acid destroyed cholera bacteria. So, to give the alleged pathogen the best chance of infecting him, Pettenkofer neutralised his stomach acid with bicarbonate first and then proceeded to drink the bacteria on an empty stomach. Apart from some mild diarrhea, *he remained well*. This result is all the more surprising considering Pettenkofer was a seventy-four-year-old man in a state of declining health, with not a tooth left in his head and glucose in his urine (a sign of diabetes).

His offsider, Rudolf Emmerich, also conducted the same self-experiment and just like Pettenkofer, *failed to contract cholera*.[27]

Asymptomatic Infection

To address the antics of Pettenkofer, Emmerich, and others like them, Koch backtracked, claiming only the first two postulates needed to be fulfilled to prove disease causation. Not only that, but Koch also then proposed the mere *presence* of a microorganism suspected of causing an infectious disease was sufficient to establish a cause-and-effect relationship.[31] His post-hoc rationalising didn't stop there, either. To further explain away his critics' anomalous findings, Koch introduced the concept of an 'asymptomatic carrier' or 'asymptomatic infection'. The idea was that pathogenic organisms could infect healthy people without producing symptoms, while still retaining the capacity to transmit to other people.[14] At face value, the concept of asymptomatic infection seems plausible, so, it is a hypothesis worth testing. But, upon closer inspection, several glaring inconsistencies become apparent.

According to Koch, a person can be 'infected' with pathogenic germs like *M. tuberculosis* and *V. cholerae* and remain completely well. Modern-day medicine states that the symptoms of a bacterial infection are either due to the pathogen directly damaging the body's tissue, or from the immune system eliminating the pathogen from the body.[32] In the case of tuberculosis, people with a 'strong immune system' can supposedly defeat the *M. tuberculosis* pathogen before it causes damage to healthy tissue.[33] Only those with 'weak immune systems' (or who are otherwise vulnerable) supposedly develop the disease.[34] Therefore, it stands to reason that individuals with 'weak immune systems' would be *highly susceptible* to developing symptomatic tuberculosis.

However, this susceptibility does not appear in reality. For example, there are currently more than *two billion* people—over a quarter of the world's population—with supposed 'asymptomatic' tuberculosis infections. These people somehow harbour a deadly pathogen inside their body, often for many years, yet never develop symptoms of the disease.[35] This is all the more peculiar given the overwhelming majority of these people live in developing countries like India, Pakistan, Nigeria, and Bangladesh.[36] These nations are some of the poorest in the world, with vast numbers of the population living in abject poverty and suffering from food insecurity, malnutrition, homelessness, exposure to poor sanitary conditions, and limited or inadequate health care. All of these are risk factors known to impair immune function, which would surely increase the risk of contracting and dying from tuberculosis.[37-40]

So, how do the most impoverished and malnourished people in the world (i.e. those most likely to have 'weak' immune function) present with asymptomatic tuberculosis? According to Koch, it was only those with 'strong immune systems' who could fight off the pathogen without symptoms. To account for this clear contradiction, modern germ theorists argue an impoverished immune system cannot mount a sufficient response, so no symptoms or disease occurs. But rather than reconciling the contradiction, this makes it worse. By this line of reasoning, highly infectious germs fail to cause disease in hosts with either strong *or* weak immune systems. It is difficult to follow this logic. It implies germs only negatively impact those who fall into some 'normal' range yet remain inconsequential to people who are exceedingly healthy or unhealthy. It seemed that Koch, in attempting to remedy his original postulates, painted germ theory into a (conceptual) corner. At the very least, germs no longer appear to be the chief causal factor in this story because they perform very little 'heavy lifting' in determining whether billions of people fall ill and die of disease.

Given the dilemmas it led to, why did Koch feel the impulse to modify his postulates immediately after developing them? In their original form, they provided a perfectly logical and rational method of establishing a cause-and-effect relationship between a specific microorganism and a particular disease. Indeed, despite their shortcomings, the postulates are still regarded as the gold standard for infectious disease causality.[41,42] Even by today's standards, the postulates are by no means redundant or obsolete. Koch's official reasons for revising them are not known, but the difficulty he encountered attempting to satisfy them and the resistance he faced in response to them likely contributed. It is also possible Koch kept running into issues because he was simply *downstream* from deeper flaws at the heart of germ theory.

Rivers' Postulates

When Koch's postulates failed to adequately demonstrate infectious diseases were caused by microorganisms, germ theorists were forced to invent a rescue device—a virus.[43] In many instances, people were found to have a specific disease (like influenza), yet the causative agent (thought to be a bacteria) was curiously absent. Contagionists had become so fixated on microorganisms, that they pre-supposed a pathogenic particle, much smaller than a bacterium, must be responsible. The introduction of this concept was convenient because it absolved researchers from producing evidence of a 'morphologically characteristic microbe'.[44] However, propelling this new idea into the mainstream was not a straightforward process. Early adopters of germ theory believed only autonomous microorganisms, like bacteria or parasites, could cause an infectious disease. At the time, it was considered *heresy* to entertain the notion that an inanimate, invisible particle, like a virus, could ever possess such a capability.[43] Furthermore, germ theory purists refused to accept any claim that a microorganism caused disease unless Koch's postulates had been fulfilled in their entirety. Though, many pointed out that viruses could never fulfil Koch's second postulate because viruses did not reproduce on lifeless media in a culture flask.[45] Instead, they only 'grew' (allegedly) inside living host cells.

So, if the medical and scientific community were to ever accept the idea that non-autonomous, inanimate, and infectious agents (i.e. viruses) caused disease, they would need to devise a new framework for disease causality. Accordingly, the American bacteriologist and virologist, Thomas Rivers, published a set of postulates in 1937. These were built upon those originally devised by Koch but were specific for establishing the cause-and-effect relationship between a virus and an infectious disease. To successfully demonstrate a causal relationship, Rivers' postulates stipulate that one must:[45,46]

1. Isolate the suspected virus from a diseased host.

2. Cultivate the virus in host cells.

3. Provide proof of filterability (i.e. separate virus particles from other contaminants like bacteria).

4. Reproduce the disease after inoculating the virus sample into a healthy host.

5. Re-isolate the same virus from the experimentally infected host.

6. Detect a specific immune response to the virus (i.e. antibodies).

Now, when Rivers' postulates were developed, very little was known about viruses. Scientists had barely scratched the surface of understanding the differences between viruses and other microorganisms, and their complex interrelationships with a living host. Not only that but the characteristics of a virus had never been described because no one had ever directly observed one in nature—a fact that was acknowledged by Rivers himself.[47] Rivers also admitted he did not fully understand the true nature of these 'obligate parasites' when he devised his postulates.[45] Early concepts of viruses were far from definitive, and they were classified as just another form of bacteria.[48] Even two decades after River's had developed his postulates, viruses remained somewhat of an enigma and were yet to be clearly defined. Then, in the late 1950s, the French molecular biologist, André Lwoff, finally distinguished viruses from other microorganisms by declaring, *"viruses are to be considered viruses because viruses are viruses"*.[49,50] Though this is painfully tautological, these kinds of ideas formed the foundations of virology as an official discipline.

Despite Rivers' limited understanding of these sub-microscopic particles, at face value, his postulates appeared to be a sound framework for establishing a cause-and-effect relationship between a virus and an infectious disease. However, in his seminal paper, Rivers drew attention to several facts which directly contradicted the very postulates he espoused. For example, he stated:

1. Different viruses can produce the same pathological presentation (i.e. identical symptoms).

2. The same virus does not always produce the same pathological changes amongst different hosts (i.e. inconsistent symptoms).

3. Inoculating a virus into a healthy host might activate an unrelated latent virus already present in the healthy host, which could cause the same symptoms as the inoculated virus.

These points cast doubt on the central premise of germ theory, which is that a single pathogenic agent (i.e. a germ) causes one specific disease. In fact, Rivers himself said, in no uncertain terms, that this premise was incorrect. In his 1937 paper, he gave the example of swine flu, declaring it was not caused by a virus, but by the synergistic effects of a virus *and* a bacterium. That is, neither the virus nor the bacterium could produce the disease alone. Apparently, both agents had to be present concomitantly. Rivers also gave an example of a particular plant disease that was supposedly caused by two viruses interacting. When researchers inoculated each so-called virus into a plant, this supposedly produced two very distinct diseases from the one being studied. Only when they inoculated both viruses at the same time were they able to allegedly recreate the disease of interest.[45] If true, and two or more interacting pathogens cause disease, then neither Rivers' nor Koch's postulates could prove causality because neither made provisions for this phenomenon.

Post(ulate) Mortem

In sum, the fields of bacteriology and virology rely on Koch's and Rivers' postulates, which, if satisfied, establish a cause-effect relationship between germs and disease. As this chapter uncovered, there are fundamental flaws in both sets of postulates. Koch not only lifted his postulates from the work of others but wasn't even able to fulfil them himself. His initial work on tuberculosis makes claims his data do not support. When other scientists were also unable to satisfy the postulates, Koch backtracked, saying some were no longer necessary and that other factors (i.e. immunity) superseded the role of germs. However, these revisions did not necessarily resolve the issues. Later, Rivers introduced postulates attempting to demonstrate the causal role of an inanimate particle he had never directly observed nor knew much about. Unsurprisingly, these suffered a similar fate at the hands of unexplained contradictions (e.g. the mismatch between virus and symptom) and complexities (e.g. supposed interactions between germs).

Altogether, the two sets of postulates are inherently problematic and potentially unfulfillable. This means no one has demonstrable 'proof' (as stipulated by Koch and Rivers) that germs cause disease. Although the tenets of germ theory rest entirely on this premise, no one can substantiate the claim due to insufficient empirical evidence. If science cannot confirm this causal story, then it cannot confidently rule out competing theories. As it stands, we do not know as much about germs as we think we do, which has many implications. For example, the weight of evidence available for disease-causing germs is disproportional to the power and reverence people attribute to this idea. Despite lacking support for its core assumptions, it constrains all walks of modern life and escapes any form of scrutiny.

Chapter 8

Unscientific Methods

The discussion in this chapter revolves heavily around science. After all, it is the best way to answer questions about bacteria, viruses, and what makes us sick. Given the burden science bears in answering big questions, and considering the reverence people pay to it, it is necessary to reflect on science as a field of scholarship and as a method of inquiry. The former is affected by many broader systemic issues that plague disciplines like medicine. The latter is hindered by more specific issues with how virologists conduct and interpret research. Thinking in this way allows us to critically evaluate ideas often considered *untouchable* while prompting us to interpret and implement scientific findings with greater caution.

This detour into science is also relevant for appreciating the extensive human experimental research reviewed in later chapters. Section two discusses experimental methods and findings at length, so a brief refresher is useful to help readers engage more fully with this material. A primer in scientific thinking will assist you in determining whether the studies make sense and are actually scientific or not.

The Sad State of Science

When people hear the word 'science' they assume it is unquestionable, infallible, ethically defensible, and—above all else—a genuine pursuit of truth. Yet, in the modern era, this assumption does not quite reflect reality. If science were a ship, its hull would be compromised and in desperate need of repair. Upon realising the extent of the damage, one might wonder how it stays afloat. The majority of scientific research findings are thought to be incorrect and between 80 to 90 per cent of pre-clinical medical studies cannot be replicated.[1,2] Scientists increasingly prioritise careers, salaries, grants, industry funding, prestige, and publications at the expense of integrity and rigour.[3] Meanwhile, the majority of funding for clinical trials comes from private companies and at least a quarter of scientists have at least one undeclared financial conflict of interest.[4,5] More alarming still, the entire budget of many so-called 'independent' medical industry regulators comes *entirely* from pharmaceutical companies.[6]

As it turns out, science is in trouble. But the problem is not with the scientific method, but rather with the way scientists (and their institutions) deviate from the method in the pursuit of some self-serving agenda. They manipulate experimental procedures to arrive at pre-determined outcomes, massage data and statistical analyses to appease those who fund their research, plagiarise the work of others, and sometimes falsify or fabricate their results outright.[7-11] Although few people want to acknowledge the extent of these problems,[12] some argue they are so widespread we should regard medical research as *fraudulent until proven otherwise*.[13] Along similar lines, other critics have argued we can no longer trust the published medical literature, nor the clinicians who draw from it.[14] What might seem like extreme views are shared by several prominent (former) editors of major medical journals,[13-15] and professors of medicine from prestigious universities, who have publicly stated the vast majority of published research in medicine is *false*.[2]

More than ever, scientific knowledge is ripe for critique and course correction. At the same time, however, the world increasingly treats scientific ideas as sacred and untouchable. This creates a paradoxical situation. On one hand, a broken system continues to career off course, producing and uncovering untrustworthy results. On the other hand, people pledge unquestioning allegiance to scientific knowledge and protect it as if it were flawless. In practice, this means the book you are reading—though perfectly justified in its scrutiny—might be dismissed by many because it challenges a preciously held understanding. It will easily receive pejorative labels like 'conspiratorial', 'heretical', and 'dangerous'. But, defending science through dismissive or destructive means is antithetical to the method itself. The best way to address challenges and uncertainty is not through nonchalance or aggression. Instead, it *is* via the scientific method. If germs are so easily proven, it should not be a difficult task to perform the necessary controlled scientific experiments to clear up any uncertainties once and for all. However, this may be easier said than done.

In 1935, physician and microbiologist, Dr Ludwik Fleck, wrote a formidable treatise on the issues plaguing science and the growing trend of conflating hypotheses with facts. He posited that, to some extent, every theory had been born out of cultural and social conditioning. This means that an idea can take hold and shape our perception of reality simply because enough people believe it to be true—even if it is based on hearsay or flimsy evidence. In specific reference to syphilis, Fleck argued that germ theory was closer to extinction than it was to fact.[16] It would seem that opposing a widely held belief is likely to encounter significant resistance or be ignored entirely, simply because it fails to conform with that of the mainstream—regardless of whether the challenge is logical and supported by sound science. So, even if robust controlled experiments were performed, they may not remedy the false beliefs instilled within society after more than a century of questionable scientific practises.

True scientific thinking is *process-based*. Issues that arise are opportunities to course correct. Rather than turning a blind eye, or seeing them as a threat, we need an approach humble enough to recognise its deepest flaws and courageous enough to confront them head-on. In the spirit of incrementally improving, we also need to openly and frequently question science without fear of reprisal. It is impossible to progress by holding on too tightly to any particular idea or practice. What we 'know' is only ever the *best available* understanding; it is a mistake to entrench what is inherently tentative and provisional. Unfortunately, many existing scientific principles like this appear to have fallen by the wayside.

The Scientific Method: A Primer

How should we, as limited beings, understand and make sense of the enormously complex world we live in? We can rely on personal experience or anecdotes, but these are biased and flawed in many ways. If we want to prove cause and effect, with high levels of certainty, and in a way that generalises, our best bet is to turn to the 'gold standard' approach: *the scientific method*. This is a logical, rational, and systematic process anyone can use to study natural phenomena. It is *iterative* (i.e. it achieves confident answers incrementally and cumulatively), *replicable* (i.e. others must be able to reproduce the method to verify or build upon existing answers), *simple* (i.e. it favours elegant answers with fewer assumptions), and *falsifiable* (i.e. it requires testable criteria to establish whether an answer is correct or incorrect). Without getting too bogged down in the finer details, the scientific method generally follows a sequence of steps:[17,18]

1. Observe a natural phenomenon.

2. Construct a hypothesis to explain the relationship between variables of interest.

3. Test the hypothesis with an experiment (involving an independent and dependent variable).

4. Analyse data to confirm or reject the hypothesis.

5. Draw conclusions.

6. If the results confirm the hypothesis, communicate them so they can be verified and replicated.

7. If the results do reject the hypothesis, construct a new one.

As seen in step three, there are two broad types of variables in a scientific experiment: an *independent* variable (i.e. the presumed cause) and the *dependent* variable (i.e. the observed effect). In an experiment, researchers ideally isolate and manipulate the independent variable under controlled conditions to observe its effect on the dependent variable. Without these two variables, an experiment cannot be considered truly scientific. The better these two variables are isolated, controlled for, and measured, the more certain the findings.

A Sunflower Experiment

To fully grasp these principles and how they relate to germs, it helps to walk through a practical example. The scientific method often starts by observing a naturally occurring phenomenon. Let's say a botanist (i.e. someone who studies plants) watches sunflowers and notices that those exposed to direct sunlight grow faster than those in the shade. Fascinated by this apparent phenomenon, the botanist wants to investigate whether sunlight affects plant growth, so they form a testable hypothesis: sunflowers grow faster in sunlight compared to sunflowers in the shade. Technically, before any further steps can be undertaken, the botanist must first verify that the independent variable (sunlight) and the dependent variable (plant growth) exist in nature by directly observing them. Completing this step is relatively straightforward because both variables are visible to the naked eye. Once confirmed, the botanist devises an experiment to test the hypothesised effect of sunlight on plant growth.

If the botanist wanted to run the most basic test, all they would need to do is put a sunflower out in the sun and watch it grow. The problem here is the botanist has nothing to compare its growth against, which undermines their ability to draw firm conclusions. That is, they do not know how much the sunflower would have grown in the shade, so they cannot determine with any certainty how much sunlight influenced its growth. Therefore, the botanist should place one sunflower in full sunlight (experimental group) and another in full shade (control group). The main variable that differs between the two sunflowers is the amount of sunlight they receive (which is the independent variable the botanist is interested in directly measuring the effect of).

Next, to ensure the best possible test of their hypothesis, the botanist should continue to control the experiment. This means reducing or eliminating the impact of other *extraneous variables* that might affect plant growth. The more controlled an experiment is, the clearer the effect of the independent variable will be on the dependent variable. Removing extraneous variables can minimise error (i.e. random variation) in sunflower growth. It can also remove *confounds* (i.e. hidden variables that also promote sunflower growth) which would make it impossible to determine whether the effect was due to the independent or an extraneous variable. So, to ensure their experiment is controlled, the botanist plants two seedlings from the same parents, into two separate but identical pots. Both pots contain the same amount and type of soil. The botanist provides the same amount and type of food and water to the seedlings, places them on identical pot stands so they are the same height above the ground and positions them as close as possible to each other outside. In this way, factors like plant species, pot, soil, food, water, air, temperature, humidity, and height do not vary markedly across the two experimental conditions (i.e. sunlight vs. shade).

Now, because this experiment adheres to the scientific method, the botanist can accurately measure the effect sunlight has on sunflower growth. After waiting an allotted time, they find the flower in the sun grows faster than the one in the shade, which confirms their hypothesis. They have successfully studied a natural phenomenon and confidently explained it by testing a hypothesis using controlled experimental methods.

Sunflower Experiments Gone Awry

One day, in a second lot of experiments, the botanist inspects the two sunflowers and notices the one in the shade isn't growing very well. The plant looks like it is dying. Its leaves are starting to turn brown, the flower petals are falling off, and there is some green-coloured sap oozing out of the stem. To explain this, the botanist hypothesises some kind of disease-causing parasite has infected the plant. As such, they collect a sample of sap from the sunflower to identify the cause of the disease.

The botanist looks at the sap under a microscope but cannot see any parasites. They remain convinced, so account for this absent finding by claiming the parasites are present, but not in large enough quantities to observe. As such, the botanist believes the only way to see the parasites is to cultivate them in the laboratory. To do this, they get a culture flask and add in fly larvae, synthetic plant growth regulator, trypsin (an enzyme), phenol red (a pH indicator), vegetable broth, and baby grasshopper blood. They also add in some pesticides, herbicides, and fungicides to prevent contamination of the experiment by any pests or other microorganisms. After mixing these substances together in the culture flask, the botanist adds a final ingredient—the sap from the sunflower. The botanist theorises that, if the fly larvae die, it must be due to the invisible parasites in the sap. After a few days the larvae do indeed die. This confirms the botanist's hypothesis allowing them to confidently claim this as proof there are parasites in the sap causing the sunflower to become diseased.

To verify this claim further, the botanist takes the culture flask mixture and examines it under a microscope. To their astonishment, they see lots of little particles that were not present in the original sap sample. These must be the parasites! Based on this deduction, the botanist believes they have successfully grown parasites in the culture. To isolate them, they then take the unfiltered mixture and put it into a centrifuge. This separates large solid debris particles from the fluid portion of the mixture (i.e. supernatant). Next, the botanist looks at the supernatant under the microscope and sees many kinds of particles of all different shapes and sizes, some of which they claim are the alleged parasites. Then, they mix a portion of the supernatant with sterile saline solution, spray it all over the healthy sunflower, and inject another portion into the leaves and stem with a syringe. After a few days, the healthy sunflower begins to die. The botanist claims this is proof that a parasite caused the sunflower in the shade to become sick, and that the parasite can be transmitted from sick sunflowers to healthy ones.

Now, take a moment to reflect on the broader scientific principles, the original sunflower experiment, and the above-mentioned procedure. In confirming their hypothesis about disease-causing parasites, how strictly did the botanist adhere to the scientific method and principles? What was the independent variable? What did they compare the effect to? How well did they control for other extraneous variables? Do you think this approach proves a parasite made the sunflower in the shade sick? Does it demonstrate a parasite can be transmitted from sick sunflowers to healthy ones? What would need to be done differently for this experiment to be considered scientific and to prove a parasite caused the disease?

Clearly, many methodological flaws in the botanist's experiment render it so uncertain as to be almost useless. Let's briefly walk through some of these to get a sense of why the second experiment is not truly scientific and why it does not prove cause and effect:

1. **It assumes rather than observes.** The botanist never detected a parasite in its natural environment—the sunflower sap. This means the existence of a parasite was assumed. Without directly observing and isolating the parasite from its natural habitat, the botanist had no reference standard to compare the particles they found in the culture flask to. They assumed the allegedly isolated particles were parasites because they weren't present prior to the sophisticated procedure (that they could well have been a byproduct of). The botanist also erroneously equates the death

of fly-larvae in an artificial medium as proof of a disease-causing parasite in a plant.

2. **The independent variable is unclear.** The botanist never truly manipulated an independent variable. Neither sap nor supernatant is independent because they both contain lots of different compounds. The parasite was also not independent because it was never properly isolated, nor was it shown to exist in the sap. As such, without an independent variable, the experiment cannot be considered scientific. It's impossible for the botanist to know which variable caused the observed effects (i.e. the death of fly larvae, and the disease in the inoculated sunflower) to occur. Was it components in the sap, additives in the culture flask (e.g. pesticides, trypsin, grasshopper blood, vegetable broth, etc.), excess shade or moisture, the unnatural injection method, the saline solution, or some kind of unexpected interaction among them? The botanist cannot be sure about any of these possibilities, let alone a parasite.

3. **The dependent variable is misinterpreted.** The botanist observes and interprets multiple effects: (a) the dying sunflower, (b) the dead fly larvae, and (c) the healthy sunflower becoming ill. It's possible a parasite produced all these effects, but because this conclusion relies on several untested assumptions at each step of the experiment, this is by no means certain. In the face of many alternative explanations, it is disingenuous for the botanist to conclude their hypothesis is the most likely interpretation of results. Experiments require both independent and dependent variables to be unambiguous. You cannot simply infer one based on the other.

4. **It misuses simplicity.** The botanist invoked needlessly complex theories to explain why the plant was dying. There are many simpler and more obvious hypotheses to rule out before leaping to invisible parasites. For example, the sunflower could have been sick because of a lack of sunlight, the presence of some other environmental factor (e.g. cold, moisture), or a biological defect. Similarly, the botanist applied unnecessarily sophisticated procedures to test their hypothesis. Instead of planting the sick

sunflower next to the healthy one to see if it too got sick, they extracted sap, brewed a complicated concoction with it, and then reintroduced it unnaturally via injection—all while making many assumptions and leaps of logic. Despite the complexity the botanist introduced (or ignored), however, they ended up oversimplifying their final interpretation.

5. **Lack of controls.** The botanist failed to use any controls. Therefore, the results could be due to random events, or a consequence of the methods and materials used in the experiment. Without appropriate controls, there is no way to tell if the outcome was influenced by factors other than the one being tested. This means no inferences can be made about the results, regardless of what they might be.

In light of the botanist's experimental woes, there is a more efficient and effective way to demonstrate the presence of a parasite in the sap of a sunflower and to prove it is the causative agent of disease:

1. First, rule out other potential causes (e.g. lack of sunlight, cold, moisture, biological defects, etc.).

2. If no other explanation is sufficient, seek to demonstrate the existence of the parasite *in nature*. In other words, directly observe it in a natural environment (e.g. the sap) under a microscope.

3. After confirming their existence, obtain a purified sample of the parasite (using filtration or centrifugation, for example). The purified parasite could then be used as an independent variable in a controlled scientific experiment to demonstrate a cause-and-effect relationship.

4. Expose the sunflower to the purified sample of the parasite via the natural route of infection. Let's say the botanist believes the parasite travels through the soil and infects the plant via the roots. The purified sample of the parasite could be added to the soil, rather than injecting the plant with a syringe, or spraying a solution on the leaves, neither of which reflect a natural route of infection.

5. Observe whether healthy sunflowers develop the exact same symptoms as the sick one while under the same environmental conditions (i.e. controlling for sunlight and other variables).

6. If symptoms occur, re-isolate the parasite from the newly infected sunflower, and visually confirm it is the same parasite used in the original inoculation.

7. Expose another healthy sunflower to the newly isolated parasite and see if it reproduces the same disease.

This process is far more logical, stepwise, and scientific compared to the original experiment performed by the botanist. If the botanist performed this experiment, it would provide evidence that parasites, not some other variable, were the likely cause of the disease. Of course, the botanist and their dying sunflower are simply a metaphor for virologists and sick people. Most of these issues apply 1:1 to the methods used in virology and, as such, the criticisms and recommendations apply equally. In realising this scenario is more real than fictitious, it might strike you as odd that contemporary scientists make such egregious errors. However, this should not come as a surprise given the slew of problems that increasingly characterise the *sinking ship* of modern medical science.

In bringing these ideas together, there are a few important points to reiterate. First, science is one of the most valuable assets in learning about ourselves and the world around us. Understanding its method and principles is helpful to be able to think scientifically. This is useful more generally in life, but also specifically for comprehending the next section in this book. Second, the initial sunflower example showed how scientific experiments, when done well, can determine a result with high levels of certainty. The follow-up example showed how science, when confused and complex, can produce specious conclusions. Though this might seem like a 'strawman' example for all its obvious flaws, it is analogous to how virologists approach their work on viruses (as will become clearer in the next chapter). It's also emblematic of the broader dilemma facing medical science, a vessel at risk of sinking from an overabundance of dubious findings. These too stem from misappropriating the scientific method.

Stepping back, these points speak to a growing disconnect between how we treat science versus how we *should* treat it. On one hand, people fiercely and rigidly defend ideas like germs and contagion—treating them as unquestionable. Yet, on the other hand, the system and methods supporting these ideas are fraught with issues. This means that, though some people might take issue with this book challenging established fields like virology and bacteriology, they really shouldn't. Rather, they need to realise their understanding is tentative and provisional, which allows them to remain humble and open to alternatives. Importantly, they must proportion their level of confidence to the weight and standard of evidence available. Coincidentally, this is much more closely aligned with true scientific thinking. Now, if this book is wrong, and virology isn't so fallible, then science should be able to easily demonstrate this fact, and people can update their understanding on this basis. If that's the case, the answer to 'Can you catch a cold?' should be simple to address. However, the fact this question still exists, despite the research done to date, might signal that it is not so straightforward to resolve.

Chapter 9

Where is the Virus?

There is a long-held belief that sodium causes hypertension because when people eat table salt, their blood pressure increases. It may come as a surprise to learn, however, that scientific evidence does not support this belief. Rather than arriving at this conclusion through controlled experimentation, scientists simply observed people's blood pressure go up from consuming salt and then assumed sodium was the culprit. Even with a fifty-fifty chance of correctly guessing the element responsible for causing hypertension, it seems scientists managed to pick the wrong one!

Sodium chloride (table salt) increases blood pressure in humans and animals. But this effect is curiously absent when people consume other sodium-containing compounds like sodium bicarbonate, sodium ascorbate, sodium phosphate, sodium citrate, or sodium amino acid chelate.[1-4] Oddly enough, sodium citrate has even been shown to counteract the hypertensive effect of sodium chloride.[1] In contrast, other chloride-containing salts like potassium chloride and calcium chloride *do* increase blood pressure.[5-7] Together, these two lines of evidence suggest it is not sodium, but *chloride* that is responsible for causing high blood pressure. This is by no means certain, though.

To definitively prove whether sodium or chloride causes hypertension, scientists would need to isolate each element and treat it as an independent variable in a scientific experiment. Now, you may be wondering why scientists haven't already given people pure sodium or chloride while monitoring their blood pressure. Surely, this would end the controversy once and for all. The problem is that sodium is highly reactive and, therefore, does not exist as a free element anywhere in nature.[8,9] For this reason, it always binds to ions, like chloride, to form a more stable compound. Due to its very nature, we cannot isolate sodium in its pure form and study it as an independent variable. Given this, how could anyone possibly claim sodium has been, or can ever be, 'scientifically proven' to cause hypertension? Technically, they can't. Of course, researchers can use salt as a quasi-independent variable, but the only conclusion they could confidently draw is that sodium chloride—not sodium alone—causes elevated blood pressure. This brings into question every single piece of health advice cautioning against the consumption of *sodium* for cardiovascular health.

So, why the detour on sodium in a book about catching a cold? Well, it is a simple way to introduce the importance of *isolating variables* and how difficult it is to establish causality without doing so. Realising that sodium cannot be isolated in its pure form puts other scientific claims into perspective. If it is so difficult to separate two basic elements from one another, then imagine the challenges associated with isolating 'virus particles' from a sea of hundreds or thousands of other substances suspended in the bodily secretions of sick people. Unlike sodium, though, scientists claim they *can* isolate viruses. However, as this chapter reveals, the process and final product are not as 'pure' as one might expect, especially considering the degree of certainty attributed to viruses on this basis.

What Even is a Virus?

Before isolating a virus, it is helpful to first understand—according to the prevailing paradigm—what viruses are and how they supposedly cause disease. A virus refers to a sub-microscopic, obligate parasite—which essentially means it can replicate itself by hijacking the machinery of the cells it infects. Each virus is allegedly comprised of genetic material housed within a tiny protein shell. They range from 20 – 500 nanometres (nm) in size,[10] which is hundreds of times smaller than the ordinary cells they supposedly infect. Unlike bacteria, which can be observed with a light microscope, viruses can only be visualised by a rather niche group of highly trained technicians with specialised pieces of equipment called electron microscopes.[11]

Though respiratory viruses are inanimate, they spread to and infect hosts in one of three ways:[12-14]

1. **Droplets** – Droplets of mucus larger than 5 micrometres (μm) are dispersed into the air by coughing, sneezing, or talking. When virus-containing droplets are inhaled, they infect the cells of the respiratory tract, oral cavity, or conjunctiva. This is considered a direct (i.e. person-to-person) airborne transmission route.

2. **Aerosols** – Droplet nuclei smaller than 5 μm can also be dispersed into the air by coughing, sneezing, talking, or breathing. These virus-containing aerosol particles are said to infect a healthy person in much the same way as droplets. Aerosol transmission is also considered a direct, airborne transmission route.

3. **Fomites** – Aerosols or droplets which contain virus particles can land on, and contaminate, inanimate objects such as door handles or computer keyboards. When a healthy person comes into physical contact with the contaminated object, they can then infect themselves or someone else by spreading fomites into mucous membranes (e.g. eyes, mouth, nose). Transmission by fomites is considered an indirect (i.e. person-to-object-to-person) transmission route.

When viruses infect a host cell via one of these transmission routes, they are claimed to cause disease.[15,16] This occurs via one of two mechanisms:[17-19]

1. **Mechanical destruction** – After a virus has infected a cell, it hijacks cellular pathways, instructing the cell to make thousands of copies of the virus. Eventually, the cell produces so many copies of the virus that it undergoes lysis, bursting open and destroying itself in the process. The copies of the virus made by this cell proceed to infect other nearby healthy cells and the process recurs.

2. **Altered physiology** – When certain types of oncogenic (cancer-causing) viruses infect cells, they supposedly alter the genetic material by causing DNA damage and mutations. These aberrations reprogram the infected cells to undergo abnormal mitosis (cell division). They also lose the ability to undergo programmed cell death (apoptosis). Rapid division of these

'immortal' cells ensues, leading to cancer.

All of this information begs the question: how do scientists know so much about the properties and behaviour of viruses? Well, through *isolation*, of course. It is therefore critical to get this procedure right because, as it turns out, much of the prevailing paradigm relies upon it. With this in mind, let's take a look at how to isolate a virus.

Virus Isolation

When the average person thinks about 'isolation', they probably bring to mind its social forms. A lonely person disconnected from friends and family. A hermit distancing themselves from society and opting to live in a remote area. A sick person removing themselves from the company of other healthy people to reduce the 'spread' of disease. In each instance, isolation means one person is separated from everyone else. Now, some people will also recall more technical forms of isolation. A pharmacologist extracting a drug from a urine sample by separating it from all other present substances. An electrician installing an isolation switch to interrupt current to a particular circuit so they can perform maintenance safely. A warehouse assembly line worker sorting through different coloured widgets to pick out just the green ones. Again, in each of these examples, isolation means separating one thing from everything else. If it isn't obvious, isolation is *subtractive*—it never means adding someone or something. Naturally, the same principles ought to apply when isolating a virus. That is, a scientist should be able to sample the bodily secretions from a sick person and pinpoint or filter out just the viral particles. But, as the next few sections reveal, virus isolation does not follow the same simple principle.

Convoluted Cell Cultures

In a process not unlike the one employed by the botanist in the previous chapter, virologists take filtered bodily fluids and introduce them to a *cell culture* in order to 'grow' or 'propagate' a particular virus.[20] This culture contains animal cells, antibiotics, growth factors, and various other substances.[20,21] When the animal cells begin to break down and die (a *cytopathic effect*), virologists consider this proof that a virus is present and define it as 'virus isolation'.[22] On the other hand, if no cytopathic effects occur, virologists do one of several things: (1) conclude no virus is present and deem isolation unsuccessful,[23] (2) use different cell lines (e.g. human embryonic kidney, nasal, or tracheal cells) until a cytopathic effect does occur,[24-26] (3) modify the materials and methods (pH, temperature, serum concentration, etc.) to induce a cytopathic effect,[27,28] or (4) inoculate healthy volunteers with crude, unfiltered cell culture material and if they develop symptoms conclude a virus was present in the culture.[24-26] Virologists rely heavily on the cytopathic effect to confirm the presence of a virus because they believe that only viruses can cause it. Yet, several studies have reported cytopathic effects in uninoculated cell cultures,[29,30] which may be caused by antibiotics,[31] and various other cell-derived components.[29,30,32] This means cytopathic effects aren't exclusive to viruses, and therefore, this standard approach specifically designed to detect viruses can't reliably do so.

Given these shortcomings, surely there's a backup plan to make this process more certain. In an attempt to add rigour, virologists studying cell cultures can supposedly quantify the *concentration* of virus particles (not just detect their presence) using plaque assays.[33] This involves adding a biological sample containing an alleged virus to host cells or aliquots of bacteria and observing the plaques that form when 'infected' cells die.[34] The plaques are viewed under a light microscope and counted manually.[33,35] Though this technique might seem like a reasonable way to measure viruses, it is also unreliable and can produce unsatisfactory outcomes.[36] One notable issue is that plaque assays require antibiotics and other additives. These substances risk damaging cell structures in a way that would completely confound results.[37] In fact, antibiotics have been shown to increase plaque surface area by up to 50-fold, undermining the validity of plaque assays.[36] This means that virologists verify an already inconsistent cytopathic effect with a procedure that is just as prone to error.

But even if these dubious methods did reliably produce cell death and plaques, there are still two major flaws in these approaches. First, does it not seem odd that the primary way to isolate a virus requires so many ingredients and additives? Cell cultures are complex concoctions. Add to this the mixture of molecules already suspended in bodily fluids and it makes for a great deal of noise and variation. With so many substances in the mix, it's impossible to know whether one or a combination of them induces cytopathic effects. What if the recipe virologists follow just so happens to destroy animal cells? It would mean they wrongly infer the presence of a virus (i.e. a false positive). Virologists might offer a simple rebuttal to this, but doing so gets them caught up in a second flaw. They *know* cell death and plaques are caused by a virus and not the other ingredients. How do they know? From isolating the virus. But how did they isolate the virus? By mixing ingredients together to induce cell death and plaques. This is, of course, circular reasoning. You cannot conclude a virus causes a cytopathic effect before you isolate one. On the flip side, you cannot isolate one by relying on a cytopathic effect because it's not clear whether the virus caused it. Pointing to an effect and attributing a cause is logically fallacious.

To escape this conundrum, virologists argue they can purify a virus from cell cultures in other ways, which allows them to pinpoint it as their true independent variable. But there are problems with this claim too. For example, influenza-like particles have been observed budding out of cells in uninoculated cell cultures. To be clear, this means virologists identified what appeared to be a virus in a culture that *should not* have had a virus in it. Then, when they inoculated that culture with biological fluids allegedly infected with influenza virus, the same particles exiting the cultured cells increased in number. 'Same', as in, the scientists described the original particles as *identical* to the influenza virus, both structurally and antigenically. As a result, when they 'purified' the influenza virus from the culture and examined it under an electron microscope, the influenza-like particles were also present.[38]

This raises several issues around claims of virus purification and isolation. First, if some other particle is present alongside what is believed to be a virus, then—by definition—it cannot be considered purified. Second, if the virus sample is not purified, it cannot be considered a true independent variable in a scientific experiment and it's impossible to determine its real effect. Third, if some non-virus particle is indistinguishable from a virus, then it becomes exceedingly difficult to identify what a virus is and confirm whether one is present. Finally, even if the two particles could be distinguished from each other, it is just as difficult to separate them to obtain a pure sample. In these ways, the possibility of an identical non-viral particle casts doubts over virologists' ability to isolate and purify a virus, even when using methods beyond cell cultures and plaque assays.

However, the challenge of pinpointing and separating viruses is not confined to a single look-alike cell. According to virologists, there are supposedly 380 trillion virus particles in the human body,[39,40] including half a dozen different families of viruses present in the oral cavity and respiratory tract of healthy individuals.[41] In people with respiratory illnesses, there may be an even greater number of different viruses present.[42,43] There are also many alleged instances where people have been 'co-infected' with both influenza A and B strains.[44-46] In this case, taking a sputum sample from a co-infected person would mean two viruses need to be separated from one another before they are added to a cell culture. If they are not separated, virologists don't know which virus particles they are working with. But conflating and confusing different viral particles with one another isn't merely some hypothetical scenario for argument's sake. Virologists admit, that when they attempt to propagate viruses in a cell culture, it *inevitably* results in a mixed population of different viruses.[47] So, while virologists say they use various methods to separate viruses from each other in co-infected cell cultures, the reality is that they *rarely* isolate viruses in their pure form because it is a 'cumbersome' and 'extremely difficult' process.[48,49] In saying that, it is debatable whether a virus has *ever been isolated* in its pure form at all.

Despite all of its issues, the cell culture method is considered the gold standard in virus isolation,[50] and continues to be used to this very day.[51,52] It appears, though, that this method struggles to achieve its primary aim: detecting and isolating viruses. It can only be used to *imply* their presence; at no point do virologists directly observe viruses in a biological sample obtained from a sick person. From a scientific perspective, this is disappointing, to say the least. Furthermore, just how these contrived cell cultures compare to real-world conditions remains to be seen. Even if they were more decisive, it would still be dubious to draw parallels between what happens in a culture flask and what transpires inside the respiratory tract of a human being. To demonstrate just how problematic and uncertain 'cultured' approaches are, the next sections walk through some historic attempts to isolate influenza and common cold viruses.

Isolating Influenza Viruses

Before the invention of the cell culture method, viruses like influenza A and B were discovered using far more crude techniques. For years, scientists inoculated rats, mice, guinea pigs, monkeys, pigs, and horses with filtrates obtained from sick people in the hope of discovering the cause of influenza. This approach provided little insight because none of the animals developed the disease. Just as this line of research was approaching a dead end, Christopher Andrewes, Wilson Smith, and Patrick Laidlaw made a discovery that would not only change the course of influenza research but also mark the beginning of modern virology.[53] Andrewes and his team inoculated eight ferrets subcutaneously and intranasally with filtered mucus secretions obtained from people with influenza. Five of the animals developed a fever, watery eyes, and nasal discharge. Another group of ferrets was inoculated with mucus obtained from healthy people. They remained completely free of symptoms. The researchers interpreted these results as proof that a virus was present in the filtered bodily fluids. The sick ferrets were then killed, and their nasal passages were scraped out, ground up with sand, and mixed with saline. This sandy, snotty emulsion was then centrifuged, and the supernatant was inoculated into another group of healthy ferrets. When these animals also became sick, Andrewes and his peers claimed the virus had been successfully 'transmitted' from one ferret to another.[54] Taken together, the results of this experiment are considered isolation of the influenza A virus.[55]

A few years later, in 1935, Andrewes, Smith, and Laidlaw conducted the first human transmission experiment with the newly discovered 'influenza A virus'. Two healthy volunteers had 1 mL of nasal washings, obtained from sick ferrets (allegedly infected with influenza), dropped into each nostril. Both men were closely monitored, yet they remained completely well. The researchers hand-waved this negative result by claiming the recipients were immune to the virus (see Appendix Experiment 32.1).[56]

In 1940, Thomas Francis and Thomas Magill isolated the influenza B virus using a very similar methodology employed by Andrewes, Smith, and Laidlaw. Mucus secretions obtained from three people with influenza were filtered and inoculated into three ferrets. Two of the ferrets remained well, while the third showed signs of respiratory distress. Francis and

Magill made a suspension from the sick animal's nasal and lung tissue and then inoculated it into groups of healthy ferrets and mice, some of which also developed respiratory distress. The researchers believed the disease must have been caused by a new virus because the animals failed to develop antibodies reactive against standard strains of influenza A. This newly 'identified' virus was classified as 'influenza B'.[57,58] In both cases of influenza, these seminal researchers were credited with discovering and isolating a novel virus, even though none of them directly observed a virus particle, or obtained anything close to a pure, isolated sample. The methods were crude, the experiments lacked appropriate controls, the disease wasn't produced in humans, and the results weren't replicated.

Isolating Common Cold Viruses

In the early 1930s, a research team led by Alphonse Raymond Dochez were conducting experiments to induce the common cold in healthy people by inoculating them with filtered nasopharyngeal washings obtained from sick people. In the days prior to receiving their inoculation, the team instilled participants' nasal passages with a solution of sterile broth, which produced cold-like symptoms. Yet, when the nine participants were inoculated with the virus filtrate several days later, just four (44%) developed a common cold (see Exp. 25.1).[59] These unexpected results led Dochez to ponder. He conveniently overlooked the fact that sterile broth induced cold-like symptoms, and instead focused on why less than half of the recipients inoculated with the filtrate developed a cold. Dochez argued that the *quantity* of virus particles in the mucus was insufficient to infect all the participants. He reasoned that, for reliable and consistent infections to occur, the virus needed to be 'grown' or 'cultured' in a laboratory setting first. Only then would there be enough virus material available to successfully infect healthy recipients.[60,61]

To propagate the virus, Dochez used chicken embryos. He injected them with filtered mucus he had obtained from a person with a cold and then incubated the embryos for up to nine days. After this, Dochez centrifuged the chicken embryo fluid (chorioallantoic fluid) to remove any debris and then inoculated the resulting supernatant intranasally into a health volunteer. This supernatant, Dochez claimed, contained the cultivated virus. Therefore, when the healthy recipient developed cold-like symptoms, Dochez and his team presumed the virus had grown successfully using their method. They proceeded to dilute the original material into different strength solutions and added these varying dilutions to more chicken embryos. It is worthwhile noting that some solutions were diluted a quadrillion times, so should have contained a negligible amount of the virus. After being inoculated, five of twelve (41%) healthy people developed colds. Based on this result, Dochez concluded that the virus had grown in sufficient quantities to infect the recipients despite achieving an infection rate *lower* than his original experiment with filtered mucus secretions.[61] Though it might seem archaic, culturing viruses in chicken embryos is a method still in use today.[62] Ironically, its application is limited as it produces 'viruses' that differ from the original 'isolate', and because a variety of substances contained within the embryo supposedly inhibit virus growth.[63,64] Despite these fundamental flaws, Dochez was credited with infecting people with a virus he never observed nor isolated.

Following in the footsteps of Dochez's work, an American virologist named Winston Price conducted landmark common cold research in 1953. He took nasal secretions from a group of nurses working in his department who were suffering from upper respiratory tract symptoms.[65] The nasal secretions were inoculated onto monkey kidney cells along with horse serum, beef embryo extract, a synthetic growth medium called '199 solution', penicillin, and streptomycin. After a few days, the monkey kidney cells began to break down and die—the all-important cytopathic effect. Observing this cell death led Price to conclude he had successfully 'isolated' the virus, which would later become known as 'rhinovirus'.[66] To determine its pathogenicity, he inoculated some of the filtered culture medium fluid intranasally, intracerebrally, and intraperitoneally into 20 newborn mice and 10 hamster pups. When none of these animals became sick, Price repeated the same procedure on six guinea pig pups and a group of adult ferrets. But these animals remained completely unaffected too.

Looking at Price's work in its entirety tells a peculiar yet familiar tale. He did not isolate and observe a pure sample of the virus, use adequate controls, transmit the disease to animals, or conduct any human transmission experiments. Yet, Price concluded he was successful in identifying the virus responsible for the common cold. Others seemed to agree because, in the years that followed, they too 'isolated' several new rhinoviruses in a similar fashion. This clearly flawed methodology led virologists to claim they had discovered more than 160 different rhinoviruses over the following decades.[67,68] Once more, suspect seminal work appears to have built a scientific 'house of cards' that others follow without question to this day.

But unconvincing discoveries didn't stop with rhinoviruses. In 1965, David Tyrrell identified a new type of common cold virus named 'B814'. To isolate this virus, Tyrrell obtained nasal epithelium and trachea tissue from aborted human foetuses and then incubated it for several days. He then added nasal washings taken from a young boy with typical common cold symptoms. When the tissue culture began to degrade, and cilia on the epithelium ceased to function, Tyrrell considered this proof that a virus was present within the mucus. He proceeded to use the tissue culture material to inoculate healthy participants, some of whom developed symptoms of a common cold. Tyrrell deemed this proof that the virus was pathogenic. He believed he was dealing with a new virus because the serum of infected individuals failed to cross react in a *complement fixation test* involving known virus antigens.[24] Normally, a precipitate would form when antibodies in a patient's serum react with antigens of a previously discovered virus. But no such precipitate formed. It is unusual that this absent antibody response was used as evidence of a new virus. Null findings are notoriously difficult to interpret with any certainty, which is why Thomas Rivers himself even stated antibody responses do not prove the presence of a virus, nor should they be considered proof of disease causation.[69]

A few years later, Tyrrell used electron microscopy (EM) to obtain the first image of particles claimed to be B814. He used a point-and-declare method, singling out indiscriminate particles in a cell culture because they had a fringe or 'crown' around their border—a characteristic that inspired its name: 'coronavirus'. While there is no doubt Tyrrell was observing a particle of some kind, it is debatable whether it was a virus. For starters, Tyrrell stated that B814 could not be purified directly from tissue fragments obtained from sick hosts because the amount of viral material and the proportion of 'infected cells' was so low. This means that, instead of obtaining a purified sample of the virus directly from the host's biological fluids and then examining it with EM, Tyrrell used a tissue culture which he merely 'believed' contained cells infected with the virus.[70] Used in this way, electron micrographs aren't particularly definitive. But they are a powerful tool that, hypothetically, should be useful for confirming the isolation of viruses, so they are worth discussing further.

Electron Micrographs

Before the invention of electron microscopy (EM), the field of virology was flying blind. There was much uncertainty about the physical properties of viruses that had otherwise only been theorised about. Without visual confirmation, scientists could not be sure that viruses even existed because they had never directly observed them. At the time, scientists did not know whether a virus was a poison, a microscopic particle, a living fluid contagium, or something else altogether. For this reason, the invention of EM marked a turning point for virology. It answered these questions once and for all because it allowed for the direct observation of virus particles...or so we are led to believe.

Although EM produces 'images', using it to confirm the presence of viral material in a sample still requires a degree of guesswork. So, even after EM had been in use for many years, it was claimed that viruses could still not be directly observed and that their existence relied purely upon *indirect* evidence.[71] Specifically, virologists assumed certain particles in infected cell cultures were viruses simply because those same particles were absent in uninfected cultures. However, after more research, they later admitted these particles were not viruses at all. Rather, they were cellular by-products that resulted from virologists adding 'infected' material to a cell culture.[72]

The promise of EM fell flat because it was *downstream* from unreliable cell culture methods. EM could only observe viruses when virologists presupposed that the particles they were looking at had been properly purified and characterised.[73] However, as discussed earlier, cell cultures were prone to all manner of problems. A particularly troubling issue was that non-viral particles—indistinguishable from virus particles—were known to be present in so-called 'purified samples' used for EM.[72,74] Furthermore, what virologists pointed to as a virus particle did not possess a distinct, readily identifiable form. This made it exceedingly difficult to differentiate a 'virus' from other materials present in the sample.[73] As such, even expert electron microscopists recommend caution whenever interpreting EM images due to how tricky it is to accurately identify viruses.[75,76] Unsurprisingly, there are numerous cases where microscopists have incorrectly classified particles as respiratory viruses. It later turned out these particles were: rough endoplasmic reticula,[77] severely altered mitochondria,[75,78] multivesicular bodies, coated vesicles,[79,80] clathrin-coated vesicles, caveolae, sub-cellular organelles,[76,81] and various other non-viral structures.[82,83] Aside from the difficulty of observing a virus on its own, virologists also admitted it was impossible to directly watch one 'grow' or 'multiply' because it can only do so intracellularly, and EM could not resolve the interior of a cell.[84] So, although electronic microscopy was supposed to be virology's saving grace, it still could not reliably confirm the characteristics and behaviour of a virus, partly from its own limitations, and partly from those it inherited from cell cultures.

Nevertheless, scientists published several studies in the early 1940s documenting how they allegedly isolated, purified, and characterised influenza A and B viruses with the aid of EM.[85-87] The process involved inoculating the fluid of a chicken embryo with the mucus secretions obtained from influenza cases. The inoculated chicken embryo was left to incubate for a few days to allow the virus to 'grow'. Next, the inoculated embryo was removed and centrifuged. This centrifuged fluid was then mixed with red blood cells from adult chickens, which allowed the alleged virus particles to 'stick' to them. To detach the virus particles, red blood cells were placed into another container and washed with a solvent. It is important to note that no one has ever directly demonstrated virus particles absorbing or 'sticking' to the surface of red blood cells using this method—it is simply presumed. Much like other virological methods, only indirect evidence supports the use of this technique.[88] Finally, the solute was ultra-centrifuged to purify 'virus particles' from it, which they then used for observation with EM.[85]

Once again, there is no doubt scientists observed and imaged particles of some description using EM. What is unclear, however, is whether these particles were those of a virus or some other substance. Indeed, other virologists have criticised this peculiar technique because it is non-specific, so any number of different particles present in the sample could theoretically bind to the red blood cells, not just the intended influenza virus.[89] In addition, it is well-established that the EM process not only produces random artefacts, but also alters the morphology of what is claimed to be virus particles.[73,90,91] So, even if the sticky blood cell gambit worked out, the scientists would still run into challenges when attempting to specify which particles are viruses and which aren't. Furthermore, not only is EM expensive and time-consuming (which limits its use), but expert microscopists are unable to clearly distinguish what they suspect are viruses from other microscopic particles, nor can they tell different viruses from the same family apart.[73,92–94] Ultimately, a technique that was supposed to reduce uncertainty has instead added to the mystery.

Addressing Artefacts

As the name implies, light microscopes use light and a series of glass lenses to magnify specimens by up to 2,000x. Biological samples are obtained from a host, placed on a glass slide and observed directly.[95] Electron microscopy, on the other hand, involves a much more complicated process but allows for magnification of specimens more than 1,000,000x.[96] First, the specimen is fixed with heavy metal salts (e.g. osmium tetroxide, uranyl acetate) and formaldehyde. Next, the specimen is dehydrated with ethanol or acetone, embedded in a resin (e.g. epoxy), and cured into a hard block. Finally, the block is cut into ultra-thin sections and stained with substances like lead citrate. Once these preparatory steps have been completed, the specimen is imaged by bombarding it with a beam of electrons inside a high vacuum.[97]

One reason for EM's ambiguity is the presence of what are known as 'artefacts'—various remnants or aberrations left behind by human intervention. The preparation process mentioned above is known to dehydrate the sample, 'shadow' it through the addition of heavy metals, and alter its structure by bombarding it with electrons. Staining procedures are also known to impact EM's ability to detect particles because the stain type, pH, and duration, can change particle concentration and morphology.[90] Additionally, during the microscopy process, particles can be damaged by the heat of the electron beam, holes can be burned through objects of interest, circular objects may appear oval in shape, and evaporation may drastically change the form and opacity of 'virions'.[91] All this is to say, electron microscopes almost certainly do not observe things *as they are*. Therefore, without ever seeing a virus particle in its natural, unadulterated state, how did virologists establish an accurate reference standard for what one looks like? There's always the possibility that electron microscopists cannot tell whether the particles they are looking at are viruses or simply artefacts arising from the techniques they employed to prepare for or perform microscopy.

Electron microscopy had only been around for a decade or so when the first images of 'so-called' influenza viruses were taken. Not long thereafter, scientists began raising concerns about the accuracy of these images, not just for influenza but for other viruses as well. In 1949, a group of researchers obtained tissue samples from healthy rodents and rodents infected with poliomyelitis (i.e. polio). They observed particles in both healthy and infected tissue samples that were indistinguishable from each other. The researchers concluded that none of the electron micrograph images of the polio virus published at that time could have possibly corresponded with a virus.[98] Meanwhile, other scientists admitted that polio transmission was not demonstrated through scientific experimentation, but rather through a process of elimination (i.e. "it doesn't seem to be X, so it must be Y"). Researchers exclaimed it was "difficult, if not impossible" to pinpoint the mechanism by which the disease spread.[99]

One year later, another group of scientists used EM to examine fluid taken from human skin lesions of a case of Pinta, a benign skin condition said to be caused by the bacterium, *Treponema carateum*. The patient was otherwise healthy, exhibiting no signs or symptoms of illness. Interestingly, the scientists observed biological structures in the sample that were morphologically identical to several other particles, including filamentous forms of influenza, polio, fowl pest, and pox viruses. This finding was so odd that the authors concluded the particles were not viruses at all, but protein fragments or artefacts originating from red blood cells.[100] The same authors also published a paper after observing virus-like particles within preparations claiming to be a purified virus sample, which suggests the samples were not pure at all.[74]

In the broader scientific literature, many other scientists have criticised the ways virologists observe viruses using EM. For example, what appear to be virus and virus-like particles may well be *normal* components present within chicken embryo fluid, or simply a natural by-product of disintegrating culture cells.[89] This possibility owes to the fact that virus particles have only ever been observed in chicken embryos and cell cultures. No one has ever seen viruses anywhere else, certainly not in sick patients or biological fluids taken directly from them. With all virus observation occurring within a contrived context, electron microscopists run two big risks. One is that they might be mistaking viruses for something inherent to the substrate and/or procedures they rely so heavily on. The other is, that even if they correctly identify particles, they might be describing and explaining phenomena that only make sense within a laboratory setting. In either case, what electron microscopists observe may have no relation to what happens inside a sick human being.

A common reason why virologists claim virus particles cannot be observed directly in the bodily fluids of a sick person is because there are not enough particles to see.[101] They assert a virus must be propagated or 'grown' in a cell culture first. Only then will there be enough virus material to visualise using techniques like EM.[102] This claim raises the obvious question, though. How many virus particles must there be in a sample to be seen with EM? According to microscopists, the minimum concentration for reliable detection using EM is between 1.0×10^5 (100,000) to 1.0×10^6 (1,000,000) particles per mL.[103] Using certain filtration techniques, some claim EM can technically be performed with a sample containing as little as 5,000 virions.[104] Putting this exception aside, the concentration of virus particles in the bodily fluids of a sick person should, in theory, be less than the lower-bound estimate (i.e. under 100,000 particles per mL). But this is not the case at all. More than one hundred and thirty billion (1.3×10^{11}) virus particles have been recorded in one mL of respiratory fluid, a number which is orders of magnitude greater than the minimum number required for EM.[105] Given this discrepancy, how can virologists argue there aren't enough virus particles to detect in bodily fluids? As it turns out, a major reason for using embryos and cultures has no validity whatsoever.

This argument makes even less sense when you consider the fact that human respiratory tracts should be the perfect environment for viruses to grow. How else would outbreaks so frequently occur? Yet, the only place a virus can be seen is in a lab after it has been cultivated in a cell culture and specially prepared for an imaging technique that just so happens to alter whatever the observer looks at. At every step, there is too much room for error. Overall, then, when looking at the best-available approach for visualising viruses, there is something seriously wrong with the picture.

Viruses & Exosomes

The discussion so far has also alluded to virus-like particles. These are also worth unpacking further because they complicate any attempt to identify and isolate viruses. Extracellular vesicles (i.e. exosomes) are particles that have similar characteristics and morphology to what virologists describe as virus-like particles. Not only are exosomes found in all human bodily fluids, they are also found in cell cultures because cells release exosomes as they are dying.[106–108] It is important to highlight that, unlike viruses, there are many papers demonstrating the purification of exosomes directly from the bodily fluids of human beings.[109–112] Curiously, viruses and exosomes are produced simultaneously by infected cells.[113,114] There are also many reports of exosomes being released from cells in cultures (including monkey kidney cells) which are of a very similar size, shape, and density to viral particles.[115,116] In fact, they are so alike, that the field of virology defines exosomes as 'non-infectious' viruses.[117]

Virologists frequently report the difficulties they face attempting to separate exosomes and viruses that co-exist in a sample. According to a 2020 paper published in a leading virology journal, a reliable method for separating virus particles from non-virus particles (exosomes) does not exist, owing to their similar morphology.[118] Another 2020 paper stated that separating exosomes from viruses is problematic because they appear to exist on a continuum.[119] In fact, exosomes and viruses are so similar they cannot be easily differentiated, so much so, that their classification is often dependent on the 'preference of the investigator'.[113] Furthermore, exosomes were only identified as biological entities in the 1980s.[120,121] So, if modern virologists are still unable to distinguish exosomes (i.e. extracellular vesicles) from viruses, and separate them from one another in cell cultures, how were they able to achieve these feats so easily more than half a century ago?

Not only are there obvious difficulties in isolating 'so-called' virus particles from exosomes, but there are also problems distinguishing different influenza viruses apart from one another. For example, influenza A and B are virtually indistinguishable when viewed under an electron microscope.[122,123] When a person is 'co-infected' with both viruses how do virologists know by looking at an EM image that they have obtained a purified sample of just influenza A or B, given the two are morphologically identical? When two or more viruses are present in a sample, molecular or antigen-based testing might miss the second agent. Altogether, these points indicate quite a muddled mess. Not only is it hard to tell different viral particles from one another,[124] but it is challenging to distinguish them from exosomes.

Is That the Best You Can Do?

Standard virological approaches are not isolation as we understand them. Despite their sophistication, none of these techniques definitively isolate a virus. There are, of course, other methods not covered here. For example, virologists regularly use centrifugal force to separate the contents of cell culture fluid containing alleged virus particles into different density gradients. This too is fundamentally flawed because there is no reference point to compare the 'output' (i.e. the particles in a particular density band) with. That is, if you've never isolated a virus to start with, and confirmed its properties, how do you verify which density band contains the virus, and then determine which particles are virions? This process is complicated further because exosomes and 'viruses' are said to be co-pelleted by centrifugation,[118] so how can they be reliably differentiated and separated from one another?

Another alternative is genomic sequencing, which similarly relies on assumptions rather than direct observations. Specifically, to sequence a virus, virologists prepare genetic material from a crude patient sample which is then analysed by a genetic sequencing instrument. The instrument then assembles the genetic fragments of unknown origin into hundreds, sometimes thousands, of possible 'outputs' in the form of genetic sequences. The presence of a virus is confirmed if one of the sequences closely matches or is identical to other 'known viral sequences'.[15,125-127] This runs into two familiar problems: (1) how did they isolate the virus to obtain the 'known' sequence to begin with, and (2) what reference point do they compare the output to? Although virologists claim they can use this technique to sequence the genome of a virus, they admit to doing so without ever having a purified sample to work with.[127]

It seems, then, that other virological techniques struggle to isolate viruses too. With all of this in mind, it probably comes as no surprise that the field of virology has no universally accepted definition of 'isolation'. Though it can mean many things to them,[20-22] none of their processes appear capable of achieving a satisfactory outcome. To hit home this point and to further ground many of the ideas discussed so far, consider the seminal work of John Enders. In 1949, Enders, along with Thomas Weller and Frederick Robbins, claimed to have isolated the polio virus from sick patients using a cell culture.[128,129] For this achievement they were awarded a Nobel Prize in 1954.[130] That same year, Enders and his colleague, Thomas Peebles, published a paper claiming to have isolated the measles virus from sick patients.[30]

To give a sense of their approach, Enders and Peebles 'isolated' the measles virus using the following steps:

1. Patients with measles gargled milk and spat it into a container.

2. Antibiotics (i.e. penicillin and streptomycin) were added to the gargled milk.

3. The mixture of milk, mucus, and medicine was centrifuged (i.e. spun at high speeds) for an hour to separate the solid and liquid components. The liquid component was labelled the 'supernatant' and was claimed to contain the virus.

4. The supernatant liquid was then spread atop Rhesus monkey kidney cells in a culture flask.

5. Many substances were then added to the monkey kidney cell culture, including bovine amniotic fluid, beef embryo extract, horse serum, more antibiotics, phenol red, and soybean trypsin.

6. When the monkey kidney cells began to break down and die (i.e. *a cytopathic effect*), it was claimed the virus particles present in the mucus of measles patients were responsible.

7. Multiple cell cultures were then mixed together and ground up with aluminium. This mixture was then centrifuged, and the supernatant was added to another cell culture. When cytopathic effects occurred in the new cell culture, this was considered successful 'serial passage' of the virus.

8. The newly inoculated cell culture was centrifuged once again, and the supernatant was examined under an electron microscope. Indiscriminate particles present in the supernatant were claimed to be the virus.

9. A control experiment was also performed by adding the same ingredients to a cell culture, except for the 'infected' mucus. This uninoculated control (which *did not* contain mucus from sick patients) broke down in *exactly the same way* as the inoculated cell culture (which *did* contain mucus from sick people).

10. Enders and Peebles admitted that whatever cytopathic agent was present in the uninoculated culture could not be distinguished with confidence from the 'virus' present in the inoculated culture.

To this day, Enders' cell culture procedure is considered the 'gold standard' for virus isolation, even though the same cytopathic effects occurred in the control sample, and their EM observation was ambiguous. This experiment is also considered proof that a virus particle was present in the original mucus sample taken from the sick patient, despite Enders never directly observing a virus particle there.

Where Does This Leave Us?

This chapter explained what viruses are, how they spread, and how they make people sick. Though isolating viruses is necessary to demonstrate they exist and spread disease, this appears difficult to achieve practically. Contrary to what most people understand 'isolation' to mean, virologists do not extract a purified sample of virus particles directly from the bodily fluids of sick people. Instead of subtracting or separating anything, they perform various forms of *addition; (1)* they introduce a cell culture, a complex concoction containing all manner of extraneous variables; (2) they introduce bodily fluids, a sophisticated solution full of unknown substances and; (3) their methods and equipment produce artefacts, which add to the uncertainty despite arising from attempts to reduce it.

Together, these sources of noise obscure virologists' ability to draw firm conclusions. Equally murky are the attempts to isolate viruses using centrifugation and to confirm their presence using genomic sequencing.

The final nail in the coffin is the fact that particles believed to be viruses are often indistinguishable (a) from one another, and (b) from other particles, like exosomes. Notable historical examples demonstrated many of these isolation issues in action. Scientists were credited with the discovery and isolation of influenza, common cold, polio, measles, and other viruses based on limited and circumstantial evidence. Each assumed or inferred the presence of viruses, rather than directly observing them.

It appears virologists are incapable of truly isolating viruses, despite their contrary claims. When such a foundational claim is riddled with uncertainty, profound and far-reaching consequences for medical science arise. It places an asterisk on any laboratory studies reporting the characteristics and behaviour of viruses. It drastically undermines the level of confidence placed on other claims about viruses, how they spread, how they cause disease, and how to stop them. In response to the question, 'Where is the virus?', it would seem virological attempts pose more problems than they resolve. One counterargument to this is that the documented real-world spread of viruses accommodates for these lab-based flaws. Surely, viruses exist and are dangerous because only contagious germs can account for seasonal outbreaks and pandemics. To address this valid position, the next section of this book reviews the findings of many studies attempting to transmit, or document the spread of colds and flu from person-to-person.

Part 2

Human Experiments

Chapter 10

The Russian Influenza Pandemic

When we hear the word *pandemic*, we typically understand this to mean a few things. First, we expect people infected with something like influenza to experience a consistent set of symptoms (i.e. one germ, one disease).[1] If symptoms differed too drastically, how would we know a disease was spreading, or if any particular individual had it? Second, we assume pandemics start in one location (i.e. an index case or patient zero) spreading outwards from the epicentre in a pattern consistent with person-to-person contact. Last, when a pandemic breaks out in a certain area, we would like to believe that medical practitioners can confirm, with little doubt in their minds, that there is a pandemic. Undoubtedly, waves of sick patients with similar signs and symptoms should present to their surgeries, clinics, and hospitals. Each of these expectations, however, was violated by a particularly peculiar pandemic—*the Russian flu*. As it turns out, this outbreak displayed several irregularities incompatible with the spread of a highly infectious and contagious influenza virus.

Origins & Oddities of Russian Influenza

The Russian influenza pandemic, also referred to as the "Russian flu" or "Asiatic flu," ravaged the world between 1889 and 1894.[2] Despite lasting more than five years and claiming over one million lives, people seldom speak about it. This is probably because it was overshadowed by the far more devastating Spanish influenza pandemic of 1918. The Russian flu outbreak is believed to have originated in the city of Bukhara in Turkestan, in May of 1889. However, there are reports that it began in many other places that same month, like the Canadian city of Athabasca.[3] By mid-October, the pandemic had reached the Russian

Empire, striking cities like Tomsk and Kazan simultaneously, which is rather curious considering they are separated by a distance of more than 2,700 kilometres.[3-5]

The pandemic moved rapidly across Russia, Europe, and the United States, and in as little as four months it had swept over the entire world.[6] It took a comparable amount of time for the Spanish (1918)[7] and Asian flu (1957)[8] to achieve the same feat. Interestingly, the SARS (2003),[9] H1N1 (2009)[10] and SARS-CoV-2 (2019)[11] pandemics were only marginally quicker, reaching every continent in just 3 months. This is odd because despite the advent of jet planes, high-speed rail, and motor vehicles, influenza takes just as long to disseminate across the Earth in modern times as it did over a century ago. Therefore, the speed at which influenza spreads is incompatible with the concept of contagion.[12]

Like other pandemics of the 19th century, the Russian flu progressed in an east-to-west fashion. Though some deny this pattern of spread,[3] it is otherwise difficult to reconcile with the concept of human-to-human transmission.[13] The Russian flu pandemic occurred in successive waves over many years, each varying greatly in severity.[3] This is odd because as a pandemic sweeps through a particular area, the infected population should develop immunity, protecting them from subsequent infections, or waves, of the same 'virus'. However, virology explains this anomaly away by suggesting; (1) people become susceptible to reinfection with the original strain due to waning immunity, and; (2) the original strain mutates, rendering previously acquired immunity useless.[14]

At this point in history, germ theory was still in its infancy, so there was considerable speculation about the cause of influenza. Doctors debated as to whether the pandemic was caused by miasma,[15] a contagious pathogenic bacterium, poor sanitary conditions, or some kind of atmospheric or meteorological phenomenon.[16, 17] Many doubted a germ was responsible for the pandemic because the very first cases of Russian flu appeared almost simultaneously in cities separated by hundreds or thousands of kilometres.[18] For example, people in Bukhara (Asia) became unwell around the same time as people in Athabasca (North America), which is perplexing because these two cities are nearly 10,000 kilometres apart. In the late 1800s, it would take weeks, if not months, to travel such a large distance, so how was the pandemic able to appear in these two places at the same time?

If the Russian flu pandemic was indeed caused by a contagious particle, it should have originated in one central location and radiated outwards. Instead, it appeared in multiple locations at the same time and spread east-to-west. Furthermore, the speed at which the disease engulfed nations was at odds with the contagion account. Quite simply, people could not travel quickly because motor vehicles were not commonplace, aeroplanes had not been invented, and embarking overseas by boat was notoriously slow. It is a mystery, then, how a germ could traverse considerable distances faster than people. The pandemic rolled across Europe at speeds of up to 650 kilometres per week, and swept across North America even faster, covering up to 1740 kilometres just as quickly. Whilst these distances are vast, even by today's standards, scholars argue that travel by rail could easily account for this rapidity.[19] However, there are extensive reports that contradict this explanation. For example, Manitoba and Quebec were struck down around the 22nd of December 1889. Such an occurrence seems strange given these Canadian provinces are separated by an expanse of 2,000 kilometres. The pandemic also ravaged Fort Macleod and Saskatchewan simultaneously, despite these military installations having no rail connections and being 500 kilometres apart. Even more inexplicable are the simultaneous outbreaks amongst remote Native American tribes that were not connected by any means of modern transportation.[20]

Some believe the flooding of the Hwang Ho River in China, in late 1889, might have triggered the Russian flu. The flooding was so extreme that innumerable human beings, pigs, rats, fowl, trees, and vegetables were swept up by the flood waters. When the flood waters eventually receded, the human, plant, and animal remains became trapped in the drying yellow mud. As the foul, decomposing matter dried out and turned to dust, it was taken by easterly air currents and deposited over Russia, which would explain the east-to-west spread. These events resulted in the Russians referring to the pandemic as the "Chinese Cold".[21]

Symptoms of the Russian Flu

Another peculiarity surrounding the pandemic was the disease's clinical presentation. According to physicians at the time, the Russian flu presented in *four* different forms: (1) a *respiratory* disease, (2) a *gastrointestinal* disease, (3) a *catarrhal* disease, and (4) a *neurological* disease.[3] The symptoms ranged from a mild respiratory illness (lasting four to five days),[22] through to a more severe disease where people experienced repeated relapses of multiple organ dysfunction, neurological symptoms, and skin rashes reminiscent of scarlet fever. If one germ really does cause one disease (a core tenet of germ theory),[1] how is it a single 'virus' presented as four distinct diseases? To get a sense of how varied the symptoms were, the following list (Table 1) provides an overview of just some of the symptoms considered to be indicative of Russian influenza.[23, 24]

Symptoms of Russian Influenza		
Abdominal pain	Dysentery	Neuralgia
Abortion	Fever	Nosebleeds
Albuminuria	Foul breath	Paralysis
Alopecia areata	Headache	Rheumatism
Anaemia	Heart failure	Rigor
Arthritis	Herpes	Scarlatina
Catarrh	Jaundice	Skin lesions
Delirium	Meningitis	Sore throat
Diabetes	Menorrhagia	Sweating
Dropsy	Nausea	Vomiting

Table 1 - Symptoms of Russian Influenza

Confusion Amongst Doctors

Many doctors described the clinical signs and symptoms associated with pandemic influenza as 'protean' (i.e. displaying great diversity or variety), 'contradictory',[25, 26] and 'chameleon-like'.[27] A doctor by the name of Egerton Fitzgerald expressed his confusion about the presentation of the disease. He reported witnessing dozens of patients with all kinds of different complaints. According to Fitzgerald, none of their afflictions were influenza, yet they had been diagnosed as such by other doctors.[23] Fitzgerald described the symptoms as being so numerous and protean that it was impossible to designate them all as cases of the Russian flu. The lack of uniformity of symptoms between patients led him to conclude that rarely were any two cases alike.[28] So, if no two people presented with the same symptoms, how could doctors be sure patients were suffering from the same disease? Furthermore, if patients weren't presenting with a distinct set of symptoms, what convinced the medical profession that a flu pandemic was even occurring?

Communication between physicians at the time indicated they were generally confused about what constituted a case of Russian influenza. A German physician by the name of Dr Hugh Hagan stated that many cases, diagnosed as the Russian flu, were something else entirely. Hagan also noted that newspapers had been reporting a high mortality rate associated with the flu, yet this conflicted with his own observations. When he inquired with fellow doctors and pathologists about their experiences, they told him they had rarely seen a patient die from the disease.[29] This suggests there was a stark contrast between what doctors were observing on the ground and what the media was reporting in news publications.

Dr Hagan was not alone in finding diagnostic errors. Doctors and surgeons from across the United Kingdom were convinced cases of dengue fever, malaria, and relapsing fever were also being misdiagnosed as the Russian flu.[5, 30, 31] The prevalence of other diseases was so great, doctors figured there must have been a coinciding pandemic of dengue fever too.[24] This sort of phenomenon has occurred multiple times throughout history and was not unique to the Russian flu. For example, cholera and influenza were both epidemic during the Black Death in 1348.[32] But were the multiple pandemics from different diseases spreading at the same time, or were they simply different presentations of the same underlying condition?

Stranger still, other medical professionals expressed their doubts about whether an influenza pandemic was occurring at all, due to the lack of sick patients. Dr David Brakenridge, physician to the Royal Infirmary, referred to it as *"The pandemic of so-called influenza"*. He found it remarkable that not a single case was admitted into his hospital wards. The city of Edinburgh, where Brackenridge was stationed, set up a special field hospital to deal with the expected influx of sick patients, yet it remained completely empty. Brakenridge even mentioned how the Royal College of Physicians put together a committee of scientists ready to study the first patient with the hope of learning more about the disease, but not a single patient was ever admitted.[33]

In the US state of Indiana, the media reported that a steady increase in the mortality rate was occurring and that the excess mortality was considerably higher than in previous years. The fact of the matter, however, was that the mortality rate was almost identical. For example, the total number of deaths in January of 1890 was 1,386, just 2% higher than the January average recorded across the previous seven years. In January of 1888, the mortality rate was 1,694—nearly 20% greater than *before* the pandemic had begun. Some doctors claimed the pandemic had been killing hundreds of people, whereas others questioned whether a single case had appeared in the entire state at all. The Marion County Coroner declared he would be willing to bet fifty dollars (over USD 1,600 in today's money) that not a single case existed in the entire city of Indianapolis. He assured any physicians who claimed they had treated Russian flu patients were simply mistaken in their diagnoses.[34]

It wasn't just physicians who had their doubts and suspicions about the inconsistencies of the pandemic. An air of mistrust began to emerge among the general population. When news first broke about the pandemic, people thought it was simply a common cold because they were able to 'fight it on their feet'. The illness was so mild, that in many instances, people believed the medical profession was needlessly trying to scare them.[35]

The Anomalies Continue

In an official government report published in 1891, Dr Henry Parsons documented an interesting case of influenza aboard a British naval vessel. The ship was carrying both sailors and soldiers. All the sailors developed influenza, yet somehow, not a single soldier became sick.[36] If a germ was the cause, how would it discriminate between sailors and soldiers? More to the point, how was an influenza virus able to infect men aboard a ship voyaging across the middle of the ocean? A virus would need to have travelled from the mainland on an air current, in sufficient quantities, and then infect the men mid-voyage. A simple counterpoint is that one of the sailors was infected *before* leaving the port and later infected the other seafarers during the voyage. While this is, of course, plausible, it does not explain why the soldiers—who were regularly in close contact with the sailors—did not contract the disease.

Many doctors believed a contagious germ was responsible for the Russian flu because individuals living in isolated communities like lighthouses, jails, and monasteries remained unaffected.[37] There were also claims that the spread of disease followed roads and railway lines, which implies human-to-human transmission was a major factor.[38, 39] These explanations, however, conflict with what doctors on the ground were routinely witnessing. For example, in large households, only one or two family members became sick while the rest remained well. In some hospitals, patients sharing wards with the ill remained completely unaffected, yet the nursing staff developed the disease.[36] In other hospitals, not a single nurse became infected despite treating countless influenza patients.[30] Commanders at Fort Tregear, deep in the Lushai Hills of India, were perplexed as to how the soldiers stationed there contracted the disease because they had barely any contact with the outside world. The only explanation they could come up with was that the germ must have infiltrated the fort by piggybacking on a contaminated letter posted by a regiment of soldiers some 2,500 km away.[40]

Meteorological Possibilities

While it is impossible to know exactly what happened during the Russian influenza pandemic, it is clear there are many unresolved inconsistencies. These, at the very least, show how doubts about the origins, spread, symptoms, and diagnosis of infectious disease are both normal and long-standing (~150 years). At the time, weather doctors attempt to explain the behaviour of the Russian flu pandemic using atmospheric or meteorological phenomena. They proposed these to address the spread of Russian influenza on several fronts. First and foremost, an atmospheric or meteorological cause could demonstrate why people in cities thousands of kilometres apart fell ill simultaneously. It could also resolve mysteries like why people living in isolation,[18] or aboard ships at sea,[41] became infected without any outside contact with civilisation.

As the Russian influenza pandemic ravaged the world, many were open to the idea it was spread by the wind, and that further investigation should be left entirely up to weather doctors.[42] Heeding these calls, Dr Edward Watson and Dr Roland Curtin sought to investigate the cause of the pandemic together. They concluded that meteorological effects like fog and a warm-humid atmosphere favoured the spread of the disease. They asserted that *"the cold we catch"* is driven by atmospheric conditions and climactic variations, and that these changes can initiate a pandemic when rapid and severe enough.[43, 44] Around the same time, a government board in Ireland corroborated this theory by publishing a report concluding pandemics are likely caused by high temperatures and a moist atmosphere, rather than some kind of contagion.[45]

Discovery of Pfeiffer's Bacillus

Despite reports pointing towards a meteorological cause, doctors sympathetic to germ theory believed there must be another explanation. Yet, very little progress had been made towards understanding what the potential pathogen might be.[46-48] It wasn't until almost three years into the pandemic, in 1892, that the German bacteriologist, Richard Pfeiffer, made a breakthrough in the quest for discovering the causative agent. He isolated small rod-shaped bacteria from the upper respiratory tracts of three dozen influenza patients, which he named *Bacillus influenzae* (Pfeiffer's bacillus).[49] Pfeiffer claimed these bacteria were found exclusively in influenza patients but not healthy individuals, prompting him to conduct further confirmatory experiments. He inoculated pure cultures of *B. influenzae* into a range of different animals including apes, rabbits, guinea pigs, rats, pigeons, and mice. When apes and rabbits developed flu-like symptoms, Pfeiffer believed he had finally discovered the cause that had proven so elusive.[50]

Pfeiffer's discovery was confirmed later that same year by two others: German physician Paul Canon, who found the same germ in the blood of influenza patients,[51] and the Japanese bacteriologist Shibasaburō Kitasato (one of Robert Koch's students), who cultured pure samples of the bacterium.[52] Several others substantiated the findings of Pfeiffer, Canon, and Kitasato shortly thereafter.[53-55] The collective work of these three scientists apparently fulfilled Koch's postulates and was, therefore, deemed a legitimate discovery.[56] Ostensibly, then, there was no reason to doubt Pfeiffer's work. After all, so many other diseases were supposedly caused by pathogenic bacteria, so influenza must be too.[57] For at least three decades, the *B. influenzae* bacterium was generally accepted as the cause of influenza,[58] despite the fact Pfeiffer, nor any other researcher, published any conclusive scientific proof to support this claim.

Though it reportedly satisfied Koch's postulations, the hypothesis that *B. influenzae* was the causative agent of influenza was based upon nothing more than pure speculation. It wasn't until the Spanish influenza pandemic of 1918 that doctors began to question whether *B. influenzae* was really the cause. They conducted several elaborate human experiments exposing healthy people to pure cultures of Pfeiffer's bacillus.[59–63] In the majority of cases, the bacillus failed to cause disease.[59–61] In a few experiments, however, it is claimed that healthy people *did* contract influenza after being inoculated with the purified bacterium.[62, 63] But how is such an anomalous and contradictory result possible? It contradicts modern germ theory, which states influenza is caused by a virus and not a bacterium.

Inconsistencies aside, the initial idea that a bacteria caused influenza led to the belief that the same must be true of the common cold. In 1894, the British physician Edmund Cautley closely examined the respiratory tracts of eight patients suffering from a common cold. In seven of the cases, he isolated a bacterium from the nasal mucus which he named *Bacillus coryzae segmentosus*.[64] Over a decade later, another British physician named Robert Prosser White confirmed Cautley's findings, isolating the same bacillus from the mucus of 17 out of 21 cases of the common cold. White undertook experiments inoculating this bacterium into guinea pigs, rabbits, and monkeys. In every attempt, he failed to reproduce the common cold.[65, 66] This demonstrates how easy it is to mistake microorganisms *present in* a disease with the *cause of* that disease.

The Russian Flu in Review

Overall, the Russian flu did not resemble a pandemic as most people understand it. Those afflicted with the disease presented with a raft of over 40 symptoms so diverse that doctors scrambled to categorise them into four broad types (i.e. respiratory, gastrointestinal, catarrhal, and neurological). The symptomology was so inconsistent that few doctors saw cases resembling one another. This (a) contributed to widespread confusion and errors regarding diagnosis, (b) led many medical practitioners to believe other diseases were spreading at the same time, and (c) cast doubt on whether a Russian flu pandemic was occurring at all. Among all the turmoil, the media sensationalised the pandemic and reported outright falsehoods (e.g. increased mortality) contrary to what physicians observed on the frontline.

If this wasn't chaotic enough, other cases defied explanation, such as instances of selective contagion in voyaging seafarers, cohabiting families, hospital occupants, and remote military personnel. Many attempted to explain the Russian flu's swift, trans-continental east-to-west spread. Weather doctors pointed to sudden, drastic, and widespread shifts in temperature and humidity. Meanwhile, germ theorists were led astray by Pfeiffer's Bacillus. Despite convincing scientific and medical minds for decades, believing bacteria caused colds and flu ultimately turned out to be a fruitless and wasteful pursuit.

Chapter 11

Contagion Trailblazers

F or hundreds, if not thousands of years, humans have been trying to solve the mystery of what causes the common cold and influenza. People have turned to volcanic eruptions, comets, earthquakes, northerly breezes, cold weather, and damp clothes to explain the cause of these illnesses.[1] The answer to this question remained an enigma until Richard Pfeiffer discovered *B. influenzae*, after which everything changed.[2] Even though Pfeiffer never proved this bacterium was the cause of influenza, his work planted a seed in the minds of medical men and scientists. They became infatuated with blaming a microscopic, contagious germ, present in the respiratory tract of sick people. Pfeiffer had done for influenza what Koch had done for cholera. He offered something tangible to search for and work with—a germ.

Presented with this new avenue to explore, doctors and bacteriologists set out to test the validity of claims made by Pfeiffer (who argued bacteria causes influenza) and Cautley (who argued bacteria causes common colds). They were curious to find out whether cold and flu germs really caused disease and whether these germs could be passed from sick people to healthy people. Initial attempts to answer these questions using animal experiments yielded little in the way of understanding the two diseases. These failures prompted those working on the problem to undertake a myriad of human experiments. What better way to put this theory to the test than by directly exposing healthy people to the bacteria-rich bodily fluids of sick people?

In this vein, hundreds of experiments were conducted during the 20th century to see what would happen to healthy people after being exposed to 'so-called' pathogens. This came in the form of saliva, snot, mucus, lung fluid, and even the blood of people suffering from influenza and the common cold. Looking back from today's perspective, it may seem odd that experiments like this would ever be allowed to take place. However, the scientific world was a very different place back in the early 1900s. There was no such thing as an ethics committee to approve and oversee the treatment of research subjects. This meant that experimental research at this point in history was unregulated (even on humans) and was akin to the Wild West—anything was allowed. As such, scientists and doctors had free reign to do whatever they wanted without repercussion (as long as it was in the name of science, of course).

Ethical safeguards only came about decades later in the 1950s and 60s.[3,4] Once ethics committees became more stringent and restrictive, contagion studies were performed much less frequently. For this reason, many of the human experiments referenced in this book are now quite old. It is essential to understand, however, that age does not render these experiments invalid, redundant, or obsolete. On the contrary, these early human transmission studies are made *even more* important by the fact that scientists can no longer conduct this sort of research. In a way, they have appreciated considerably in historical and medical value because they put the claim of sick-to-well transmission directly to the test.

The Pioneers of Human Transmission (1798 – 1900)

The earliest attempts to induce illness in healthy people—by exposing them to the bodily fluids of sick people—go quite far back. For instance, in 1798, Renée Desgenettes (protégé of Napoleon Bonaparte and physician-in-chief of the French army stationed in Egypt) performed an experiment on himself many would consider a death sentence. After liberating a fortress from the Ottoman Empire, the bubonic plague broke out amongst the ranks of the French army.[5] To quell the soldier's fears about the contagiousness of the plague, Desgenettes dipped a lancet into the suppurating wound of a 'bubo' (a term used for a person with the plague). He then pricked himself in the groin and armpit with the contaminated lancet. To the bewilderment of the soldiers, Desgenettes remained completely well, allaying the fears of any despondent or weary troops that the plague might be contagious.[6,7]

To further dispel any doubt French soldiers might have had about the contagiousness of the plague, Napoleon Bonaparte himself grabbed the corpses of soldiers who had died from the disease with his bare hands and lifted them about. Needless to say, Bonaparte remained unaffected. This was around the same time the French had won the 'Battle of the Pyramids'. Following the victory, Bonaparte, Desgenettes, and their staff occupied the quarters at Murad Bay, where sixty enemy soldiers had died of the plague just days prior. Despite living within the confines of the pestilent quarters for some time, not a single Frenchman inhabiting its walls contracted the dreaded disease.[8]

In 1835, Antoine-Barthélémy Clot, better known as 'Clot-Bey', a physician and sergeant major in Napoleon's army, performed an experiment similar to that of Desgenettes. Clot-Bey took the blood of a 'bubo' and injected it into five Egyptian prisoners. Only one prisoner became unwell, which Clot-Bey argued was not a consequence of the injection, but because the man had been living in a pestilent plague-ridden hospital for three days prior. Clot-Bey proceeded to inject himself six separate times with the blood of another 'bubo'. When he failed to fall ill, Clot-Bey then injected himself with the pus taken directly from the open wound of another man dying of the disease. Like Desgenettes, Clot-Bey remained completely unaffected.[9]

Throughout the 1800s, at least 50 self-inoculation and human-to-human transmission experiments (like that of Desgenette's and Clot-Bey's), were performed. These looked at a range of other infectious diseases to gain a deeper understanding of how (or whether) they are transmissible.[10] Although somewhat crude by modern standards, these experiments largely failed to reproduce the disease under investigation,[11] bringing the entire premise of contagion into question. Not only did these experiments provide valuable insights into the (non)contagious nature of various diseases, but they also paved the way for others to conduct subsequent investigations into human-to-human disease transmission. Indeed, these earliest human trials likely served as inspiration for transmission experiments that began in the early 1900s to pinpoint the cause of infectious diseases like the common cold and influenza.

Early Human Transmission Experiments (1900 – 1950)

It took nearly a decade after Pfeiffer discovered *B. influenza* for the first human experiments on influenza to take place. In 1906, Davis isolated the *B. influenza* bacillus from a patient with whooping cough (Appendix Experiment 1.1). He mixed a pure culture of the bacillus into a saline solution and then smeared it over the throat, tonsils, and nasal membranes of one healthy volunteer. Within 48 hours, the recipient developed a cough, headache, and fever. According to Davis, however, the symptoms did not match whooping cough or influenza.[12] They appeared to be some other form of sickness entirely.

In 1914, Walther Kruse conducted two experiments exposing 48 healthy male volunteers to nasal secretions he obtained from two cases of the common cold (Exp. 2.1).[13] He was not convinced that bacteria were the cause of the malady and believed something else present in the mucus was to blame. Eager to prove this theory, Kruse decided to mix the nasal secretions obtained from common cold patients with saline and then pass this mixture through a 'Berkefeld' filter. Now, to clarify, Berkefeld filters are essentially a cylinder made from diatomaceous earth. Firing at extremely high temperatures produces a hardened material consisting of thousands of overlapping micro-pores capable of removing particles larger than 2 - 5 microns in size. When a mixture of saline and mucus passes through a Berkefeld filter this removes bacteria and other impurities, but supposedly allows viruses to pass through. As such, this filtering technique can yield a sterile virus 'filtrate'.[14–16] This is essentially the same as using paper to filter coffee grinds out of coffee while allowing the smaller active ingredients (like caffeine) to pass through. In Kruse's first experiment, four out of 12 participants (33%) developed symptoms of a common cold when exposed to the filtered mucus. In his second experiment, 15 out of 36 (42%) became ill (Exp. 2.2).[13]

Two years later, in 1916, George Foster conducted a similar set of experiments. In the first, he too passed the nasal secretions of three cases of the common cold through a Berkefeld filter and then immediately dropped it into the nasal cavities of 10 healthy participants using a pipette. Nine of the 10 healthy participants (90%) developed common cold symptoms (Exp. 3.1). In Foster's second experiment, he mixed nasal mucus with ascitic fluid, tissue broth, rabbit kidney tissue, and petroleum jelly. This mixture was then incubated for several days and passed through a Berkefeld filter. Foster then dropped the sterile filtrate into the nasal cavities of 11 healthy men. Every single man developed symptoms of the common cold (Exp. 3.2).[17]

The following year, Herman Dold conducted three experiments exposing healthy people to the filtered nasal secretions obtained from patients with a common cold. In the first experiment seven out of 17 healthy participants (41%) developed symptoms of the common cold within 72 hours of inoculation (Exp. 4.1). It is worth noting a separate group of 15 healthy participants served as controls. They worked, ate, and slept in the same quarters as those who were experimentally infected. However, none of the controls developed a cold. In Dold's second experiment, just one out of the 40 healthy participants (2.5%) became unwell (Exp. 4.2) and, in a third, two out of three participants (67%) developed common cold symptoms (Exp 4.3).[18]

The experiments conducted by Kruse, Foster and Dold were the first to cast doubt on the hypothesis that bacteria caused the common cold. Their results convinced the medical profession that influenza was not caused by Pfeiffer's bacillus, despite several cases of bacteriologists purportedly developing influenza after accidental exposure to the bacillus in laboratory settings.[19,20] From their use of Berkefeld filtration, Kruse, Foster, and Dold assumed there must be an 'invisible' substance or particle present in the filtered mucus which caused symptoms in the healthy participants. To them, there could be no other explanation—some unknown pathogen in the mucus was making people sick. Even though they had no idea what that substance might be, they called it a 'filter passing virus' or 'filterable virus'.[13]

At this point, the definition of a virus was rather ambiguous. Filterable viruses were originally thought to be small bacteria.[21] The term 'virus' could have also been referring to the Latin word meaning 'poison' or 'toxin',[22] or *contagium vivum fluidum*', which is Latin for 'living fluid contagium'.[23] All of these definitions were listed in dictionaries for hundreds of years.[24] Similarly, the word virus could have been referring to the Greek term 'imii' which means *'to throw the arrow, the poison, the toxin'*.[25] What were Kruse, Foster, and Dold referring to exactly?

A poison, a replication-competent, obligate parasite, or something else? They certainly did not know. It was simply an idea in their minds.

A Curious Case of Pesticide Inhalation

During his work, Dold made a very interesting observation. The head nurse working at the hospital where he was performing his experiments opened a box of pyrethrum-based insecticide powder (Exp. 4.3). She accidentally inhaled some of the fine powder and, according to Dold, *"an amazing effect was observed"*. Almost immediately, the nurse began to sneeze heavily, and within a matter of hours, she had developed an acute cold, which lasted almost an entire week. To see if these results could be replicated, six other people working in the hospital were exposed to the insect powder in a similar fashion. Two of the six individuals began sneezing immediately after breathing in the insecticide and went on to develop typical colds. These results led Dold to conclude that the common cold might actually be caused by the inhalation of chemical substances.[18]

This case raises a question about what caused the cold symptoms observed in Kruse, Foster, and Dold's experiments. They assumed the presence of some kind of invisible 'infectious agent', but it could also have been a *chemical substance* retained in the filtered mucus, or simply the consequence of *local irritation* after having a foreign substance squirted into the nasal cavity. There is experimental evidence to show that introducing various substances into the nose (like insect powder, saline,[26] beef broth,[27] and egg yolk suspensions[28]) can cause common cold symptoms. Because Kruse, Foster, and Dold did not test for the presence of other substances, nor introduce inert inoculations as controls, they could not rule out the possibility that these other factors might be at play.

More broadly, the lack of testing and control in these experiments did not go unnoticed. Not only were these shortcomings highlighted in the medical literature, but calls were made for Kruse, Foster, and Dold to try again with more rigorous, scientifically valid methods using proper control groups.[29] Though properly designed and controlled experiments would leave the results much less open to interpretation, the three scientists never followed up their initial work.

The Hidden Role of Inflammatory Mediators

Given the alternative explanations, why did Kruse, Foster, and Dold assume a virus was the only thing present in filtered mucus capable of causing symptoms? There are countless substances much smaller than virus particles in the nasal mucus of people suffering respiratory illnesses. Such substances include inflammatory chemicals like prostaglandins, interleukins, cytokines, lysozymes, lactoferrin, hyaluronan, mucins, fibrinogen, and immunoglobulins.[30-32] Undoubtedly, there are many experiments showing respiratory tract symptoms occur when people are inoculated with mucus secretions obtained from sick people, but not when they are inoculated with mucus from healthy people.[33-35] However, researchers often conclude this effect is due to the presence of a virus, while ignoring the role of inflammatory mediators and non-chemical irritants.

Studies have found that during a cold or flu, mucus membranes release inflammatory mediators like histamine and bradykinin. For example, histamine is known to be present in the nasal secretions of people with common colds.[36] It has also been shown to cause respiratory symptoms like nasal congestion, sneezing, and a sore throat when experimentally inoculated into the respiratory tract of healthy individuals.[32,37,38] Critically, this inflammatory chemical is small enough to pass through a Berkefeld filter.[39] Bradykinin is also present in the mucus of people with a cold or flu, with concentrations increasing up to 30x the normal level during respiratory illness.[40] When inoculated into the respiratory tracts of healthy people, bradykinin has been demonstrated to cause flu-like symptoms, including rhinitis (i.e. nasal congestion and irritation, sneezing, runny nose, itchy nose, etc.), increased respiratory mucus secretions, pharyngitis (i.e. a sore throat), cough, and a sensation of rawness in the airways.[38,41-44] Again, bradykinin is magnitudes of times smaller than a 'virus',[45] so it stands to reason it would also pass through a Berkefeld filter.

These inflammatory chemicals are responsible for *producing symptoms* like a cough, sore throat, and runny nose.[46] Though most people consider these symptoms to be the 'problem', they are merely the body's response or answer to the problem. Knowing this, our forefathers regularly used 'snuffs' to promote the flow of respiratory secretions as a means of restoring health.[28] Why does the body need to release these chemicals and produce symptoms? In many cases, flu-like symptoms arise to eliminate alleged 'pathogens', toxins, foreign particulate matter, and other irritants from the respiratory tract.[47–50] People routinely experience various cold and flu-like symptoms after inhaling allergens (leading to hay fever) and other seemingly innocuous substances. Several medical papers have acknowledged the inhalation of non-infectious agents can produce a clinical illness *indistinguishable* from that of an 'infectious' cold.[28,34,51] Of course, viewing symptoms as *adaptive* and *homeostatic* opposes the mainstream notion that cold and flu symptoms are disease states induced by a virus to facilitate its spread to other hosts.[52] Clearly, allergens, pollutants, and toxins do not cause symptoms to 'spread' inhaled irritants to other people. Introducing foreign materials simply produces an eliminatory response by the body—one that is inherently difficult to differentiate from colds and flu.

Kruse, Foster, Dold, and other scientists conducting similar human experiments at that time (or earlier) were ignorant of these facts. Unfortunately, these substances were only discovered and inoculated into people's respiratory tracts decades after the early experiments by Kruse, Foster, and Dold, and the belief in contagious viruses had taken hold. It's likely their conclusions (and perhaps even their methods) would have changed if they knew the mucus of sick people contains inflammatory chemicals and other irritants capable of inducing flu-like illness. It's also possible they may have discovered this fact themselves had their original experiments strictly adhered to the scientific method. Could it be that these inflammatory mediators, and not 'viruses', are responsible for the observed symptoms in human experiments exposing healthy people to the bodily fluids of sick people? Clearly, further research is required to answer this question.

The Early Bird Catches No Worm

To briefly summarise, the mystery of the common cold and influenza has persisted throughout history. Perplexed, people once looked to major environmental and celestial events in an attempt to explain their afflictions. Though they also suspected contagion at times, notable examples like Napolean and his protégé promptly allayed fears when they were unable to catch or transmit the bubonic plague after directly exposing themselves and others to it. Likewise, in the 1800s, around 50 other experiments failed to reproduce the diseases that researchers exposed themselves or others to. It wasn't until the discovery of Pfeiffer's Bacillus that scientists were inspired to look for disease-causing pathogens. Though a bacterial explanation for colds and flu was ultimately incorrect, it catalysed the next line of research on human transmission during the 1900s.

In search of a smaller culprit, Walther Kruse, George Foster, and Herman Dold all used Berkefeld filters to remove bacteria and other large materials from their filtrate. Using their 'filtered virus' method, they were able to make people sick (to varying degrees). However, none of these researchers accounted for the fact that their results were confounded by the potential presence of other equally tiny substances. As it turns out, their experimental methods were not rigorous enough to test for or remove foreign contaminants. Likewise, they did not adequately control for the fact that sick secretions contain inflammatory mediators which are known to produce cold and flu symptoms. For these reasons, the evidence that Kruse, Foster, and Dold gathered is insufficient to support their conclusion that an invisible pathogenic virus caused the symptoms they observed. This same caveat casts doubt on other human transmission studies that failed to rule out the effect of allergens, pollutants, toxins, and inflammatory mediators as alternative explanations for symptoms.

Chapter 12

The Spanish Influenza Pandemic

The Spanish influenza pandemic of 1918-19, aptly named due to its prevalence in Spain, and because it was the first country to publicly report the disease, is one of the most notorious pandemics of modern times.[1] Over two years, between 50 and 100 million people are said to have died,[2-4] and an estimated 500 million people fell ill.[5] Despite its scope and impact, the exact origin of the pandemic is shrouded in mystery. It is believed the pandemic originated in several different areas, making it almost impossible to determine where it truly began.[6,7] There are reports of the first cases occurring at multiple sites: a British Army post in France in 1916,[8] somewhere in China towards the end of 1917,[7] the Sing Sing prison in New York in late February of 1918, and the Fort Riley military base in Kansas in early March that same year.[3] After the first cases broke out, the pandemic spread across Asia, North America, Europe, and Africa, before doubling back through the same regions—all within a matter of months.[7]

Three Peculiarities

Just like the Russian influenza pandemic of 1889, there are several peculiarities surrounding the Spanish flu. The first being its unusual pattern of spread. The pandemic was said to have appeared in Boston and Bombay on the same day, despite these cities being separated by more than 12,000 kilometres. Stranger still, the flu somehow took over three weeks to travel the 300 km from Boston to New York, and more than a month to spread a mere 60 kilometres from Joliet to Chicago.[1,9] This pattern of spread seems inconsistent with human-to-human contact.

Even in desolate places, the dissemination of the disease seemed rather peculiar. In 1919, the Governor of Alaska, Thomas Riggs, wrote a report to the U.S. Senate detailing the situation that was unfolding there.[10] To prevent the spread of the disease, Riggs ordered the seaports closed. The very last ship to dock in Nome before the winter set in, was the Victoria, a steamship carrying mail and 30 passengers.[11,12] Although the passengers were in a good state of health after the 11-day voyage, they were examined by three different doctors before disembarking. Once on dry land, they were placed in hospital quarantine for another five days.[11,13] Every precaution was taken to protect the townsfolk, even the mail was *fumigated* for 10 hours before being collected by the postal service.[11] Despite these measures, the people of Nome soon became ill. Apparently, the quarantined passengers were 'asymptomatically infected', spreading the disease throughout town upon their release.[11,12,14] At this time, the weather conditions were some of the worst in living memory.[9,10] Travel was incredibly difficult and restricted entirely to snow-ready dog teams. The terrain was unforgiving, the days were short, and the temperature was freezing. This meant even experienced travellers could cover no more than 50 kilometres on a good day.[9,10] To put things in perspective, some towns were so remote, that even in optimal conditions it took over a month for news to arrive that WWI had ended.[15] Yet, the pandemic still managed to sweep across the state, allegedly carried by mailmen and hunters as they went from town to town.[12] Despite having a population of just 50,000 people, who were thinly dispersed across a vast area of wilderness roughly the size of Europe,[9] Alaska suffered one of the highest mortality rates per capita of anywhere in the world.[14]

The second peculiarity is that there were three waves of Spanish flu in the first year alone. The pandemic spread back and forth across the Earth for the first time in the spring of 1918; a second time in the autumn just a few months later; and a third time in the winter of 1918-19. A fourth and final wave occurred between late 1919 and mid-1920.[7,16] The waves were relatively brief, lasting just three or so months, disappearing for three months, and then returning for the same amount of time.[17] Many considered it unusual that distinct waves could re-occur in such a short timeframe, especially when it took more than three years for the same number of waves to hit during the Russian influenza pandemic.[18,19] This is atypical of influenza more generally, which normally hits during a single season each year.

The third peculiarity is that about half of the people who died of Spanish flu were young adults, specifically males between 20 and 40 years of age. This is rather unexpected considering mortality rates in previous and subsequent pandemics were highest among children and older adults.[20,21] Though the scientific and medical communities put forth different explanations (e.g. the 'cytokine storm' hypothesis), none were properly substantiated, so this anomaly remains a mystery.[20] Another piece of puzzling information is that civilian and military healthcare workers such as doctors, nurses, and ambulance officers had mortality rates lower than any other occupation.[22-24] How did front-line workers evade the most infectious and lethal form of flu the world had ever seen, despite regular close contact with sick and dying patients? Given their heightened risk, it is miraculous they were found to have *the best* chances of surviving the pandemic.

Unusual Symptomology

Even in the face of these three peculiarities, the most perplexing aspect of the pandemic was the great disparity of symptoms experienced by those struck down by the disease. Much like the Russian flu, doctors described a wide variety of 'strange' and 'inconsistent' forms of Spanish flu (Table 2). These forms were protean enough to convince doctors there must be multiple pandemics of different diseases occurring simultaneously.[25] In fact, the symptoms were so unusually diverse, that doctors were mistaken into thinking the Spanish flu was the bubonic plague,[26] while others misdiagnosed it as typhoid fever, dengue fever, or cholera.[27,28]

There were at least four different types of Spanish influenza described in the literature: (1) a *normal* form indistinguishable from the seasonal flu, characterised by typical symptoms (e.g. chills, fever, headache, sore throat, nasal congestion) lasting 3 to 4 days, (2) a *severe* form characterised by more significant respiratory symptoms (e.g. pneumonia and bronchitis), (3) a *gastrointestinal* form characterised by respiratory symptoms plus nausea, vomiting and diarrhoea, and (4) a *phthisic* form resembling tuberculosis (i.e. coughing up blood).[29] As stated previously, germ theory subscribes to the premise that 'one germ causes one disease'. If this is true, then how is it possible the same influenza virus could cause such a broad and varied array of symptoms?

Symptoms of Spanish Influenza[26,30-33]		
Adrenal insufficiency	Endocarditis	Heliotrope cyanosis
Anorexia	Enlarged liver	Mahogany Spots
Blood nose	Enlarged spleen	Muscle aches
Bloody sputum	Fatigue	Nausea
Conjunctivitis	Fever	Pulmonary oedema
Constipation	Frothy sputum	Skin rash
Coryza	Gastrointestinal bleeding	Sore throat
Delirium	Hair loss	Tachycardia
Diarrhoea	Headache	Tracheitis
		Vomiting

Table 2 - Symptoms of Spanish Influenza

In addition to varying considerably in *form*, the Spanish flu also appeared to vary dramatically in *severity*. During the first wave, doctors from around the world reported the pandemic could not be influenza because the symptoms were so mild.[19] However, subsequent waves struck with much greater intensity. In September of 1918, Colonel William Welch, who was stationed at Camp Devens in Massachusetts, examined the lungs of a dead soldier and stated the disease must be a new kind of infection or plague.[33] Similarly, a pathologist for the United States Public Health Service remarked that the lungs of the dead were unlike any other form of pneumonia he had ever come across.[34] Every day, hundreds of people dropped dead in the street, despite waking up completely healthy just a few hours prior.[35] To confuse matters even further, a very well-known medicine manufacturer of cold and flu remedies (who are still manufacturing the same product to this day) published newspaper advertisements claiming that authorities were in agreement the disease was nothing more than an old-fashioned flu masquerading under a new name.[36]

The worst cases of Spanish flu started as what seemed like any normal bout of the flu. Before long, mild symptoms like dyspnoea would rapidly progress to bronchitis and then pneumonia. By the time people had been rushed to hospital, they already had dark 'mahogany' spots on their cheekbones—the beginning of cyanosis (i.e. skin colour changes from lack of blood oxygen). The spots on the cheekbones soon expanded over the entire face, before spreading to the rest of the body in just a few short hours.[37,38] Cyanosis—a hallmark symptom of the Spanish flu—may have been caused by thick, purulent, yellow sputum blocking the airways.[38] Some described it as '*the most vicious type of pneumonia that has ever been seen*'.[39] The cyanosis was very distinct in that the whole body would turn a deep blue-purple colour,[4,39] making it impossible to tell dark-skinned people apart from light-skinned.[40,41] Hence it was often named 'Black Flu',[42] or 'Purple Death'.[43,44]

In the most extreme cases of Spanish flu, people bled from the ears, eyes, mouth, and nose.[27,45,46] People's hair and teeth fell out and, in many instances, their bodies emitted a strange smell reminiscent of musty hay or straw,[47,48] symptoms which are atypical of influenza.[19] Few were lucky to survive once they had become cyanotic, as they often developed right-sided heart failure.[38] The main symptom of Spanish flu was haemorrhagic tracheobronchitis (respiratory tract inflammation & bloody sputum), which appeared suddenly and was often fatal.[49] It was not uncommon for people to die within as little as 24 hours after the onset of symptoms. However, the average time of death was around 10 days—a consequence of a so-called secondary bacterial pneumonia 'superinfection'.[50–52]

Chemical Warfare

The Spanish flu was also unique in that it coincided with WWI. In the Summer of 1918, American troops approaching the Western Front slowed to a crawl after experiencing an unprecedented number of casualties among the ranks. More than 43,000 had already died by that point, not due to combat, but because of pandemic influenza. Such losses were by no means insignificant, amounting to 80 percent of the total number of combat deaths recorded for the entire war.[53] Indeed, the Spanish flu crippled military efforts by incapacitating up to 40% of the United States Army and Navy personnel with illness.[54]

As previously mentioned, there is much debate as to where and how the pandemic began. Some historical records point to the first cases emerging from military posts, such as a British base camp at Étaples in Northern France during the winter of 1916, or a British barracks in Aldershot in March of 1917.[55] Coincidentally, at these two bases, more than 100,000 soldiers were stationed in treacherous and unsanitary conditions. Inhabitants huddled together in cramped tents pitched on ground contaminated with thousands of tonnes of chemical warfare agents known as 'battle gas'.[8] Battle gas had been deployed by German forces as early as 1915 and was used unforgivingly throughout the entire duration of the conflict.[56] Living in such conditions would have undoubtedly had deleterious effects on even the most robust and battle-hardened soldiers.

During the Great War, over 150,000 tonnes of chemical warfare agents were produced worldwide, with approximately 125,000 tonnes being deployed on the battlefields.[57] These gasses could persist in the environment for weeks, possibly months, after being deployed because they were heavier than air and not readily soluble in water.[58,59] The gasses were so poisonous, doctors were forced to evacuate entire wards if a man was brought in still wearing contaminated clothing. The gas residue on the affected individuals' clothing readily dispersed into the air and would irritate the eyes of medical workers, making it impossible to see.[60]

Despite its widespread use, the military was tight-lipped about battle gasses and shared little to no information about the consequences of human exposure with doctors on the front line. The only way for doctors to learn about the horrific effects was by treating victims in the field.[61] They frequently encountered the most widely used battle gas, *phosgene*. This weapon was preferred because it was easy to manufacture, rapidly fatal at high concentrations, and exceptionally hard to detect. Upon detonation, phosgene gas was usually colourless and odourless—a true invisible enemy.[62] However, it could present as a pale-yellow or pale-green cloud,[63] with some reporting it had a smell reminiscent of musty hay, or freshly mown grass.[62] Of the 90,000 men who died from exposure to battle gasses during the war, 85% were killed by phosgene.[64] Military forces also employed mustard, chlorine, and lewisite gasses, but did so far less than phosgene because these were not typically colourless or odourless. This made them much easier to detect and evade. Alongside phosgene, the military implemented lacrimatory gasses—also known as 'blue gas'—throughout the war. Although not fatal, blue gas was originally thought to be fine enough to pass through a gas mask filter, causing violent irritation of the respiratory tract. The intention was to force soldiers to remove their gas masks, after which the enemy would deploy more lethal gasses like phosgene. It was soon realised, however, lacrimatory gasses could not penetrate gas mask filters, nevertheless, they were still widely used for strategic purposes.[56]

Although inhaling large quantities of phosgene was almost instantly fatal, it could take up to 24 hours for victims to succumb to their injuries. To make matters worse, there were no effective treatments available for gas poisoning apart from oxygen therapy, which afforded only a minor reprieve. Records from an open-air hospital in Boston showed that patients with access to fresh air, sunlight, and hygienic facilities fared much better than their counterparts in enclosed wards.[54] This contrasts markedly with the experience of frontline doctors and nurses who could do little more than comfort soldiers while they suffered an agonising death. Gas-afflicted men who felt better after laying down for several hours would often die within minutes of getting up and moving about.[60,65] Other victims ripped their clothes from their bodies as they asphyxiated to death,[37] with some even committing suicide to escape the unbearable suffering.[56]

Symptoms of severe gas poisoning were initially mild, presenting as a flu-like illness, before progressing rapidly over several hours to bronchitis, pneumonia, and pulmonary oedema (an acute-respiratory-distress-like syndrome). Eventually, those severely poisoned with gas would die.[59,66–69] Dyspnoea and cyanosis were hallmarks of gas poisoning. Men clutched their chests as they gasped for air. They coughed up blood and frothy yellow sputum as their bodies turned a deep blue-purple colour—a serious condition known as 'heliotrope cyanosis'.[60] The cyanosis was so pronounced, that many medical practitioners feared the black death had returned.[60,70–72] Despite the wide range of serious side effects, the lethal effects of poison gas were primarily due to respiratory failure and right-sided heart failure.[48,73,74]

In instances of mild phosgene exposure, it could take up to 48 hours or longer for symptoms to develop.[61,75] Mild cases presented as a flu-like illness with delayed onset of symptoms including, but not limited to a persistent cough, bloody and frothy yellow sputum, sneezing, general weakness lasting several weeks to months,[76] irritated eyes and throat, chest tightness, pulmonary oedema, nausea, vomiting, headache,[77,78] a runny nose, sinus pain, shortness of breath,[79] hair loss,[32] and heliotrope cyanosis.[80] In moderate to severe cases, exposure to battle gasses rapidly eroded the mucous membranes of soldiers, resulting in bleeding from the eyes, mouth, and nose.[79,81]

Something in the Air

Medical personnel believed poor living conditions, the stress of war, and exposure to chemical agents all lowered soldiers' immunity, making them more susceptible to infection with the Spanish influenza virus (H1N1).[55,82] Though this is a plausible story, many other doctors at the time were unconvinced that military flu deaths were largely attributable to the pandemic. This is because, as the first gas victims began arriving at field hospitals, attending doctors could not help but draw parallels between the pathology of Spanish influenza and battle gas exposure.[3,55,83–85]

When pathologists examined the lungs of soldiers poisoned with phosphene gas at autopsy, they were astonished to find that damage to the respiratory tract was remarkably similar to that of Spanish flu victims.[19,86–88] Meanwhile, at world-leading universities, bacteriologists and pathologists also noted how closely the effects of influenza resembled poison gas inhalation when they examined tissue samples obtained during autopsy.[89] Even revered influenza experts acknowledged how reminiscent the lesions of Spanish flu infection were to poison gas inhalation.[90] After the war had ended, doctors continued to learn about the effects of phosgene gas. They found that, when it was inhaled by soldiers, phosgene mixed with water vapour in the lungs to form hydrochloric acid, resulting in significant tissue damage. In follow-up animal experiments, they showed that inhaling hydrochloric acid produced lesions in the lungs *identical* to those observed in patients who died of pandemic influenza.[91] It's no wonder, then, why people described the pandemic as an 'attack' or 'invasion' that was *"as dangerous as poison gas shells"*.[92] As illustrated in table 1.3, the symptoms of battle gas victims align very closely with those of Spanish flu patients. The two presented in a way exceedingly difficult to distinguish from one another.

The conflation of gas and flu is worsened by the fact they coincided in history. That is, the Spanish influenza pandemic occurred around the same time that companies were mass-producing and shipping chemical warfare agents for armed forces to deploy extensively on the front lines. As previously mentioned, over 150,000 tonnes of poison gasses were produced worldwide during WWI.[57] Of this, 68,000 tonnes were produced by the Germans, 36,000 tonnes by the French, 25,000 tonnes by the British and 2,500 tonnes by the Americans.[93,94] Soldiers were regularly afflicted with phosgene poisoning and, therefore, the potential for a flu misdiagnosis was significant. Unsurprisingly, there was also a higher incidence of Spanish influenza among employees working at phosgene gas manufacturing facilities, but not for workers at facilities manufacturing other types of battle gasses, who were largely unaffected.[95] Much like the military, it is possible that workers poisoned by phosgene gas in manufacturing plants were also misdiagnosed with the Spanish flu.

Symptoms	Spanish Influenza	Gas Poisoning
Bloody sputum	✓	✓
Dyspnoea	✓	✓
Flu-like symptoms	✓	✓
Hairloss	✓	✓
Heart failure	✓	✓
Heliotrope cyanosis	✓	✓
Musty-hay body odour	✓	✓
Pulmonary oedema	✓	✓

Table 3 – Common Symptoms of Spanish Influenza & Gas Poisoning

Beyond exposure from battlefields and supply chains, there are other ways battle gas might have caused illness in distant locations. On the 9th of March 1918, a noxious pale-yellow gas cloud emanated from the Fort Riley military base in Kansas. Two days later, the first reported outbreak of Spanish flu in North America occurred at that very base. The official story states the yellow-cloud was the result of manure being burned, of which nine-thousand tonnes per month were produced by the innumerable horses stabled there. Just as the manure was being incinerated, a sandstorm kicked up, blowing the stinking cloud across the base and surrounding areas.[96] The cloud was claimed to contain an equine virus that infected the soldiers stationed there. Strange occurrences like this weren't restricted to military installations. There were claims that German forces had been infiltrating allied countries around the world releasing 'airborne agents' in cities and ports. In September of 1918, Lieutenant Colonel Philip S. Doane—the head of the Health and Sanitation Section of the Emergency Fleet Corporation—announced that the outbreaks of Spanish flu in the United States may have been a result of covert German military operations. He suspected German submarines had deployed spies along the coastline under the cover of night, who would then release 'flu germs' in theatres or other crowded places. According to Doane, the Germans had already achieved this in Europe, so it was not unreasonable to think the same thing could happen on American soil.[97]

Indeed, eyewitness accounts from civilians described camouflaged German ships sneaking into ports of major American cities under the cover of darkness and releasing 'greasy looking gas clouds' into the air that wafted ashore.[98] Similar claims were also made by media outlets in Brazil. For example, a prominent newspaper in Rio de Janeiro reported that Germans had put 'germs' in bottles which were then dropped into the ocean near the coastlines of allied countries. The bottles were then carried ashore by the current, dispersing their contents onto innocent civilians unfortunate enough to pick them up.[99] Of course, it is impossible to confirm what these clouds and bottles contained, or if such events ever actually transpired. However, if these reports are true, it seems more plausible from a technological and logistical standpoint to release poison gas instead of flu germs, especially given the fact both afflicted people in the same way.

Many pertinent questions remain unanswered concerning the relationship between poisonous phosgene gas and Spanish influenza. First, if doctors could not tell one from the other, to what extent was gas poisoning mistakenly attributed to the flu? The highest Spanish flu mortality was recorded among males aged between 20 and 40 years—those most likely to have been exposed to chemical weapons in combat. Second, why did doctors, nurses, and those transporting the 'infected' have the lowest mortality rates of any profession? It's possible 'sick' soldiers were frequently dying of gas poisoning—not influenza—meaning healthcare workers caring for them were being exposed to poisoned people, not infected people. Given that poisoning isn't contagious, the lack of disease transmission in such cases could have been confused as 'immunity' or 'asymptomatic infection'. Third, and finally, why was the Spanish flu orders of magnitude deadlier than every other influenza before or after it? This influenza killed up to 100 million people, which is significantly more than the Russian flu three decades prior (up to one million deaths) and the Asian flu four decades later (slightly over one million deaths).[100] Coincidentally, the worst year of the pandemic was 1918—the final and deadliest year of the war, occurring in a narrow window in history where phosgene gas was widely dispersed into the atmosphere. Though these questions are difficult to resolve a century later, the connection between gas and flu is nonetheless interesting to ponder.

Cure or Curse?

A final point deserving brief mention relates to the way Spanish flu was medically treated. Some argue an influenza virus simply cannot explain the vast differences in symptom form and severity, as well as the great disparity in the case-fatality rates (which ranged from 0.58% in some areas and up to 10% in others).[101] This suggests other factors might have been at play. In September of 1918, the United States Navy and the Surgeon General recommended people take aspirin as a symptomatic treatment for the Spanish flu.[102,103] Historical evidence suggests that, during the pandemic, aspirin was readily handed out 'like candy' to anyone looking for symptomatic relief.

Nowadays, the current recommended dose of aspirin is around 4,000 mg per day. During the pandemic, however, doctors prescribed anywhere from 8,000 – 15,600 mg per day, resulting in widespread aspirin poisoning across the general population. These doses are equivalent to taking twenty-five, 325 milligram aspirin tablets within 24 hours.[104] The symptoms of aspirin poisoning include lung damage, pulmonary oedema, respiratory failure, and pulmonary haemorrhage—all symptoms characteristic of the Spanish flu.[101,105] Again, how much of a role did aspirin poisoning play in the scope and severity of (what was reported as) pandemic influenza? It is plausible that widespread and indiscriminate aspirin use contributed to illness and mortality at this time, despite being relatively overlooked.

The Spanish Flu in Review

Once again, the world witnessed another influenza pandemic mysteriously emerge and evaporate. Though the Spanish flu is notorious, it is odd we cannot verify something as simple as its point of origin due to distinct geographical locations reporting outbreaks at the same time. During the outbreak, experts were baffled by the characteristics and behaviour of this atypical flu. First, they struggled to comprehend its *spread*, occurring halfway across the world, yet taking over a month to go from one nearby city to another. It also conquered regions like Alaska despite low population density, vast distances, and oppressive weather conditions limiting travel. Second, they struggled to explain its *recurrence*. The Spanish flu came in waves covering the earth three times within a year (followed by a fourth shortly thereafter). This is unusual for influenza, which typically arises once a year within a narrow window. Third, they struggled to account for its *victims*, who were primarily young males aged 20-40. Though it was the deadliest flu in history, those who would normally be most susceptible to influenza (i.e. children and older adults) were relatively unaffected. Similarly, even those who treated victims (i.e. medical personnel) were the least likely to die despite the highest risk of repeated exposure. Much like the Russian flu, the Spanish influenza pandemic presented particularly unusual symptoms that varied so tremendously that they convinced doctors the plague or other fevers were breaking out. The fact that doctors needed to categorise the breadth of symptoms into four types (i.e. normal, severe, gastrointestinal, and phthisic) is at odds with the one germ, one disease dictum. The symptoms also varied extraordinarily in severity. Ranging from nothing more than a typical bout of flu to killing sufferers within a matter of hours.

This chapter also uncovered the previously overlooked role that poison played in causing people to fall ill and die during this same period. The most notable instance likely went unnoticed due to the considerable overlap between the symptoms of phosgene battle gas and the presentation of Spanish flu. Though it is hard to know all the facts due to the secretive nature of chemical warfare, phosgene mimicked the Spanish flu so closely in presenting patients and autopsies that medical professionals struggled to tell them apart. Nevertheless, the association between the two appears to be broader than many realise, both coinciding most prominently at a specific moment in history (circa. 1918). The hidden role of poisonous gases might help explain why mortality was highest in soldiers, lowest in healthcare personnel, and why the Spanish flu was extraordinarily deadly. Another notable instance where poison likely played a role was through widespread aspirin consumption. People took excessively high doses, as prescribed, out of fear for their health. Yet, this led to their demise and afflicted them with a symptom profile that also happened to overlap significantly with that of the Spanish flu.

Taken together, the Spanish flu was particularly difficult to define, diagnose, and describe the behaviour of. This uncertainty means we know much less about the nature of the Spanish flu than modern recounts imply. It has a mysterious origin, inexplicable peculiarities (e.g. *spread*, *recurrence*, and *victims*), as well as a highly abnormal symptom profile that was inconsistent in *who* it spread to and *how* it affected them. All the while, the story is made murkier by the overlooked role of toxic compounds. Though a germ-based explanation seems to provide a simple explanation of what happened, it fails to account for these inconsistencies and exceptions, leaving many unanswered questions.

Chapter 13

Investigating Influenza

F rom the outset of the Spanish flu pandemic, doctors and scientists desperately wondered what the cause might be. Strangely enough, it seems they did not consider the effects of war or overzealous usage of various remedies as potential causative or contributing factors at the time. Instead, medical professionals were steadfast in their belief that an infectious agent was to blame, despite a lack of proof. They didn't even know exactly how the disease was transmitted between people. One thing was certain, though. Experts doubted Pfeiffer's bacillus was the culprit because it was found in less than one percent of patients and inoculating healthy people with the bacillus did not recreate the disease.[1,2] Identifying the cause of the Spanish flu was not only important for the war effort but also for quelling fears in the general populace. As a matter of urgency, doctors and scientists undertook many human experiments with the hope of identifying the causal agent. As this chapter will demonstrate, the woeful Spanish flu experiments eventually transitioned into equally unsuccessful influenza research.

Failure as a Motivator

Shortly after the pandemic broke out, John Nuzum and his colleagues conducted three human experiments exposing healthy volunteers to the mucus secretions and ground-up lung tissues they excised from influenza patients. Of the seven participants who volunteered themselves for this experiment, *none* developed the Spanish flu (Exp. 5.1 & 5.2).[3] In another self-inoculation experiment, Hugo Selter attempted to infect himself and his assistant with the nasopharyngeal washings of five influenza patients. Again, neither of the two men developed influenza (Exp. 6.1).[4] René

Dujarric also conducted a similar self-experiment by injecting himself with the blood of four influenza patients. His attempts, too, were met with negative results (Exp. 8.1).[5] So, despite how important and urgent it was to find an explanation for Spanish flu, initial attempts to transmit the disease came up empty.

It was at this point that efforts to experimentally infect men with Spanish influenza escalated. As the pandemic intensified, so too did the desperation of scientists tasked with understanding its cause. This was exemplified in the work of investigators like Charles Nicolle and Charles Le Bailly, who conducted a series of four risky experiments reserved for only the bravest of volunteers. The researchers collected mucus secretions from influenza patients. Then, using a pipette, they dropped these secretions into the conjunctiva and nasal passages of a monkey. After a few days, the monkey developed a fever, at which time they extracted a blood sample. Nicolle and Le Bailly then injected the freshly drawn sample of monkey blood subcutaneously into one man and intravenously into another. In the face of such a bold procedure, both men remained well (Exp. 7.1). In response to this null result, the researchers took mucus secretions originally sampled from the influenza patients and injected it subcutaneously and intravenously into two healthy people (Exp. 7.2 & 7.3). Only one developed mild flu-like symptoms a few days later. After falling ill, this infected man proceeded to share living quarters with several other healthy individuals, all of whom remained completely well. That is, not a single case of transmission occurred (Exp. 7.4).[6]

These experiments also failed to transmit Spanish flu infections. The one exception who became unwell did so with many caveats, so it does not prove a pathogenic microbe was involved. As discussed in Chapter 11, many other substances present in mucus secretions are capable of producing flu-like symptoms (e.g. inflammatory mediators). As such, even this single positive result is unreliable and, therefore, does not constitute strong evidence to support a virus as the cause.

Military Might

As the curtain closed on the theatre of war, the United States military and the United States Public Health Service focused some of their post-war efforts towards unlocking the secrets of influenza. Just when the

Spanish flu reached its peak, the military conducted a barrage of human experiments to determine the cause and mode of disease spread. They hoped the experiments would yield valuable insights into influenza so that an effective treatment, or at least a better management strategy, could be developed. With high hopes, the U.S. Navy devised an extensive series of experiments at military quarantine hospitals on Deer Island,[7] Angel Island,[8] and Gallups Island.[9]

The experiments involved more than 160 sailors, who volunteered to participate in one of 25 human experiments conducted over six months. The U.S. military took the matter very seriously, partnering with and involving more than 50 of the highest-ranking naval officers, the Surgeon General, as well as various scientists and medical doctors from the Laboratory Corps, Pathology and Bacteriology Division, Zoology Division, Pharmacology Division, Chemistry Division, and Special Details. They also consulted professors from several leading universities from around the country to ensure the experiments adhered to the highest standards. For these reasons, the human contagion experiments conducted by the U.S Navy and Public Health Service are arguably the most comprehensive, thorough, and well-controlled human transmission studies ever undertaken in the history of medicine. The next three sections outline the experiments conducted at each of the three islands, respectively.

Deer Island Human Transmission Experiments

The U.S. Navy conducted human influenza transmission experiments on Deer Island in November and December of 1918. The men subjected to these experiments were all volunteers from the naval training station located on Deer Island, Boston. There were 62 men in total, ranging in age from 15 – 34 years. All men were in excellent physical condition and were willing participants. Of the 62 subjects, 39 reported they had never previously contracted influenza at any point during their lives. Eight of the 62 men had been ill the previous flu season with non-specific symptoms that may or may not have been influenza. At the time of these experiments, an epidemic of influenza had broken out at the naval base on Deer Island.[7]

Spanish flu patients from the Deer Island Naval Hospital, as well as mainland military hospitals, were used as sick donors. The healthy participants were enlisted sailors stationed at the naval hospital for the duration of the experiments. This allowed for the sailors to be carefully monitored by medical staff for any changes to their condition. The Deer Island researchers conducted a total of eight separate contagion experiments, which are briefly outlined below. For more specific details, please refer to the summary tables included in Appendix 1: Experiments 9.1 – 9.8.

Experiment 1: Six healthy sailors were inoculated with a pure culture of Pfeiffer's bacillus obtained from a case of the Spanish flu. *All men remained well* (Exp. 9.1).

Experiment 2: Unfiltered mucus secretions were taken from 16 influenza patients and sprayed into the nasal passages and throats of 20 healthy men. Some of the unfiltered mucus was also swallowed. *None of the men fell ill* (Exp. 9.2).

Experiment 3: Unfiltered mucus secretions from four influenza patients were instilled into the eyes and nasal cavities of 10 healthy sailors. *All men remained completely well* (Exp. 9.3).

Experiment 4: Nineteen healthy men had their nasal passages and throats swabbed with mucus transferred directly from 10 influenza patients. *None of the men were adversely affected* (Exp. 9.4).

Experiment 5: Filtered mucus secretions obtained from three influenza patients were injected subcutaneously into 10 healthy sailors. *Every single man remained well* (Exp. 9.5).

Experiment 6: Blood was drawn from five sailors suffering from pandemic influenza and then immediately injected subcutaneously into 10 healthy men. Apart from some localised muscle soreness at the site of the injection, *none of the healthy recipients became ill* (Exp. 9.6).

Experiment 7: Ten healthy sailors were taken to the Chelsea Hospital Naval Quarantine Ward where 30 men were being treated for influenza. Each of the ten volunteers sat next to the bed of a sick man. They spoke with each other in close proximity for two to three minutes. The sick man was directed to breathe five times and then cough five times directly into the face of the healthy volunteer, while the healthy volunteer breathed in. The healthy volunteer then proceeded to move to the bed of a second patient and repeated the entire process. Each volunteer repeated this procedure with 10 different sick patients. The total exposure time was between 30 - 50 minutes. *None of the healthy participants became sick* (Exp. 9.7).

Experiment 8: Pfeiffer's bacillus was isolated from 13 influenza cases and cultured. One billion bacteria were sprayed into the nose and throat of 19 healthy men. *None of the men developed influenza* (Exp. 9.8).

In sum, across the eight different U.S. Navy experiments on Deer Island, *none* of the 62 participants directly exposed to influenza patients or their bodily fluids became unwell.

Angel Island Human Transmission Experiments

While the experiments on Deer Island were happening, the U.S. Navy simultaneously conducted a second series of experiments at the Angel Island Quarantine Station in San Francisco. The healthy participants were all sailors from the naval training station, Yerba Buena. There were 50 men in total, all of whom had been quarantined for one month prior to the experiments. Of the 50 men, only five had fallen ill with influenza in the previous season and 46 had suffered from influenza at some point in their lives. The age of the men ranged from 18 to 23 and they were all in very good physical condition. As summarised below, the Angel Island researchers performed eight distinct contagion experiments. Again, please refer to the summary tables included in Appendix Experiments 10.1 – 10.8 for more detail. Naval doctors carefully monitored all volunteers to observe any response following each experiment.[8]

Experiment 1: Filtered and unfiltered mucus secretions obtained from a young girl suffering from influenza were instilled into the nasal passages of six healthy men. *None developed influenza* (Exp. 10.1).

Experiment 2: Filtered and unfiltered mucus secretions obtained from an infant with influenza were inoculated into the nasal passages of eight healthy sailors. *None of the men developed influenza* (Exp. 10.2).

Experiment 3: The lung fluid from a case of influenza was used to culture Pfeiffer's bacillus. A solution containing the bacteria was sprayed into the mouth and nose of four healthy men. *All remained well* (Exp. 10.3).

Experiment 4: A young *male* hospital apprentice with influenza had his nasal cavity washed out with saline into a container. He also coughed up lung fluid and spat it into the same container. The unfiltered fluid was then sprayed into the nasal cavities of 10 healthy sailors. *Not a single case of influenza developed in any of the men* (Exp. 10.4).

Experiment 5: A young *female* nurse with influenza had her nasal cavity washed out with saline into a container. She also coughed up lung fluid and spat it into the same container, which was then mixed with saline. This solution was sprayed into the nose and throat of four healthy men. *All remained well* (Exp. 10.5).

Experiment 6: The mucus obtained from the young female nurse in experiment five was dropped into the eyes of two healthy sailors. *They both remained well* (Exp. 10.6).

Experiment 7: The mucus from experiment five was also injected subcutaneously into the arm of one healthy sailor. *He remained well* (Exp. 10.7).

Experiment 8: Blood was collected from a female nurse with influenza. It was mixed with sodium citrate and injected intramuscularly into one healthy sailor. *He remained in good health* (Exp. 10.8).

Overall, during eight U.S. Navy experiments on Angel Island, *none* of the 50 healthy volunteers developed influenza after exposure to the bodily fluids of sick patients.

Gallups Island Human Transmission Experiments

The final series of contagion experiments conducted by the United States Navy and United States Health Department occurred at the Gallups Island Quarantine Station in Boston, in February and March of 1919. The volunteers (49 in total) came from the naval detention camp located on Deer Island, Massachusetts. They ranged in age from 19 – 36 years and were in very good physical condition. Two of the men had contracted influenza in the previous flu season. The rest of the 47 men had not suffered from influenza in the previous season, suggesting they were unlikely to be immune. The Gallups Island researchers carried out nine different contagion experiments (see summary tables in Appendix Experiments 11.1 – 11.9 for further detail).[9]

Experiment 1: Bacteria isolated from influenza patients were cultured and mixed with a solution of broth. This formed a thick solution, which was then sprayed and dropped into the nasal passages and throats of 10 healthy sailors. *None of the men became ill* (Exp. 11.1).

Experiment 2: Mucus obtained from a case of influenza was sprayed and dropped into the nasal passages of 10 healthy sailors. One man developed symptoms diagnosed by the medical doctors as a 'syndrome somewhere between influenza and a sore throat'. *He completely recovered in little over a week with no complications* (Exp. 11.2).

Experiment 3: Millions of Pfeiffer's bacillus and *Staphylococcus aureus* bacteria were sprayed and dropped into the nasal passages and throats of ten healthy men. *None developed influenza* (Exp. 11.3).

Experiment 4: Nasal and bronchial mucus from one case of influenza was instilled into the nasal passages and throats of ten healthy men. *They all remained well* (Exp. 11.4).

Experiment 5: Nasopharyngeal washings were collected from four influenza patients and mixed with milk. Four healthy men drank the snotty-milky solution. *None developed influenza* (Exp. 11.5).

Experiment 6: Nasopharyngeal washings were obtained from ten healthy men recently exposed to cases of influenza. The mucus was then sprayed into the nose and throat of four healthy sailors. *Every volunteer remained in perfect health* (Exp. 11.6).

Experiment 7: Mucus secretions obtained from a case of influenza were sprayed into the nasal passages and throats of ten healthy sailors. *One of the men developed influenza-like symptoms. The other nine men remained unaffected* (Exp. 11.7).

Experiment 8: Unfiltered mucus from three influenza cases was sprayed and dropped into the nose and throat of nine healthy men. *One of the men developed symptoms of influenza. The other eight sailors remained well* (Exp. 11.8).

Experiment 9: Mucus secretions from a case of influenza were sprayed and dropped into the nasal passages and throats of fourteen healthy men. *None of the men developed influenza* (Exp. 11.9).

Taken together, the nine U.S. Navy experiments on Gallups Island produced *two* cases of influenza, and one case of an influenza-like-illness, in 49 healthy volunteers by exposing them directly to the bodily fluids of sick patients.

Making Sense of Military Experiments

Understandably, the doctors and scientists who conducted the above experiments were at a loss as to why only two (1.2%) out of 161 men developed influenza and one (0.6%) developed an influenza-like illness across 25 independent experiments. They could not explain this anomalous pattern of results. Specifically, they offered no explanation as to what the causative agent of the Spanish flu might be, nor could they say with any confidence how it was transmitted. Despite their most diligent attempts, it was all but impossible to infect healthy men with influenza.

Though some might argue the three positive cases prove the disease is contagious, there are several caveats to consider here. First and foremost, it seems dubious to claim experiments demonstrate contagion when they failed to achieve it in over 98% of cases. If a drug (e.g. painkillers) only worked in 1-2% of patients, it would be branded a failure and taken off the market. Second, a contagion claim relies entirely on cases confined to one of the three islands, which means the illness could have conceivably occurred via some 'naturally acquired' source present in that particular shared environment. To have any weight, then, transmission would need to have consistently occurred *across* the three separate locations. Third, claiming contagion relies on *assumption* because no infectious agent was ever identified or isolated. Though the results could be interpreted as viral in origin, this would need to be verified before researchers could draw a firm conclusion about what truly caused these few men to become unwell. Fourth, it is a stretch to classify these two positive cases and one questionable case as Spanish influenza because their symptoms did not resemble any of the hallmarks of the disease (e.g. cyanosis, haemorrhage, pneumonia, or heart failure). Fifth, and finally, due to the lack of adequate control groups, it's difficult to conclude whether the illness was caused by an unidentified substance in the mucus (e.g. virus, toxin, inflammatory mediator), a nocebo effect (i.e. becoming ill because they expected to), or something else entirely.

Taking a step back from these specific limitations, it is rather perplexing that 158 men did not fall ill and die when directly inoculated with sick people's secretions, considering the Spanish flu is claimed to be the most infectious (~500 million cases) and deadly (~50-100 million deaths) influenza pandemic in human history. How can such a contradictory finding be explained? Two counterarguments appear most tempting to apply here. One is that the sailors' *immune systems* were strong enough to prevent them from contracting any illnesses. However, this seems implausible after comparing the radically different infection and fatality rates between the experimental sample and what was recorded in the general populace. In 1918, the global population was approximately 1.8 billion. If up to 500 million people were infected, this means 28% of the world's population experienced Spanish influenza. This figure is orders of magnitude larger than the 1.2% rate observed in the experiments and means 45 of the participants should have been infected (instead of three). Of course, this 28% occurred over multiple waves, but even with a conservative halving (i.e. 14% infected) or thirding (i.e. 9% infected), this is still too stark a difference to account for by immunity (especially given the second counterpoint below). Even using the most conservative estimate of 50 million global infections (2.8%), this is still more than double the experimental infection rate.

The other appealing counterargument is *weakened pathogenicity*. Perhaps experiments conducted at the end of the war exposed participants to a less infectious or severe viral strain. This possibility quickly becomes implausible when accounting for a few important data points. First, cases at the time were pathogenic enough because they happened to kill doctors and sick donors involved in the experiments. Second, the population itself (i.e. young male soldiers) had the greatest susceptibility to severe infection and death. This means they should have observed substantially *higher* rates of infection, severe illness, and death than the general population. The overall fatality rate for Spanish influenza was between 2.7% and 5.4%, which includes 'safer' low-risk groups (i.e. youths and the elderly).[10] Despite this, both statistics are markedly higher than the mere *infection rate* in experiments involving only members of a high-risk group.

Additional Spanish Influenza Experiments

Following the United States Navy and Public Health Department's landmark experiments, many other research groups ran studies to better understand the Spanish flu. The following section runs through five of these attempts: (1) Yamanouchi's, (2) Michelli, Sata, and Schofield's, (3) Lister and Taylor's, and (5) Wahl, White, and Bloomfield's.

Yamanouchi's Experiments

A group of Japanese researchers led by Professor Tamotsu Yamanouchi published some rather interesting results in June of 1919. They took lung fluid from 43 influenza patients, combined it into a single concoction, and then mixed it in a flask with saline—an isotonic called 'Ringer's solution'. They then inoculated this mixture into the nasal passages and throats of 24 healthy recipients (Exp. 12.1). Eighteen of the participants (75%) developed symptoms of influenza, including fever, headache, sore throat, back pain, and a cough. Some of the mucus was then injected subcutaneously into eight other people, seven of whom developed influenza (87.5%) (Exp. 12.2). Finally, the blood of influenza patients was injected into six healthy subjects, all of whom developed influenza (Exp. 12.3).[11]

At first glance, these are much more convincing contagion ratios. How were these researchers able to induce illness in their participants so easily where others had failed? Digging deeper into the experimental methods provides some important context. Crucially, the Yamanouchi procedure did not include *control groups* (for comparison), *random sampling* (to represent a general population), or *participant blinding* (to 'hide' the experimental aims and conditions). This opens up many alternative explanations that make it difficult to interpret the reported results with any level of clarity or confidence.

One issue with a lack of *control groups* was that mucus samples were mixed with Ringer's solution (an isotonic solution), which on its own produces a long list of adverse effects in humans, including coughing, sneezing, nasal congestion, and difficulty breathing.[12] Without a control group to compare against (i.e. one that received saline, or a solution of non-virally infected lung fluid), it's impossible to rule out Ringer's solution as a potential cause of the symptoms experienced by the volunteers in this study. One issue with *non-random sampling* was that all volunteers were the friends and colleagues of the researchers. Aside from being a questionable practice, it means experimenters cannot draw general conclusions applicable to a broader population, regardless of the outcome they produce. Without a randomly selected sample, the findings only apply to people who match the specific characteristics of those tested. One issue with *blinding* was that participants could easily figure out (or even be told) what the experiment was trying to achieve and, in turn, respond consciously or subconsciously to these 'demands'. Therefore, without blinding it's impossible to rule out the influence of internal states like desire or expectation, which are known to produce 'nocebo' effects (i.e. experiencing harm because you expect to). The risk of confounding results is even higher given the participants were friends and peers who had an existing relationship with the research team.

Another obvious oversight made by Yamanouchi's team was they never identified the virus, nor did they isolate it and use it as an independent variable. This is problematic because the solution they injected people with contained the combined bodily secretions of 43 sick people. Under what circumstances would someone in the real world be exposed to such drastic conditions? Clearly, the design of these experiments lacks 'external validity'. That is, the results are difficult to apply to settings or circumstances *beyond* those tested because they use a mode of exposure too far removed from what would occur in nature. At best, all they could say with certainty is that injecting the bodily fluids of dozens of people into a healthy person will make them sick—which is perhaps not all that surprising. Overall, then, Yamanouchi's overwhelmingly positive results end up crumbling under scrutiny. They provide shaky and tenuous evidence to support the claim influenza is caused by a contagious virus.

Michelli, Sata, & Schofield's Experiments

Another factor that casts doubt over Yamanouchi's findings is the fact they contrast substantially with those found by other researchers undertaking human-to-human transmission experiments around the same time. A notable example is that of Ferdinando Michelli and Giuseppe Sata, who were unable to infect *any* of the 18 healthy participants enrolled in their study (Exp. 13.1 & 13.2). This is despite injecting them subcutaneously with filtered mucus secretions or unfiltered blood.[13] While Yamanouchi's transmission rate was 87.5% using this method, Michelli and Sata's was 0%. Another point of comparison is that of Frank Schofield who, using similar methods, conducted four separate experiments exposing eight healthy people to the mucus and blood of influenza patients. Like Michelli and Sata, all of Schofield's attempts failed (Exp. 15.2 – 15.4). The only exception is when he injected himself and two of his research assistants with unfiltered blood. After self-inoculating, Schofield and one assistant developed an influenza-like illness (Exp. 15.1).[14] Notwithstanding the clear risk of experimenter bias here, the sheer number of substances present in unfiltered blood completely confounds this outcome. It also goes without saying, that injecting blood directly into a vein, in no way, shape, or form reflects a natural mode of transmission. Therefore, Schofield's two positive cases do not constitute high-quality evidence for a contagious virus.

Lister & Taylor's Experiments

Frederick Lister and Edward Taylor conducted a rather elaborate series of experiments involving 25 healthy participants. They shipped 11 healthy men to a remote island 500 miles away from their home—a place spared from the grip of the Spanish flu. The researchers proceeded to filter 'infected' mucus secretions and inoculate this material into the nasal passages of the healthy men. Like so many other influenza trials, all subjects remained well (Exp. 16.1). Lister and Taylor also attempted to infect nine other men with pure cultures of Pfeiffer's bacillus (Exp. 16.2). One of these men developed influenza, which is an odd finding given that Pfeiffer's bacillus is undoubtedly *not* the cause of influenza. In a final experiment, two out of five men (40%) developed an influenza-like illness after Lister and Taylor sprayed their nasal passages with mucus secretions obtained from influenza patients (Exp. 16.3).[15] Overall, three out of 25 participants (12%) developed influenza symptoms. One of these can be immediately discounted on account of its bacterial origin. The remaining two cases reflect a total infection rate of 8%, which isn't particularly convincing on its own given the brute-force efforts to make subjects sick. Any confidence in this result is once again undermined by similar methodological shortcomings (e.g. no controls or blinding; no observed and isolated independent variable). Also, the fact that inoculated bacteria produced one-third of observed influenza symptoms exemplifies how flawed methods can influence results in profound ways. With this possibility in mind, and without accounting for the limitations, it is entirely speculative as to what caused the two volunteers' symptoms in Lister and Taylor's experiments.

Wahl, White, Lyall & Bloomfield's Experiments

During this period, Harry Wahl and his two colleagues, George White and Harold Lyall also conducted some human transmission experiments. They ground up lung tissue samples from a deceased influenza patient, centrifuged them, and then sprayed the supernatant into the nostrils of two healthy men. Both healthy subjects remained well (Exp. 17.1). The three researchers then inoculated pure cultures of Pfeiffer's bacillus into the respiratory tracts of seven men, yet they all remained completely healthy (Exp. 17.1 & 17.2).[16] In a comparable study, Arthur Bloomfield attempted to infect 14 healthy men, yet not a single one developed the flu (Exp. 19.1).[17] Just like the previous studies, Wahl, White, Lyall, and Bloomfield's experiments stack more null results on the pile.

Post-pandemic Experiments

Although dozens of these human experiments were conducted during the Spanish flu pandemic, scientists and doctors made very little progress towards understanding its cause. Indeed, by the time the pandemic had ended in April of 1920, the field of medicine was no closer to understanding the secrets of influenza than before it had begun. Opinions among doctors as to the cause and mode of transmission of the disease were divided. Some theorised that a filtrable virus was the cause,[18] whereas others were still adamant that Pfeiffer's bacillus was responsible.[19] Meanwhile, research into the common cold had all but ground to a standstill during the pandemic because understanding the Spanish flu was far more pressing. Consequently, this all but halted any progress toward understanding the aetiology of the common cold for some time.[20]

Schmidt's Experiments

This hiatus persisted until October of 1920, when Paul Schmidt published the first series of post-pandemic human experiments investigating the common cold and seasonal influenza. In the first experiment, Schmidt collected mucus secretions from 16 influenza patients, which were mixed with saline solution and then filtered. One drop was inoculated into both eyes of each of the 196 healthy participants. Twenty-one (10.7%) healthy volunteers developed colds, while three (1.5%) developed influenza (Exp. 20.1). In the second experiment, 84 healthy men were inoculated with the filtered mucus secretions obtained from 12 influenza cases. Five (5.9%) developed influenza and four (4.7%) developed a common cold (Exp. 20.2). Schmidt's final experiment was different in one critical way. He inoculated 43 healthy men using only a physiological *saline* solution. Despite an absence of infectious material, a remarkable eight men (18.6%) developed common colds (Exp. 20.3).[21]

These results are particularly important because they highlight the capacity of an inert substance, like saline, to produce the common cold. What's even more surprising is that subjects receiving saline developed colds at a significantly higher rate (18.6%) than those who were inoculated with the mucus secretions of sick people (<10.7%). How is it that inert inoculations can not only induce a so-called 'infectious disease', but outperform active inoculations in doing so? There are, of course, a few possibilities here. It could be due to a nocebo effect, a chemical or irritant effect from introducing a foreign substance into the upper respiratory tract, or some combination of both. One other curious observation that can easily fly under the radar in Schmidt's experiments is how the mucus of *influenza* patients caused the *common cold*. According to modern virology, these are two distinct illnesses caused by separate viruses. So, how then, did healthy people in Schmidt's studies develop an infectious disease entirely different from the one they were exposed to? This could be a product of researcher error (i.e. Schmidt misdiagnosing the cases), or it could imply some other factor is driving people's symptoms.

Other Notable Experiments

Following Schmidt's lead, many others returned to human transmission experiments from 1920 to 1932.[22-26] Despite renewed efforts, these continued to follow the same trend, such that the majority of transmission experiments were completely unsuccessful and/or contributed little towards advancing our understanding of influenza or the common cold. For example, Anna Williams, Mary Nevin, and Caroline Gurley, failed to infect any of the 45 healthy participants they inoculated with the bodily secretions of cold and flu patients (Exp. 22.1).[23] Likewise, Robert Robertson and Robert Groves were unable to infect 100 healthy volunteers who they exposed to filtered mucus secretions of the common cold (Exp. 23.1).[24] Similar results were presented by Oscar Costa-Mandry, Pablo Morales-Otero, and Jenaro Suarez, who failed to infect 18 healthy men with unfiltered and filtered influenza mucus secretions (Exp. 29.1).[26] Anatoly Smorodintseff and his colleagues inoculated 72 healthy participants with the aerosolised lung tissue of mice experimentally infected with influenza. Just 14 of the 72 recipients (19.4%) developed mild flu-like symptoms. Without ever having a pure sample of the virus, or ever observing a single virion, the researchers concluded a virus was the causative agent (Exp. 33.1).[27] This experiment might seem like proof that influenza is contagious, however the methods (inhaling aerosolised mice lung tissue) do not reflect the natural mode of transmission. A lack of adequate controls and an independent variable also make the results difficult to interpret.

Call Off the Investigation

Inspired by dire circumstances, scientists and doctors searched frantically for the cause of Spanish influenza by conducting a series of studies that exposed healthy volunteers to the bodily secretions of sick people. When initial attempts failed miserably to demonstrate contagion, it heightened the intensity with which experts sought to explain the notoriously infectious and lethal influenza pandemic. Despite this desperation, subsequent trials fared no better in making people ill. Even the well-funded and sophisticated efforts of the U.S. military only managed to reproduce influenza symptoms in under two per cent of subjects. Other motivated researchers couldn't help but follow the same trend—their efforts were null and void.

Across this program of influenza research, two sets of experiments are worth noting for their ironic contribution. Instead of supporting the contagion story, their search attempts actively thwarted it. The first was Yamanouchi, whose team was able to produce an influenza infection rate greater than 75%. Though remarkable on its face, this work was fatally flawed. It achieved these results without the use of control groups, random samples, participant blinding, or a truly independent variable. Perhaps unsurprisingly, no other study came close to producing the same infection ratios. It seems, then, that the most compelling evidence for contagious influenza is tied to the least reliable experimental methods. The second notable irony came from Schmidt, who observed a substantially higher rate of flu symptoms for an *inert* substance (i.e. saline) than for an *active* substance (i.e. sick secretions). This result poses a serious dilemma for human transmission studies. It means that in any instance where experimenters have mixed bodily fluids with other seemingly neutral or inactive ingredients, they can no longer be sure which one caused symptoms. If scientists wish to claim an infectious virus makes people sick, they must show that symptoms occur at a rate over and above whatever inert substances they use. Unfortunately, most transmission experiments do not include control groups to allow for this, so it's simply impossible to draw firm conclusions from them.

All in all, these human transmission experiments present quite a conundrum. Without a doubt, they are among the best studies available to confirm whether infectious germs cause influenza. Yet, at the same time, reviewing this program of research leads to two rather doubtful takeaway points. First, in aggregate, it simply does not support a contagion model. Most studies find no infection and, when they do, the positive case ratios are dismally low. Second, it is so fundamentally flawed that, *even if* the studies consistently achieved infection—and *even if* the rates were as high as Yamanouchi's—it would be difficult to place trust in the results. The methodological rigour is too grossly inadequate to claim viral transmission occurred. With all this in mind, it is quite astonishing then that modern scientists and doctors are now so convinced of a contagion model. When these human transmission experiments first emerged, the scientific community was understandably sceptical, given the consistent negative results alongside unimpressive and flawed positive results. This body of work prompted experts at the time to sincerely doubt that invisible 'filter-passing agents' such as viruses caused Spanish and seasonal influenza. So, what's changed? One might assume scientists have since conducted additional and improved human-to-human contagion experiments. This, however, is most definitely not the case, so the source of their confidence is puzzling.

Chapter 14

Chasing Colds

In 1940, the United States helped establish an infectious disease hospital for the British Military in Salisbury, England. Consisting of 22 prefabricated huts, this 125-bed hospital provided medical care to civilians suffering from infectious diseases during World War II. It also investigated infectious disease outbreaks in the local area.[1] By 1946, after the war had ended, the hospital was donated to the British Government and became known as the Common Cold Research Unit (CCRU). This unit was tasked with identifying the causative agent of the common cold and with finding a cure. The CCRU consisted of 12 flats that could house up to 30 volunteers for 10 days during research trials. To entice volunteers, the unit advertised research opportunities as all-expenses-paid holidays and would reimburse participants £1.25 per day for their time. Upon arrival, volunteers were quarantined from each other and inoculated with either a 'cold virus' or a placebo. These interventions were usually administered in a single- or double-blind fashion. This means volunteers, and sometimes even researchers did not know whether inoculations contained the so-called virus or placebo. Once inoculated, recipients' symptoms were then observed and recorded by the resident virologists. During the observation period, volunteers could watch TV, play games, read books, and make telephone calls. They were also allowed to go hiking, provided they maintained a 'safe distance' of 30 feet from anyone else they encountered.[2]

For the first six and a half years, virologists at the CCRU tried to infect 20 different animal species with common colds, including rabbits, guinea pigs, rats, mice, cotton rats, hamsters, voles, squirrels, ferrets, kittens, pigs, hedgehogs, and several species of monkey including baboons, sooty mangabey, brown capuchins, red patas, and green monkeys. Their attempts were entirely unsuccessful.[2,3] After failing to transmit the common cold from one animal to another, researchers began conducting human experiments, the results of which were no better than the animal experiments that had preceded them.

Although most of the human experiments conducted at the CCRU were rather crude in their approach, some were more sophisticated. In one of these more rigorous experiments, researchers inoculated a group of healthy participants with 'experimental colds'. They took 0.5 mL of a virus-containing solution—grown in a laboratory using chicken embryos—and instilled it into subjects' nasal passages. Before developing symptoms, the researchers divided participants into groups and exposed each group to a pair of healthy people. Inoculated participants and healthy pairs stayed in a room together for 10 hours. This exposure aimed to see if colds were infectious during the incubation period. *None of the eight healthy participants became sick.* Then, a few days after the inoculated participants developed symptoms, the four with the worst symptoms were exposed to 11 healthy people. Only one healthy person developed a cold as a result (Exp. 39.1). When nine healthy participants were exposed to people with experimentally induced colds, just one (11.1%) developed mild symptoms (Exp. 39.2 & 39.3). In a later experiment, five healthy people were exposed to a person with a naturally acquired cold, but *they were unaffected* (Exp. 39.4).[2,4]

Needless to say, virologists were perplexed as to why these initial attempts were unsuccessful at transmitting colds. They wondered if people living in isolated communities might be more susceptible to infection.[3] To test this idea, the CCRU virologists conducted one of the unit's most elaborate experiments in 1951. They sent 12 healthy volunteers to a remote island in the Hebrides—where no one had lived for over a decade. The volunteers had enough supplies to last three months, allowing them to remain completely isolated and free from any physical contact with the outside world. The volunteers were divided into three groups of four and lived in abandoned dwellings for 10 weeks. It was at this point, that the CCRU sent six participants with experimentally induced colds to the island. Like before, virologists induced experimental colds in volunteers by inoculating their nasal passages with fluid from tissue cultures.[4]

In their first trial, virologists wanted to see if colds could be transmitted indirectly via 'fomites' (i.e. when droplets contaminate objects). So, one group of healthy volunteers vacated their accommodation, while the six participants sick with experimentally induced colds proceeded to smear their nasal secretions all over items and surfaces inside the dwelling. Then, the sick participants vacated the premises before the healthy participants returned. In this way, four healthy participants were deliberately exposed to a contaminated living environment. Yet, *none* of them became unwell (Exp. 40.1).[4]

In a second trial, virologists wanted to see if colds could be transmitted directly via aerosols and airborne droplets. So, the sick participants interacted inside a room with a different group of four healthy participants. Despite being coughed and sneezed on for three hours, *none* of the healthy participants became sick (Exp. 40.2). Similarly, a new group of people with experimentally induced colds were brought to the island and spent a total of six hours with a group of healthy participants. *All remained well* (Exp. 40.3). In a longer experiment following a similar format, a group of healthy people lived with infected participants for four days. Even with this extended exposure period, *none* of them fell ill (Exp. 40.4).[4]

After failing to transmit experimentally induced colds to healthy participants, the research team decided to see what would happen when healthy people were exposed to a person with a 'naturally acquired' cold. They found a farmer on a nearby island who had developed a 'natural cold' five days prior and brought him to the island where the experiments were taking place. The sick farmer interacted with each person in one of the groups for two hours. *Three* out of four people in the group developed a cold (Exp. 40.5). Immediately afterwards, the farmer was exposed to another group of four healthy participants for nearly four hours. *None* of the healthy participants in the second group developed a cold (Exp. 40.6).[4] Now, although this experiment can be construed as evidence a cold is contagious, many alternative explanations would need to be ruled out to confirm person-to-person transmission took place.

After more than a decade of searching for common cold viruses, the CCRU had made little progress towards identifying the cause of a cold or discovering a cure.[5] Their limited success was not for lack of trying, and researchers soon realised finding the answer was far more difficult than originally thought. Staff virologists at the CCRU admitted that one of their biggest challenges was giving people colds.[6] But why was it so hard to give people colds under experimental conditions when common cold viruses are considered 'highly contagious' and 'easily spread' from close contact?[7-9] Demonstrating such an ordinary phenomenon should be a straightforward process. After all, isn't it commonplace for children to bring home a cold from school and infect their whole family with little more than a sneeze? Virologists should have been able to replicate this scenario with relative ease yet were met with roadblocks at every turn.

A Critical Review

The lack of scientific evidence concerning the cause and mode of spread of the common cold did not go unnoticed. In 1950, a critical review of the experimental evidence concerning the common cold was published. The authors expressed their disappointment about how little progress had been made toward understanding the common cold in any regard. Their appraisal concluded;[10]

1. No clear-cut definition of the common cold existed.

2. The relationship between subjective symptoms and objective findings was lacking.

3. There was no way to clinically diagnose the common cold.

4. The variability in the symptoms was very broad.

5. The cause of the illness was unknown.

6. The disease could have been caused by many different factors.

Due to these facts, the reviewers doubted whether any objective study on the common cold could ever be performed.[10] How could anyone study it in a meaningful way without satisfying such basic requirements?

The difficulties in demonstrating common cold contagion persisted even after the critical review. This can be seen, for example, in a 1952 study that tested whether the common cold was transmitted via aerosols and droplets. Researchers at the CCRU divided a room in half with a partition made from a large blanket. They left a one-foot gap between the edges of the blanket and the walls, floor, and ceiling to allow for airflow between both sides of the room. They also placed a fan strategically inside the room to ensure good air circulation. In each experiment, five or six healthy participants sat quietly on one side of the partition, doing something innocuous like reading or knitting while they waited. Meanwhile, a group of four or five people with 'natural colds' entered the room on the opposite side of the partition and talked, played games, sang, and shouted for two hours. To saturate the air with 'infected' respiratory particles, the researchers also induced sneezing in sick participants by administering sneezing powder (i.e. o-dianisidine hydrochloride). Over five days, a total of 25 healthy people and 22 sick people participated in five separate experiments. After all was said and done, just *two* participants (8%) developed colds (Exp. 41.1).[11]

The same researchers ran a similar set of five experiments a short time later. This time, instead of being separated by a partition, groups of healthy and sick people with 'natural colds' were allowed to interact directly with one another. They played card games, ate lunch, and conversed at close range with each other for two hours. The sick participants coughed, sneezed, and blew their noses 'violently' at regular intervals throughout the interaction. Even after this 'all-out' attempt, only three out of the 32 healthy participants (9%) developed colds (Exp. 41.2). But the experiment didn't end here. At the end of each of the five experiments, all participants vacated the room and a new set of five healthy subjects entered. These 'fresh' participants were encouraged to handle the objects (e.g. cups, plates, cutlery, playing cards) used by the sick participants over the previous two hours. Using this indirect method, only *two* of the 25 healthy participants (8%) developed colds (Exp. 41.3). Interestingly, the researchers themselves questioned whether the small number of positive cases were attributable to the experiment because at least one of the volunteers who fell sick had shown signs of a common cold in the days prior to commencement.[11]

Later studies also sought to determine whether the common cold might be spread indirectly by fomites (i.e. surfaces covered in microorganisms). The researchers gave healthy subjects handkerchiefs that were contaminated with the mucus of sick people. The healthy subjects used the handkerchiefs for 24 hours, yet *no one* became ill (Exp. 41.7). Similar experiments involved healthy people wiping their noses with gauze contaminated with the mucus of sick people, while other experiments involved people stuffing their noses with gauze soaked in undiluted nasal washings. Just *two* out of 27 people (7.4%) developed colds in these trials (Exp. 41.8, 41.10 & 41.11).[11]

In the search for cold contagion, a glimmer of hope emerged when 26 out of 89 people (29.2%) developed symptoms after wearing oxygen masks that delivered a steady stream of air containing 'cold germs' for up to five minutes (Exp. 41.5).[11] While the researchers considered these positive results as proof that a virus caused the common cold, they ran into the same old trap as so many before them. Not once did they use a control group, so they cannot rule out alternative explanations. It's entirely plausible that factors such as the nocebo effect, the concocted solution the 'germs' were suspended in, conditions of the inhaled air, or some other unrealised factor played a role. Researchers should be particularly wary whenever they produce an effect that is substantially different from other attempts—especially if they cannot account for *why* it happened. A ~30% positive case rate is many times greater than other studies at the time (e.g. those listed above are 9% or less). Such major methodological oversights, along with discrepant findings, make it difficult to interpret the results of this experiment with a high degree of certainty.

Scientific Vandalism

By the mid-1950s, the CCRU had accrued a decade and a half of research findings. Much like these other experiments, however, they were no closer to identifying the cause of the common cold, let alone finding a cure. Between 1952 and 1953, a total of 292 participants were inoculated with cell culture material allegedly containing cold viruses, yet only 15 (5%) developed colds.[12] Consequently, the unit was on the verge of being disbanded. They made a last-ditch effort in 1957 to turn things around by appointing a new director by the name of David Tyrell—a young British virologist credited with discovering and isolating the coronavirus (see Chapter 9).[5] Under the management of Tyrell, virologists at the CCRU all of a sudden began 'isolating' cold viruses left, right, and centre using tissue and cell culture methods.[13,14] By the time the CCRU closed its doors in 1989, more than 1,000 papers had been published detailing the discovery of several coronaviruses and more than 100 common cold viruses.[5,15] Nearly 20,000 individuals from across the world participated in experiments at the unit. Of those who were inoculated with 'cold viruses', between one-third and one-fifth developed a cold. Though it outperforms many earlier studies, this 'success rate' still seems awfully low considering they were transmitting a *concentrated* form of highly infectious and contagious particles. Nevertheless, closing the CCRU down was considered 'scientific vandalism' by the field of virology because of the significant contributions it had supposedly made towards shedding light on this seasonal malady.[6] Arguably, though, the CCRU's track record seemed quite underwhelming, considering the amount of time, money, and resources that were devoted to understanding the common cold. Instances, where they did successfully transmit experimentally induced colds, hold little clout due to one glaringly obvious oversight—a lack of experimental control.

Losing All Control

Without adequate methodological controls, scientists simply have no way of knowing which variable induces the symptoms they observe in subjects. By bringing someone into a laboratory and delivering foreign substances into their body, it might irritate and inflame mucous membranes, set off an allergic response, elicit a nocebo effect, or introduce some other unknown factor.[16] It is therefore scientifically inappropriate to conclude symptoms are from germs without controlling for these other possibilities. Doing so renders any experimental result meaningless.[17]

Saline is an inert control commonly used as a placebo in medical science. Large trials involving thousands of volunteers have produced colds in 10% of participants from inoculating saline.[18] This positive case rate is higher than many common cold studies that attempted to expose participants to germs. So, what is going on here? How can sterile salt water possibly cause a cold? Well, as far back as the 1930s, researchers established that directly irritating a mucous membrane would disturb the structure and function of respiratory tissue.[10,16] When inoculated into the sinuses, saline can act as an *irritant*—one that the body produces a defensive cold-like response to deal with. Also, the psychological literature shows that participants inevitably form an understanding of the researchers' hypotheses and how they as a subject should respond. When inoculated into the sinuses, then, saline can act as a nocebo *trigger*—one that catalyses information and expectation in the form of a cold-like physiological response (which makes sense, of course, when under observation at the Common Cold Research Unit). Now, these are only some of the possible pathways, but the fact of the matter remains. Even inert substances, like saline, can induce symptoms of a common cold.

If an experiment cannot outperform a saline inoculation, then it would certainly struggle to demonstrate contagion. But, although saline is better than nothing, it is still less than optimal. The quality of a control increases the closer it matches whatever it's being compared to. Ideally, the only difference between an experimental condition and a control condition should be the *active ingredient* (e.g. a germ). As such, it would be far better to use a mucus sample that contains all the same materials, except for the virus. With this in mind, common cold researchers should collect filtered mucus secretions from people suffering from non-viral related respiratory illnesses, such as allergic rhinitis, sinusitis, or bronchitis. Comparing with these is a prerequisite for concluding whether colds are caused by a germ or not.

The reason we know more complex controls are necessary is that, just like saline, experiments have induced common colds in healthy people by inoculating them with mucus samples obtained from healthy people. In one study, 28 healthy volunteers were inoculated with the nasal washings taken from healthy people who did not have colds. Six (21%) of the 28 healthy individuals developed colds.[2] This result suggests there are indeed other substances present in healthy mucus capable of causing a cold or flu. What's more, the number of positive cases might have been even higher if the researchers collected mucus samples from patients sick with non-viral respiratory diseases. Such a result would suggest that it is some other non-viral material in the mucus of sick people that causes cold-like illness. Though this seems great in theory, there do not appear to be any contagion experiments published in the literature using such a methodology.

In some rare instances, control substances other than saline have been used, with very telling outcomes. In one experiment, 65 volunteers were inoculated with 'viruses' grown in chicken embryos. Of these, 15 (23%) developed colds and 20 (31%) developed 'doubtful' colds (i.e. very mild symptoms). Meanwhile, when 57 healthy participants in the control group were inoculated with chicken embryo fluid that had not been 'infected' with a 'virus', eight (14%) developed colds and another eight (14%) developed 'doubtful' colds.[2] Whilst it might be tempting to attribute the difference in the number of colds between these two groups to a 'virus', the chicken embryos were not inoculated with a pure virus. Rather, they were inoculated with filtered nasopharyngeal washings obtained from sick people which contains all kinds of different substances—making it impossible to know what caused the recipients symptoms. A similar experiment inoculated healthy volunteers with normal chicken embryo fluid that did not contain an alleged virus. The healthy recipients developed common cold symptoms including nasal irritation, sneezing, nasal obstruction, hyperaemia, swelling of the nasal mucosa, headache, and an elevated body temperature.[19] There are also reports of people developing a blocked nose, sneezing, and a headache after being inoculated with sterile broth. They became self-convinced of having developed a cold despite never having been exposed to a virus.[20]

It seems a wide range of different substances can cause cold and flu-like symptoms following inoculation. This fact led several authors to conclude the symptoms caused by filtrates are an *allergic* response, rather than a viral one.[16,21] In 1922, Dr Victor Vaughan, Professor of Hygiene and Chairman of Medical Sciences for the National Research Council, Dr Henry Vaughan, Commissioner of Health for the city of Detroit, and Dr George Palmer, an epidemiologist at the Department of Health in Detroit, published a medical textbook for physicians, medical students, and healthcare workers. In this textbook, they explained that the symptoms resulting from the sick-to-healthy inoculation of filtrates are caused by an allergic reaction to non-viral proteins suspended in the mucus. In their professional opinions, when these proteins were introduced into the nasal passage, they caused local sensitisation and inflammation. Vaughan and his co-authors concluded that introducing any substance containing proteins into the upper respiratory passages had the potential to cause reactions including common colds, epidemic coughs, and acute coryzas (upper respiratory symptoms). They also stated that exposure to cold temperatures can compromise the integrity of respiratory tract tissue by impairing the natural cleansing mechanisms and increasing the permeability of the mucous membranes to inhaled proteins, thereby increasing the risk of 'catching a cold'.[21]

Blinding Them With Science

Another factor that must be accounted for, not just with the studies conducted at the CCRU, but any human transmission study, is *blinding*. In scientific experiments, employing double-blinding ensures neither the researcher nor the recipient knows anything about the nature of the intervention.[22] If either party were privy to which intervention was being employed, it could have a significant impact on the validity of the results. Double-blinding reduces the risk of *experimenter bias* (e.g. how they treat participants; how they clean and analyse their data; and how they interpret and write up the findings). It also minimises the effect of *participant reactions* (e.g. placebo or nocebo; whether they chose to stay in or leave the study; what information they divulge). Studies without adequate blinding lose their ability to draw confident conclusions about what caused the observed effects.

This is an ever-present issue for inoculation experiments because blinding is not as simple as withholding information. Even though many of the experiments at the CCRU were technically double-blinded, people regularly pick up on more than what they are explicitly told. So, although researchers concealed which intervention (active or control) participants were allocated to, there is still a chance those participants reacted in a consistent way not attributable to the 'active ingredient'. It could be the case, for instance, that participants were more likely to suspect they have been inoculated with a cold for the simple fact they attended a large, state-of-the-art facility called "The Common Cold Research Unit". It is well known that the more elaborate and impressive an intervention appears, the greater its placebo or nocebo effect.[23-25] Participants weren't blind to the fact they were at this research facility to be experimented on and that there was a good chance of being inoculated with 'cold germs'. The problem is this knowledge, and the effect it produces just so happens to move in the same direction as the experimenters' hypothesis that germs cause colds. What this means is that even though participants were blinded, they could still have responded to a range of other contextual cues in a way that systematically biased the results.

It is plausible, then, that CCRU subjects manifested more common cold symptoms than they would have otherwise because they were primed to believe they had been exposed to a virus. Official-looking people—who were desperately trying to understand the common cold—subjected participants to very elaborate experiments and invasive procedures using high-tech equipment within a purpose-built laboratory. Implying such a large amount of information could produce a nocebo effect that accounts for a non-trivial portion of the positive results obtained by the CCRU. It would be fascinating to compare CCRU outcomes against trials where subjects were paid to attend the 'Everyday Immunity & Resilience Institute' and inoculated with cold and flu germs, whilst believing they had been administered a substance that would make them impervious to sickness. There are, of course, problems with this design too, but at least it would produce an effect in the opposite direction to what the researchers desire. The science must account for limitations like these to be more certain. Just the possibility of alternative explanations is enough to cast doubt on the CCRU's findings.

To ground this criticism, consider the situation at the CCRU by 1950. Over a decade, across the experiments using filtered and unfiltered nasal secretions, they had inoculated somewhere in the vicinity of 231 subjects and confirmed 137 cases of the common cold.[26] Though this 55% case rate dwarfs most others listed in this chapter, the researchers expressed disappointment, doubt, and caution towards it. They lamented the fact that, despite their best efforts, what appeared to be an impressive result turned out to be a 'will-o'-the-whisp' (i.e. something impossible to grasp). They admitted their current techniques were uncertain and difficult to interpret. From a germ perspective, they regarded 55% as a failure—to the point where they disliked using human subjects due to how *resistant* they were to catching colds. This was despite giving participants enormous doses via unnatural means, like in one trial where subjects were inoculated with the combined nasal washings of 26 sick people.

But the reasons to question the 55 per cent case rate go even deeper. The CCRU paid volunteers for ten day's holiday, travel expenses, accommodation, and spending money. This meant that those who self-selected to volunteer were non-random and, therefore, might vary in some systematic way. For instance, they might be poor and desperate, stressed and in need of a reprieve, or hypochondriacs seeking assurance and validation. At the very least, the rewards were likely to elicit a desire to reciprocate—something that would make a volunteer even more eager to contribute to the scientific enterprise. The incentives also enticed many CCRU volunteers to return for their second, third, and fourth visits (some even came up to nine times).[27] Testing the same people over time might reinforce various learned responses. As such, volunteers may have been conditioned to experience symptoms based on what happened in the *previous* trial(s). To make matters worse, participants also kept a record of their symptoms, which the CCRU admitted *"naturally influences the doctor's decision"* to count them as having a cold or not. From the perspective of scientific rigour, these are big problems. Combining self-selection, repeated exposure, and self-monitoring creates all sorts of biases that could easily inflate case numbers. Another factor researchers failed to account for was 'Leisure Sickness', where people fall ill with colds and flu shortly after going on holiday.[28,29] Volunteers could have been primed to experience this phenomenon because the CCRU advertised the opportunity in the media as a 10-day, all-expenses-paid vacation. This 'marketing strategy' might have inadvertently impacted the trial results.[27,30]

The Chase Continues

In chasing down the cause of and cure for the common cold, many experimental efforts came up empty-handed. Despite colds being 'highly infectious' and 'readily transmissible', studies consistently produced poor positive case rates. Even the Common Cold Research Unit—a dedicated facility with colds as their sole focus—was almost shut down after nearly two disappointing decades of research. A scathing scientific review hit home these woes by pointing out how the common cold was ill-defined, difficult to diagnose, and severely lacking in causal evidence. As always, some studies did manage to induce positive cases, but these were hampered by poor scientific rigour. Among other problems, these trials frequently omitted appropriate controls and blinding procedures. This opens them up to a litany of confounds and alternative explanations which, ultimately, cast doubt over their conclusions.

A saving grace for common cold research was David Tyrell's cell culture approach, which took the CCRU from faltering to flourishing in a short time. This drastic change, however, begs the question: if colds are so common and contagious, why could virologists only identify and transmit them by using such a complex and artificial procedure? As it turns out, even after 'concentrating' a lab-grown virus in this way, the CCRU was only ever able to produce symptoms in about one-third of participants, at most. But, considering the fact their methods are (a) disconnected from reality, (b) littered with problems (see Chapters 8 and 9), and (c) susceptible to experimenter and participant biases, then common cold researchers may well need to continue their chase.

Chapter 15

Challenging Contagion

People come into contact with sick individuals, and then, all of a sudden, fall ill with similar symptoms. This is such a frequent occurrence that nearly everyone has seen or experienced it in their lifetime. Despite its regularity, we cannot simply intuit what is going on here because there are invisible processes at work. In almost all cases, though, modern society reverts to a one-dimensional explanation for sickness: an infectious particle spreading from person-to-person. This model of contagion is so ubiquitous that no one in their right mind thinks or dares to question it. They assume such a widely held idea has the full weight of scientific evidence behind it. Furthermore, they also build an affinity for the model because it helps them make sense of real-world experiences. As this chapter reveals, however, neither of these is completely true. Not only is there a substantial deficit in the contagion science, but many historical events exceed the explanatory power of the contagion model. To challenge contagion, the following sections unpack even more scientific studies and recount inexplicable outbreaks in unthinkable places.

The Current Misunderstanding

In the scientific world, contagious viruses are currently accepted as the cause of the common cold and influenza. Scientists say that viruses transmit from a sick person to a healthy person in one of three ways: droplets, aerosols, or fomites.[1,2] Though this appears to be a straightforward claim, there is a lack of scientific evidence to support it.[3,4] As it stands, virologists don't know how viruses are transmitted, let alone cause disease. They even readily acknowledge their uncertainty in many review papers on the subject, though skirt around the issue using vague language.[1,2,5] So, rather than admitting they are unsure, virologists say things like they "believe virus transmission occurs via large droplets",[6,7] but that they are "still unclear how different modes of transmission contribute to respiratory illness".[8] Reading between the lines, this kind of wording hints at how little virologists truly understand about viral contagion. By contrast, if they were confident in the data, they would instead say things like, "decades of controlled experiments repeatedly and consistently demonstrate that respiratory illnesses spread from person-to-person via droplets, aerosols, and fomites".

But virologists do not and cannot say things like this because it's not what the data show. Systematic reviews on the topic are more explicit and conclude airborne transmission is *unlikely* to be of any significance in the spread of contagious respiratory illnesses,[9] and that there is *no evidence* to show any disease is transmitted through large respiratory droplets.[10] Several studies have highlighted the lack of evidence supporting the transmission of respiratory viruses like rhinovirus[11-14] and coronavirus via fomites.[15,16] Other reviews have revealed an absence of scientific data showing aerosol transmission of well-known pathogens such as SARS-CoV-1 and SARS-CoV-2,[17] and that demonstrating such a phenomenon is *notoriously difficult*.[18] These uncomfortable truths were reiterated, in no uncertain terms, by a separate group of researchers who stated that there is no direct evidence for the transmission of SARS-CoV-2 via any route, whether it be fomites, direct contact, droplets or aerosols.[19] It seems, then, that when it comes to viral contagion, what scientists currently accept—and insist upon—is not what they can demonstrate.

This gap in current understanding exists even after a century or so of research into viral contagion. During this considerable timespan, society has invested an enormous amount of economic and human resources to no avail. But if respiratory illnesses so obviously spread from person-to-person via close contact, why has it been so difficult for virologists to objectively prove this? As previous chapters revealed, the one thing that human transmission experiments *should* demonstrate is the same thing that eludes them: viral contagion. The bottom line is that this core mechanistic pillar of germ theory *does not stand up to scientific scrutiny*. In the search for influenza transmission routes, a 2003 literature review could not find a single published study delineating human-to-human contagion.[20] A similar review, conducted a few years later, was also unable to find any conclusive evidence demonstrating the transmission routes of influenza. On this basis, the authors of the review concluded that sick-to-well transmission is *not* how influenza spreads.[21] In line with this, other researchers have found that the natural spread of respiratory illnesses is 'incredibly difficult' to replicate under experimental conditions.[22–25]

Close Contact

This lack of evidence demonstrating contagion is rather strange because viruses are supposed to spread readily via droplets, aerosols, and fomites. Indeed, according to the current understanding, cold and flu viruses are 'highly contagious' and can easily be transmitted between people,[26,27] so much so, that even a few seconds of fleeting contact is claimed to be enough to make someone ill.[26,28] Logically, if viral transmission occurs so often 'out in the wild', then it should be trivially simple to recreate it under controlled conditions when people are put in close contact with one another. This is because putting people in close contact should maximise their risk of catching a cold or flu. However, nothing could be further from the truth. It turns out that experiments directly exposing healthy people to sick people failed to adequately demonstrate that illness is transmissible. This is despite setting up optimal conditions for contagion to take place, and actively striving to make it happen.

In a series of immersive studies conducted in the 1930s, Kerr and Lagen housed healthy participants with other people who were sick with naturally acquired colds. Both groups lived together in climate-controlled, pressure-regulated, and air-locked rooms. The well and the ill ate together, played cards with each other, and drank from the same glasses. Cold sufferers even sneezed directly into the faces of the 19 healthy volunteers. Remarkably, *none* developed colds, even after a lengthy observation period of six days (Exp. 31.1). Taking a more direct approach, Kerr and Lagen also conducted other experiments where they squirted the nasal secretions of sick people directly into the conjunctiva of healthy participants (Exp 31.3). Again, all 15 healthy participants remained completely well.[29]

Buckland conducted a series of human trials in 1965 attempting to transmit the common cold. In the first experiment, 20 groups, consisting of a single healthy participant and up to two sick donors, lived in complete isolation together for nine days. Just one of the 20 healthy volunteers developed 'questionable' symptoms of a common cold (Exp. 58.1). In the second experiment, six sick people coughed and sneezed into bags. Then, eleven healthy participants immediately inhaled the air directly out of the bags, yet none of them became unwell (Exp. 58.2). In a third experiment, eight healthy participants attended 'sneeze parties', where they spent one hour, twice a day, for three days, playing card games in a room with sick participants who were coughing and sneezing profusely. All eight volunteers remained completely healthy (Exp. 58.3).[30]

Similar attempts were undertaken by Gwaltney in the 1970s, with mixed results. In the first of three experiments, one person with a cold sat at a table for 15 minutes with either two, three, or four healthy participants. The sick person was encouraged to talk loudly, sing, cough, and sneeze with the intention of expelling droplets, aerosols, and fomites. A total of 12 healthy participants were exposed to six different donors, yet *none* of the healthy participants developed a cold (Exp. 65.2). In the second experiment, 10 healthy participants were housed in a large room for three days with six people suffering from colds. The room was divided with wire mesh to prevent any physical contact between sick and healthy subjects. The sick donors were allowed to cough and sneeze freely. No fresh air was introduced into the room to maximise the amount of 'infected air' inhaled by the healthy volunteers. Again, not a single healthy volunteer developed a cold (Exp. 65.3). In Gwaltney's third experiment, six sick donors blew their noses directly into their own hands. Fifteen healthy volunteers then touched the sick donor's hands for ten seconds each. They then proceeded to 'self-inoculate' themselves by touching the mucosal surfaces of their eyes and nose. Nine of the fifteen healthy volunteers developed cold symptoms (Exp. 65.4).[31]

In total, Gwaltney recorded 9 out of 37 participants (24%) falling ill from his experiments. This result emerged entirely in the third experiment, which appears to show 'self-inoculation' with fomites. However, there are a few caveats worth taking into account here. First, experiments one and two found no droplet, aerosol, or fomite transmission, so overall contagion was inconsistent at best. Second, the way Gwaltney diagnosed colds is potentially questionable. He scored each possible symptom on a scale from 0 to 3: zero for *absent*, one for *mild*, two for *moderate*, and three for *severe*. The list of potential symptoms included sneezing, headache, malaise, chilliness, nasal discharge, nasal obstruction, sore throat, and cough. Gwaltney considered recipients to have caught a cold if they achieved a minimum symptom score of six total points. This cut-off seems arbitrarily low, considering he derived the symptom scoring method from another experiment where a minimum score of 14 was required to indicate a cold.[31] In addition to achieving a score of six, Gwaltney also required participants to have a subjective impression that they were suffering a cold *or* report a 'runny nose' for at least 3 out of 5 days during the observation period.

To help give a sense of what a 'positive cold' looked like in practice, here is an example. One of the donors had a symptom score of seven. They had 'scant' nasal secretions and sneezed only once during the three-day experiment. Despite so few symptoms and no detectable virus in their nasal mucus (by the author's admission), this participant was categorised as having a 'positive cold'. Now, if your nose was barely runny and you sneezed only *one time* in three days, would you say you have a cold? What if you then tested your mucus and it came back negative? Probably not. So, when diagnostic tools produce false positives like this, it calls into question the other confirmed cases reported in experiment three. If it's uncertain whether donors or recipients were actually sick, this undermines the ability of this study to confidently claim contagion.

Of course, every study has its flaws, so it is important to pay attention to the overall body of evidence that accrues over time. Toward this end, D'Alessio contributed to the corpus of contagion knowledge by conducting a series of five separate experiments in 1984. In two trials, groups of four or five healthy participants sat at a table with two or three people suffering from colds. They all played cards and conversed freely, yet *no one* developed a cold (Exp. 66.1 & 66.2). In another trial, five pairs of healthy people spent 12 hours per day, over three consecutive days, in a room with two sick donors. Just one of the 10 healthy participants developed symptoms suggestive of a cold (Exp. 66.3). D'Alessio conducted two other trials where healthy people kissed sick people for upwards of one minute. Out of 16 healthy participants, only one developed mild symptoms (Exp. 66.4 & 66.5).[32] Ultimately, then, D'Alessio's findings do not make up for Gwaltney's failings because they do not support a contagion account. It seems the overall body of evidence for flu transmission does not stack up.

More recently, a human transmission experiment involving 127 participants attempted sick-to-well transmission of influenza. The researchers inoculated a total of 52 healthy participants intranasally with cell culture fluid allegedly containing an influenza virus. A remarkable 42 of these participants (81%) developed flu-like symptoms, which might seem like evidence of contagion—at least, at first glance. As no adequate controls were used, it is unclear whether these participants became ill from a virus, a substance present in the cell culture fluid, a nocebo effect, or something else altogether. The 42 'infected' volunteers were then directly exposed to two groups of healthy participants with different levels of protection. The *protected* group consisted of 40 participants who all wore face shields and sanitised their hands every fifteen minutes. They were only allowed to touch their face with a wooden spatula. The *unprotected* group consisted of 35 healthy participants who did not wear any protective gear nor sanitise their hands. They were allowed to touch their face freely. This experiment took place under controlled, household-like conditions, for four days. Only one person in the *unprotected* group became infected and all participants in the *protected* group remained well (Exp. 70.1).[6] Of the 75 healthy people exposed to sick people, just one (1.3%) developed symptoms. In conclusion, it appears that, despite initial appearances, the lab-induced cold was impotent. Regardless of their protection level, it did not readily transmit to the exposed groups.

These kinds of failed transmission experiments can also be found hiding outside the peer-reviewed literature.[33] In one unpublished study, 20 healthy participants failed to develop colds after being exposed to infected donors separated by a double wire barrier, which prevented direct physical contact.[34] There are countless other experiments with similarly negative results that have also remained unpublished.[33] Now, there are many reasons why such studies might not proceed to peer review and publication. It is often the case that null results—like those found in the above-mentioned study—get rejected by journals who prefer to publish novel or ground-breaking projects that are much more exciting than those showing nothing happened. Over time, rejecting null results contributes to a widespread publication bias known as the 'file drawer' problem, which seems to be getting worse in the medical sciences (e.g. in studies on infection and immunity).[35,36] This is a technical point, but it suggests that studies showing positive outcomes are likely to be over-represented in the literature, and, as such, scientists can easily fall into the trap of overestimating the power and prevalence of things like contagion.

There are two key points to take away from this scientific commentary. The first is that despite the large number of failed transmission studies, there are probably *many more* experimental findings that never saw the light of day. The second, which flows from this, is that we can only know the 'true' state of the science—the complete picture—by accounting for unpublished effects. Together, these two research realities mean cold and flu contagion is, at best, shrouded in uncertainty. In the meantime, it is only possible to point to and draw conclusions from publicly available work.

In all this talk of null results, several contagion studies claim to have been successful.[13,14,37-39] For example, for some healthy participants, fomites were able to 'infect' them. That is, they touched contaminated objects and then touched their eyes, nose, or mouth. However, they did not become infected by aerosols or droplets.[31,39] Yet, in other experiments, healthy participants were unaffected by fomites, and only became infected (allegedly) by aerosols and droplets.[13] Unfortunately, the conflicting nature of these results only thickens the fog of uncertainty. The three modes of contagion are unreliable. To make matters worse, there are often methodological limitations that make experimental results difficult to interpret if people do happen to fall ill. In the studies mentioned thus far, only two used donors with 'natural colds', while the rest used donors with experimentally induced colds. None of the studies exposed people to an isolated, purified virus, nor did they use adequate blinding or control groups. Poor methods make it impossible to determine whether positive cases were due to a virus, environmental factors, suggestibility, false positives, or some other contaminant. Bringing this all together, there is a double-barrelled argument against contagion. Barrel one is loaded with null findings, which are extensive despite being under-represented. Barrel two is chock full of inconsistent positive findings plagued with confounds and errors. When aiming down the line, it starts to look like contagion is cannon fodder.

Outbreaks in Isolation

Even outside the laboratory, contagion still gets blown to smithereens. Beyond the dry experimental data, reports of real-world scenarios also bring up tough questions and cast doubt on the spread of common colds and influenza. The most noteworthy instances are those where people have contracted illnesses in extremely isolated settings. For context, viruses like influenza are supposedly contagious for about a day prior to the onset of symptoms and for seven days after symptoms develop.[40] Exceeding the eight-day timeframe should make it technically impossible to catch a cold or flu. In everyday settings, this narrow window is always open because there are plenty of new people as sources of infection. But how would the window stay open when groups of people live together without any contact with the outside world for months or years at a time? Throughout history, numerous influenza outbreaks have occurred aboard sea-faring ships and among groups of Antarctic explorers. In such isolated and enduring circumstances, sick-to-well transmission becomes utterly useless in explaining outbreaks.

Disease on the Seas

In September of 1781, influenza attacked the crew of an East Indiaman on its voyage between Malacca and Canton. When the ship left the port in Malacca, no influenza was present there and the crew was in good health. Somehow, the outbreak onboard began in the middle of the China Sea at the same time influenza had broken out with great intensity in Canton, a considerable distance away.[41]

A year later, in 1782, influenza ravaged a British fleet of warships under the command of Admiral Richard Kempenfelt. At the end of May, almost four weeks after setting sail, influenza broke out among the crew, despite no contact with the outside world. The illness struck with such intensity that the entire fleet was forced to return to port by the middle of June.[42,43] Earlier that same month, Lord Richard Howe set sail for a long voyage to the Dutch coast with a large fleet under his command. The entire crew was in perfect health upon their departure. Towards the end of the month, however, influenza started breaking out among the crew, despite no contact with the mainland for many weeks. The fleet was forced to return to Portsmouth, arriving home on the 4th of June.[44]

In another historic case, a French mail steamer set sail from Marseilles to Alexandria in 1847. At the time of departure, there was no flu in Marseilles and the crew were free of disease. By the time the ship reached the middle of the passage to Alexandria, influenza broke out among the crew. Oddly, this coincided with an outbreak ravaging the citizens of Alexandria on the Mediterranean coast, far off in the distance.[42]

In 1857, influenza broke out on the 'Monarch' while sailing from the most Northern part of Peru to the city of Valparaiso, Chile. Of the 690 men aboard, 191 (27.7%) developed influenza. At the time of the outbreak, the ship had been sailing for 20 days without any outside human contact. That same year, an outbreak occurred aboard the British warship 'Archane' while cruising off the coast of Havana, Cuba. The ship's crew began falling ill at precisely the same time as the people living in Havana, despite having no outside human contact and being at sea for a considerable length of time. Of the 149 sailors aboard, 114 (76.5%) developed influenza.[42,45] One more instance occurred again in 1857 aboard the ship 'Juno'. Long after the vessel had set sail, 131 of the 200 sailors (65.5%) were struck down with severe influenza. Then, in 1891, sailors aboard the 'Wellington' somehow fell ill with influenza 74 days into their journey from London to New Zealand, despite no outside contact with the mainland.[45]

Antarctic Anomalies

From floating on water to standing on ice, cold and flu outbreaks are even more remarkable when they afflict Antarctic explorers. In 1901, Captain Robert F. Scott of the 'Discovery' led the British Antarctic Expedition to conduct scientific research at the South Pole. The crew of 48 men were completely isolated from all outside human contact for two and a half years. During this time, two common cold outbreaks and one influenza outbreak occurred. In the first instance, the entire expedition developed severe colds, long after they had been completely isolated on the frozen continent. The cause was attributed to 'cold germs' hidden in a bale of woollen clothing which the men were exposed to after unpacking it. In the second instance, the majority of the crew developed severe colds after they had pulled up the carpet in one of the huts for cleaning. Again, 'cold germs' had supposedly been lying dormant in the carpet for months on end, and dispersed into the air when the carpet was disturbed. In the third instance, an influenza outbreak occurred in three men who had left the camp on an inland expedition. The men had to cut their journey short after just a few days and return to camp. They had become so ill with what they believed was influenza, yet the entire crew was in perfect health upon their departure from the base camp.[46]

In 1928, Admiral Richard E. Byrd was given command of the U.S Navy's Antarctic expedition. The fleet consisted of three ships and two planes. They established a well-equipped base called 'Little America' atop of the Ross Ice Shelf.[47] After a year of complete isolation from the outside world, an influenza outbreak occurred among Byrd's men stationed at the base. Much like their predecessors, they attributed the cause to opening a box of clothing that must have been carrying 'flu germs'. A similar event was reported by the Antarctic explorer Lincoln Ellsworth, who made four expeditions to the Antarctic Circle between 1933 and 1939. During one of his trips in November of 1935, Ellsworth and his pilot ran out of fuel, forcing them to make an emergency landing near Little America. This occurred long after Byrd and his men had returned to civilisation, so Little America was unmanned. Due to a radio malfunction, the men were stranded in complete isolation until the middle of January 1936.[48] Despite the lack of human contact for over two months, both men were suffering from common colds when they were eventually rescued.[49]

Another outbreak of the common cold occurred among a group of twelve British Antarctic explorers in 1969. The men were dropped off at a base on the 18th of March, where they lived, worked, and slept together in huts. For 17 weeks they remained in good health until the 14th of July, when one man developed a severe cold. Over the next two weeks, eight of the 12 men (66.6%) developed typical colds while two others (16.6%) experienced 'sneezing attacks'. Mucus samples were collected from the sick men and sent to the Common Cold Research Unit in England. The pooled secretions were inoculated into 10 healthy volunteers, only one of which developed something resembling a cold. Another seven healthy volunteers were inoculated, yet none developed any symptoms. The CCRU undertook a range of experiments to try and find an infectious agent, but they all failed. The leading theory is that one man must have been harbouring an undetectable virus in their respiratory tract.[50]

Breaking Down the Outbreaks

In these extreme scenarios, sea- and snow-bound crews experienced cold and flu outbreaks while far away from civilization. Not only were the men protected by the ultimate form of social distancing, but they evaded sickness for longer than contagion could feasibly take place (i.e. the eight-day window). Therefore, explaining every one of these cases in terms of sick-to-well transmission is quite a feat. It invokes multiple mechanisms, requires improbable circumstances, and relies on unfounded assumptions. Broadly, there are three ways a virus could have sailed the seven seas or sleighed around the South Pole: through the *air*, on a *surface*, or in a *person*. Let's consider each, in turn.

First, for a virus particle to travel freely through the air and successfully land on the mucosal membranes of someone in such a remote location seems exceedingly improbable. Outright, it's unlikely to account for most, if any, of these cases. The downside to granting this possibility is it contradicts other core practices in virology, such as the need to grow viruses in cell culture to make them potent enough to infect a host. If such a procedure is necessary, then surely a sparse dose of particles floating haphazardly in the air would never deliver an infectious enough dose. Also, granting such aerial superiority flies in the face of epidemiological recommendations like social distancing or isolating. If there is a reasonable chance that stray viral particles can hurtle across the planet and infect someone floating through a vast ocean or bunkered down in a desolate ice shelf, then what good would it do to keep 1.5 metres away from someone or shelter in place?

Next, for a virus particular to travel on surfaces seems more reasonable. Fomites could certainly land on a surface stowed in luggage or equipment and then later transmit through physical contact. The main problem with this possibility is that viruses do not remain active indefinitely. Influenza is claimed to 'survive' just 48 hours on hard environmental surfaces.[51] This timeframe drastically shortens for porous surfaces like textiles or fabrics, especially wool, which is anti-microbial. So, this sort of explanation is perfect for the first two or three days of a journey. After this, its plausibility falls off a cliff. This aligns with a common understanding that, after the first few weeks of complete isolation, people living in Antarctica should never develop respiratory tract infections due to the simple fact no one and nothing is around to infect them.[52]

Last, for a virus particle to travel within a person's system seems the most tenable. A sick person boards a ship or sets foot in the base and begins emitting droplets, aerosols, and fomites. This would be human-to-human transmission at its finest if it weren't for the timeframes. In none of the listed cases did any man fall ill within the first eight days, so sickness didn't disembark with them. At a stretch, it might be possible to continually 'juggle' a virus from person-to-surface and then back to a person. This is not only a low-probability feat, but it would mean someone is falling ill every few days to keep the chain unbroken. This pattern of spread simply does not match any of the aquatic or arctic scenarios. What's more, even if this mode could somehow explain the spread, it would almost poke fun at virological approaches that have attempted for decades to successfully transmit colds and flu. In a comical irony, sending people off to the farthest reaches of the planet and exposing them to the faintest hint of a virus seems to produce much higher contagion ratios than deliberately crowding people together and inundating them with viral material in a sealed laboratory setting.

Is it Catching on Yet?

To quickly wrap up, this chapter presents a serious challenge to contagion by questioning whether viral droplets, aerosols, and fomites can reliably spread infectious diseases. Lab-based scientific experiments tell two parallel stories. One is a tale of null findings that, due to the growing 'file drawer' problem, are likely to be under-represented in the medical science literature. As such, there are probably many more unpublished studies that reported *no contagion* yet will forever stay hidden. The second story is a tale of problematic positive findings. While some research claims to have successfully transmitted cold and flu cases, it did so inconsistently and in the presence of methodological shortcomings. For such hyper-infectious pathogens, it is odd that virologists have had such a difficult time demonstrating person-to-person transmission. Overall, then, the weight and standard of evidence in favour of contagion is neither clear nor compelling—it leaves much to be desired. In addition to floundering support for the spread of cold and flu cases in the lab, a contagion perspective is also unable to make adequate sense of outbreaks in the real world. The unique conditions of oceanic voyages and Antarctic expeditions pose quite a conundrum. In such isolated and enduring circumstances, it's difficult to conceive of plausible ways a cold or flu virus could be transmitted through the air, on surfaces, or in people to cause an outbreak. Using contagion to account for these historical events also creates a *double-bind*, where any feasible explanation seems to conflict with other virological or epidemiological principles. All in all, it appears viral contagion is having trouble catching on.

Part 3

Catching Colds

Chapter 16

No Pathogen Required

M ost people believe the only way a disease can be transmitted from one person to another is via an infectious organism. There are at least three broad reasons for this. First, they live in ignorance and don't even realise this is a belief worth questioning. Second, even if they are aware, they don't have the necessary information to mount a serious counterargument against this belief. Third, even if they are aware *and* informed, they don't have any reasonable alternative viewpoints to fill the chasm left by their newfound disillusionment. So far, this book has focused primarily on reasons one and two. It has prompted readers to examine their preconceptions, while outlining historical and scientific arguments against contagion. But, if viruses aren't causing colds or flus, then what is? What are other plausible ways to account for these illnesses? This chapter begins to answer these questions and it addresses reason three by introducing potential psycho-physiological (or 'mind-body') mechanisms. Specifically, it uncovers the *nocebo* effect, which is known to cause disease states and, therefore, could potentially explain apparent cold and flu outbreaks. Evidence for nocebo comes from many instances throughout history where people have fallen ill without an infectious pathogen being present. Naturally, these occurrences are deceptive because they have all the hallmarks of an infectious disease. Instead of a germ, however, it seems individual and collective psychology are operating behind the scenes.

The Nocebo Effect

The placebo effect—Latin for *"I will please"*—refers to beneficial or positive effects that arise from a treatment containing no active properties. In contrast, the nocebo effect—Latin for *"I will harm"*—refers to deleterious or negative effects that arise from a treatment containing no active properties.[1] Because there is no identifiable ingredient involved, placebo and nocebo are generally considered psychological phenomena, meaning people can make themselves healthy or sick with their minds alone. The effects of placebo and nocebo are so common and potentially powerful that they affect outcomes in almost all human research. For this reason, scientists fight a constant battle to control placebo and nocebo effects when determining the true impact of an intervention. One way to do this is by 'blinding' participants and researchers—concealing the nature of the experimental procedures given.[2] This reduces the likelihood they will respond based on expectation or suggestion.

Though it might be tempting to dismiss placebo and nocebo as irrelevant and inconsequential 'noise', hundreds of scientific studies have documented the ways people can create and reverse illness with nothing more than the power of their mind. For example, a 1981 study reported an intriguing case of nocebo in 34 college students.[3] Researchers attached an electrode to the head of each student and then led them to believe it was going to deliver an electrical impulse capable of causing headaches. Even though no electrical current was ever administered, 71% of the students experienced headaches.[3] This implies that the mere expectation of exposure to something potentially harmful is enough for people to experience an ailment.

A more recent experiment conducted in 2002 compared the effects of genuine and placebo surgery on 180 patients with knee osteoarthritis. The real treatment involved a standard arthroscopic surgical procedure, whereas the fake treatment involved a small, superficial skin incision behind the knee (made to appear as though they received surgery). Despite receiving a sham procedure, the placebo group experienced the *same* reductions in pain and improvements in knee function as those who underwent real surgery. Importantly, both groups were blinded to the nature of the treatment they had received until 24 months after the trial. This blinding appeared to work because, when asked which treatment they thought they had received, only 13% of people in either group guessed correctly.[4] This means people can feel better by simply being led to believe a legitimate medical procedure has been performed on them.

In another quirky case, a young man involved in an anti-depressant medication trial burst through the doors of an emergency department requesting urgent medical assistance. He exclaimed, *"Help me, I took all my pills"*, before collapsing on the floor and dropping an empty prescription bottle as he fell. Hospital staff began treating the drowsy, lethargic man, who admitted taking 29 pills in an attempted suicide. He presented with low blood pressure (80/40 mg/Hg), elevated heart rate (110 bpm), diaphoresis (sweating), rapid breathing, and a tremor. To try and flush out his system, the staff administered six litres of intravenous fluids over 4 hours. At this point, one of the lead researchers of the trial arrived at the hospital. To everyone's surprise and relief, they determined the man had been placed in the trial's placebo group. This means the 'medication' he attempted to overdose on was not an anti-depressant at all. It was merely a course of *sugar pills*. Upon hearing this news, the man's condition normalised within 15 minutes, and he left the hospital soon after.[1]

Expectations and suggestions can even affect the development and treatment of conditions as serious as cancer. In 1983, a group of British researchers divided over 400 cancer patients into three groups during a placebo-controlled chemotherapy trial. Two groups received different forms of chemotherapy, while the third received a saline placebo. Of the 130 patients receiving the saltwater treatment, 40 (31%) developed alopecia (hair loss), 45 (35%) experienced drug-related nausea, and 28 (22%) developed drug-related vomiting.[5] These are all typical side effects of chemotherapy, *not* symptoms of cancer. As such, these results are a testament to the power of nocebo. Simply believing they had received chemotherapy—and understanding what this treatment typically entailed—was enough to induce dramatic side effects. These cancer patients vomited, experienced malaise, and lost their hair because they expected to.

Although this is quite a remarkable occurrence, mind-body manifestations can be expressed in even more extreme ways. In 1992, a medical journal published a perplexing case study of a man diagnosed with metastatic oesophageal cancer that had spread throughout his entire body. The man, his family, and the doctors were all convinced he would soon be dead. In fact, he was given only a matter of months to live. Sure enough, shortly after receiving his grave diagnosis and dire prognosis, the man passed away. The autopsy, however, did not find a single tumour, apart from a small two-centimetre nodule on his liver. In response to this inexplicable finding, his doctor admitted, *"I do not know the pathological cause of his death"*. Medical professionals therefore speculated that the man was 'killed' by the expectation of cancer, rather than by the cancer itself.[6] If true, then a mere diagnosis is enough of a noxious agent to afflict someone with a deadly condition. In this case, a lethal strain of nocebo.

Another mind-boggling cancer case involved a man known only as "Mr Wright," who had been diagnosed with lymphosarcoma—a form of cancer that affects the lymph nodes and bone marrow. Doctors gave him just months to live because of the numerous, orange-sized tumours that riddled his body.[7] Mr Wright had heard promising things about an experimental substance derived from horse serum, known as 'Krebiozen'. Convinced that injections of Krebiozen would save his life, he requested them from his doctors. Not long after commencing the equine treatment, Mr Wright's tumours began to shrink dramatically. So much so that he returned to a state of good health for several months. That was, however, until he heard the news that debunked Krebiozen by showing it could not fight cancer. Mr Wright's tumours promptly returned, and his condition began to deteriorate rapidly. In an effort to save his life, the doctors treating Mr Wright presented an argument in favour of Krebiozen, suggesting it was indeed an effective cancer treatment. The only issue, they claimed, was that the original dose he had received wasn't strong enough. On the basis of this cover story, the doctors began administering regular injections of saline, all the while telling Mr Wright he was receiving high-dose Krebiozen. Miraculously, the cancer completely disappeared soon after the placebo treatments began. In a twisted turn of events, months later, a peak medical body stated conclusively that Krebiozen was useless. Shortly thereafter, Mr Wright's cancer returned once again, and within a few days of being admitted to the hospital, he passed away.[8]

Altogether, these cases show how psychological processes have the power to promote and undermine health. Nocebo can affect circulation, respiration, perspiration, and other physiological systems outside of conscious control. It can induce a wide array of symptoms, including headaches, nausea, vomiting, and hair loss. Perhaps the most remarkable is its ability to induce and reverse tumour growth, which indicates that mind-body mechanisms are a matter of life and death. Given the scope and severity of the effects listed (which is by no means exhaustive), it is well within reason to assume nocebo can cause a cold or flu. But rather than simply assume, it is possible to demonstrate this outright via numerous cases where this very phenomenon has occurred. Furthermore, it is even possible to go one step further and discuss how nocebo itself can spread from person-to-person. The following sections do just this.

Nocebo Contagion

Though it's not common knowledge among the general population, doctors have known for more than 100 years that the nocebo effect is capable of causing influenza and the common cold. After the U.S. Navy's inconclusive human experiments at the height of the Spanish influenza pandemic, news outlets around the country were quick to jump on these failed attempts to transmit the disease. Several newspaper articles recounted the elaborate studies and then remarked on how baffling the negative results were. The journalists also offered the confused scientists a word of advice on how to combat the disease. Essentially, they recommended that if people eliminated their *fear* of the disease, there would not be a single case of Spanish influenza in the entire country—for people could not catch something they did not fear.[9]

It's not unusual for media to spout unsolicited and ill-informed recommendations, but these news reports happened to echo the sentiments conveyed by public health officials at the time. Throughout the pandemic, Chicago's director of public health was aware that interfering with the morale of the public could be counter-productive, stating, *"It is our job to keep people from fear. Worry kills more than the disease".* These sorts of phrases were repeated countless times by media outlets throughout the pandemic. This suggests that at least some people understood the insidious role fear could play if left unchecked.[10] Indeed, the consequences of fear were reinforced by esteemed medical doctors like William Kerr, who stated in a published journal article, *"Acute colds are nasty, but the element of fear in the presence of the miserable sufferer is one of our modern bogies".*[11]

In 1930, a curious observation made by Alphonse Raymond Dochez, Gerald Shibley, and Katherine Mills validated this sense of caution against unmitigated fear. One participant in their study was told he had been inoculated with the filtered mucus secretions obtained from a person with a cold. In reality, though, he had received a test injection of sterile broth. The following day, a nurse commented in passing how peculiar it was he hadn't developed a cold. Convinced he had been inoculated with the virus, the man developed a severe cold that evening. He reported sneezing, coughing, a sore throat, and a blocked nose. The following morning, the researchers told this participant the inoculation he received was nothing more than sterile broth. His symptoms subsided within the hour.[12] Documented evidence like this is very important because it proves people can manifest a common cold through fearfulness alone. Critically, it also shows how the authority of scientific and medical professionals legitimises fear.

This relationship between the mind and cold susceptibility was also reported by George Jackson and his colleagues in 1960. They conducted a large-scale study involving thousands of participants (n = 2545) over many years. In the active experimental group (n = 2028), about 30% of participants developed colds when inoculated with filtered mucus secretions. Surprisingly, in the control group (n = 517), about 10% developed colds after being inoculated with a sterile saline solution. This result indicates that at least one out of every 10 colds was purely psychological. But there is more to these findings. The authors discovered that, across conditions, participants who doubted they would develop a cold after being inoculated were *less likely* to develop one. Conversely, those who believed they would develop a cold after being inoculated were *more likely* to fall ill. They also found that participants with lower levels of concern, stress, or worry in their lives—who were more optimistic about their future and had a positive attitude towards health—were less likely to develop a cold following inoculation.[13] This means mental effects were at play even in the active group.

Building on these ideas, a similar study published in 2003 found that people inoculated with an experimental cold were far less likely to become sick if they tended to experience positive emotions, like happiness.[14] A similar study conducted in 2006 found that people with a positive emotional status (i.e. higher self-esteem, better self-reported health, optimism, purpose, etc.) were less likely to develop symptoms when experimentally infected with a cold, compared to people with a negative emotional status (i.e. lower self-esteem, worse self-reported health, pessimism, lack of purpose etc.). In participants who did develop symptoms, those with a positive emotional status experienced far milder symptoms compared to those with a negative emotional status. The authors theorised that emotional status impacts the production and expression of inflammatory mediators (i.e. histamine, bradykinin, etc.), which determines the severity of symptoms.[15] Taken together, these studies indicate how critical mindset is in protecting or endangering people's health.

Nearly two decades on, psychological research continues to support the role of mindset. For instance, a 2020 paper detailed the results of a longitudinal study that tested whether someone's risk of contracting the flu increased based on their thoughts about it. Specifically, the social scientists found that the more a person *expected* to develop flu symptoms (measured at timepoint 1), the more they *reported* experiencing influenza-like symptoms later (measured at timepoint 2). The significant association between anticipated and actual symptoms is evidence of a 'self-fulfilling prophecy'. In other words, what people believe influences what they receive. This, of course, aligns with the nocebo effect by showing how preconceived ideas can make people more likely to fall ill.[16]

The Mind Virus

Given that these negative beliefs weren't instilled by social science researchers, it is worth thinking about where they originate and how they perpetuate. This requires a deeper discussion of personal and social psychology. In general, humans are motivated to form an understanding of the world via sources of information they trust. Learning starts at a young age, from parents and teachers, and then continues into adulthood through health professionals, mainstream and social media, as well as political and scientific institutions. Over time, the entire population hears the same contagion story and sees it play out repeatedly, which conditions people to believe they can 'catch' a respiratory illness simply via close contact with others who are sick. This story sticks in the mind because repetition makes it familiar, authority makes it credible, and fear makes it critical. In turn, this understanding influences how people then think and behave. For instance, anyone coughing or sneezing becomes a threat to avoid and shun. Meanwhile, other compulsive behaviours—like washing hands, spraying disinfectant, isolation, and wearing masks—become worrisome obligations. Also, the concern is not just confined to contracting invisible germs, but it also extends to spreading them. Even while ill, people will devote their limited mental energy to prevent passing their cold or flu on to someone else. Overall, then, the belief in contagion originates from trusted authorities who repeat and justify it to others. It is kept alive by fearful everyday folks who unknowingly think, say, and do things that perpetuate this story.

These ideas manage to persist across time because people rarely encounter an opportune moment to sit down and examine them. The contagion story exists either in a 'dormant' state that sits outside of awareness, or in a 'critical' state that hijacks attention. As a result, it is typically only front of mind in two dire situations. One is during *individual illness*, which occurs when encountering another sick person and then falling ill a few days later. In this localised instance, it's difficult for any individual to see past the germ narrative because they feel unwell and don't have all their faculties available, so it's easier to invoke well-known contagion principles to make sense of what happened. Joining the dots seems so obvious too—someone else was sick and then they got sick. It is hard not to conclude another's germs infected them because the direct experience appears to align with what society has always said. As a result, falling ill—one of the few fleeting moments where contagion comes to the fore—becomes an opportunity to reinforce rather than interrogate the germ narrative. Other motivators are comfort and certainty; returning to a familiar tale feels satisfying and allows people to feel like they know what's going on. Consequently, the contagion story continues to evade scrutiny. It hides in the shadows until someone gets sick, at which point it strengthens ever so slightly in their mind.

The other dire situation where this story re-awakens is during *collective illness*, which occurs during seasonal outbreaks and pandemics. Each year, new cold and flu seasons propagate across the Earth and cause government agencies, public health bodies, educational institutions, and news media outlets to ramp up repetitive, authoritative, and fear-based messaging. These trusted sources warn the populace to take precautionary measures to protect themselves and others. They advise the public to stay home if sick, wash their hands, cover their mouth and nose when they cough or sneeze, and minimise close contact with others. Also, the topic of sickness often pervades casual conversation, so even friends and acquaintances intensify the signal. Altogether, these sources of influence reinvigorate a story that might otherwise start to fade from memory.

Occasionally, everything escalates to new heights and the seasonal 'recommendations' become urgent pandemic mandates. This heightened crisis state also gives license to a raft of never-before-seen measures like social distancing, wearing masks indoors and outdoors, checking in at venues for infection-tracing purposes, and receiving multiple injections to permit access to public spaces. Now, remember that humans are already capable of falling ill through their own self-influence, so imagine the potency of social influence at such scope and scale. All day, every day, everywhere, to everyone, from the highest of authorities, with the worst of consequences. This comprehensive and relentless barrage lends even more cultural weight to the contagion story, making it nearly impossible to pry oneself away from and see beyond.

Without a doubt, these sorts of individual and collective scenarios light the spark and fan the flame of the nocebo fire. They make people sick (or at least cause them to fare worse) via expectation and suggestion. Yet, despite the mounting evidence for nocebo, society continues to pay *no* mind to the power *of* the mind. They never suspect this ever-present possibility (or any others) because they are preoccupied with a one-dimensional explanation. An obvious (though cynical) reason people downplay nocebo is that it's much more palatable to blame something or someone else for your ailments, rather than your own psychology. But this is just another instance in a broader pattern of *externalising* the problem. People look outwards to germs, authorities, and society for the cause and solution to their suffering. This mindset stops them from ever taking important matters, like health and wellbeing, into their own hands.

Arguably, this adds another layer to the nocebo effect—people receive what they believe, which is that they are helpless victims in need of rescue. Taking personal responsibility is important not just for psychological reasons but also because outsourcing one's safety during the most recent pandemic completely backfired. What were supposed to be credible explanations and protective measures ended up profoundly undermining the population's health and well-being. Germ-based public health initiatives clearly derailed people's ability to consume wisely, exercise regularly, socialise freely, sleep soundly, and think constructively.

Ironically, attempting to curtail the outbreak thwarted the very lifestyle factors that would otherwise keep people strong, resilient, and alive. The population became fatter, weaker, lonelier, more tired, and neurotic.

Though lifestyle may seem like a separate point from placebo and nocebo, the two are intimately related. This is because healthy living keeps people well via two pathways: (1) *directly* by regulating physiological and biological systems in the body, and (2) *indirectly* by giving people the psychological 'subject matter' they need to manage their mindset. Put simply, when someone looks after themselves, this give them grounds to challenge negative expectations and cultivate positive ones (e.g. "I won't get sick. I'm doing all the right things, so I have the best chance of staying well"). Any progress they make allows them to further affirm their hope and optimism, forming a positive feedback loop and giving them psychological inertia. This mentality and the momentum it generates is particularly powerful because it turns people into active agents who are empowered to shape their destiny, rather than passive victims awaiting an inevitable demise. Moreover, the same psychological processes and trajectories also apply to groups. So, when *many* people look after themselves, this creates a social platform to do even more than any single person could do alone. Groups can band together, affirm one another, provide social support, and construct a helpful shared story that allows them to persist in the face of adversity (e.g. "We're all doing the right things and, therefore, we will make it through together").

A critical point to highlight in all of this is that placebo and nocebo aren't psychological 'ghosts in the machine' completely divorced from how the mind normally works. Expectation and suggestion are ordinary mental processes that all humans engage in and respond to. Furthermore, the mind and the body are not separate—they are parts of an integrated whole. What happens to one will inevitably affect the other. In addition, human minds are not separate—we are social creatures who live increasingly interconnected lives. In the modern world, we are constantly influencing and influenced by others. All this is to say that mind-body power is not some abstract enigma that exists 'out there' in the ether. It is the personal and social power available to all human minds. The key implication here is that we all have the capacity to create positive or negative trajectories for ourselves and others. The limits of placebo and nocebo are still unclear, but the overall phenomenon is certain: for better or worse, the mind operates based on whatever it currently understands or believes. So, what is the story you are telling yourself? What is the story others are telling you? What story are you telling them? These narratives indicate the mental models that are structuring our reality. Clearly, they can support or thwart our well-being. They can help or hinder society. Therefore, it's critical to reflect on what you currently believe and to carefully consider how you and others continue to shape that understanding, moment to moment.

The reasons that mind-body processes like placebo and nocebo seem so mystical and magical are threefold. First, they can be subtle, often occurring outside of awareness. Second, they can take place unintentionally without conscious control. Third, they seem extraordinary due to the hand-picked case studies and experimental findings, which are at odds with most people's comparatively mundane day-to-day experiences. The reality, however, is that the underlying psychology that produces placebo and nocebo is constantly unfolding in everyone in some way. So, even though it goes unnoticed, these positive or negative effects compound into meaningful change given enough time, repetition, intensity, or legitimacy. For this reason, it's difficult for people to realise the individual or collective trajectory they are on until they look back and see the overall change from where they started.

A Call to Action

In conclusion, people regularly fall ill in the absence of pathogens. One potent yet overlooked mechanism is *nocebo*, which describes a psycho-physiological ('mind-body') process that makes people unwell through expectation and suggestion. It can arise internally through self-influence, or externally through social influence. Nocebo can also manifest in many different forms, from headaches to hair loss. It can also manifest to varying degrees, from subtle symptoms through to death. It can occur in multiple ways simultaneously and set off a cascade of other processes that propel people down troublesome trajectories. Based on findings in the published literature, it is entirely feasible that nocebo could cause cold and flu symptoms. Its ability to spread is tied to the belief in contagious germs. This mind virus 'infects' through lifelong conditioning, lies dormant, and then emerges only at critical moments, where it feeds on basic human motives like familiarity, trust in authority, and fear. During personal and collective crises, the contagion story grows in strength, yet people never consider the potential for nocebo, let alone the capacity for the prevailing germ narrative to produce nocebo.

Ultimately, the contagion story is a deleterious double-whammy. It ushers people down a harmful psychological path and it increasingly hinders their ability to live a healthy lifestyle (which, as discussed, has direct and indirect flow-on effects). It is also inherently victimising because it encourages people to externalise problems and solutions, rather than take personal accountability. Instead, every human needs to realise that the capacity for placebo and nocebo exist within them as normal psychological processes. The untapped power of the mind is available to everyone. But, to capitalise on this, we must pay careful attention to the mental models we and others operate on. Over time, what we expect and what others suggest will manifest—in the mind, body, and world. We receive what we believe. So, let's examine our beliefs to ensure they take us where we want to go.

Chapter 17

Social Contagion

The previous chapter alluded to social influence as a key mechanism through which nocebo originates and perpetuates. To fully grasp how cold and flu outbreaks might spread from person-to-person without a pathogen, it is necessary to unpack two phenomena in more detail using specific examples. The first is social contagion, which refers to instances where some aspect of a person's psychology or physiology is transmitted to another. This might involve an exchange of *mental content* (e.g. specific attitudes, ideas, and beliefs), *psychological processes* (e.g. ways of thinking, feeling, and behaving), or *physiological states* (e.g. weight, hormones, and appetite). Although people are always influencing one another in their day-to-day interactions, social contagion tends to affect large groups of *susceptible* people in short periods without conscious effort. This makes it *appear* to spread just like a contagious disease.[1,2] In fact, the models used to explain social contagion are inspired by germ-based principles. If each person transmits to more than one other person, an epidemic will arise from the exponential growth rate.[3]

This naturally escalates into the second phenomenon, which is mass hysteria. Also known as mass psychogenic illness, this form of hysterical contagion refers to a set of signs and symptoms that spread rapidly across a group of people in the absence of any known cause (i.e. a pathogenic microbe). In a way, mass psychogenic illness is an extreme case of nocebo brought about by rapid and extensive social contagion. Together, social contagion and mass hysteria offer a serious alternative account of colds and flu because they are difficult to distinguish from other causes of disease like bioterrorism, toxin exposure, or so-called pathogens.[4] The mere belief that people might have been exposed to something dangerous is sufficient to cause an epidemic illness. On the flip side, the same phenomena can also explain the spread of helpful or positive changes, which the germ model cannot.

A Survival Mechanism?

A leading theory is that social contagion is a form of automatic or spontaneous mimicry that evolved to serve an adaptive function for animals living in groups.[5-7] The basic idea of social contagion is that members of the same species will attune to and readily adopt one another's internal states. They do this to acquire some form of survival benefit.[5,8] Mimicking other people, even when it seems detrimental to do so, promotes trust and cooperation because one of the ways humans identify friends from foe is through *similarity*. It is important to be on the same page as others because this makes you 'one of us' instead of 'one of them'. Also, experiencing the same psychological or physiological states can prepare allies to face a common enemy together. This is why animals that live in groups are far more likely to adapt to changes or issues in their environment. Only one or two individuals need to notice something is wrong for the necessary response to communicate rapidly and invisibly through the rest of the group.[9] For example, if a meerkat sees a lion stalking in the nearby grass, it can silently transmit its fear and stress to the rest of the mob, who are nearby. This triggers a collective and simultaneous fight-flight response, which confers a considerable survival advantage. With everyone aligned and ready, vulnerable animals can reliably coordinate with one another to evade a predator's attack.[10,11] Though humans no longer have natural predators, it appears we have retained many socially contagious signalling and regulatory mechanisms.

Contagious Yawning

Yawning is a classic example of social contagion in humans. When one person in a group yawns, other people also tend to yawn. This effect is more pronounced in groups of people who share a close bond, like friends and family members.[12] Although scientists don't know why yawns spread, they suspect yawns might synchronise and coordinate group behaviour.[13] For example, a yawn could allow group members to cool their brains down when the air temperature is elevated.[14] Other experts theorise that yawning might also serve as a way to demonstrate empathy,[15] signal boredom, or even equalise pressure in the middle ear while also conveying air pressure changes to other members of the group at the same time.[16] Though this is an innocuous example, yawning shows how humans can subconsciously send, receive, and interpret socially contagious cues.

Contagious Obesity

Social contagion, however, is not limited to fleeting bodily reflexes; it extends to much more profound and complex activities. As of 2020, 40% of the world's population is overweight or obese. This figure is on the rise and predicted to surpass 50% by 2035.[17] Though obesity clearly relates to physical inputs (e.g. food) and outputs (e.g. exercise), social contagion also helps to explain how obesity is rapidly increasing in prevalence. This metabolic condition appears to spread from person-to-person, just like a cold or flu.[18,19] One large study of over 12,000 people found that individuals were 57% more likely to become obese when a close friend or family member became obese. By mapping body mass against geographical location, the researchers found that weight increases *ripple outwards from central nodes* in a social network.[20]

In light of this pattern of spread, some doctors see obesity as biologically contagious, going so far as to claim it is caused by a virus.[21] Though it may seem counter-intuitive, some virologists argue obesity is caused by person-to-person transmission of the alleged human adenovirus 36.[22] This theory has gained such widespread acceptance that the term 'infectobesity' was coined to explain the exponential increase in weight gain amongst western populations.[23,24] If true, this would give a whole new meaning to the term 'obesity epidemic'. However, one reason to seriously doubt this theory is the time course of excessive weight gain. That is, it has only been happening for a few decades. If an alleged adenovirus increases body fat, then where has it been hiding for the past several thousand years when virtually no one was overweight, let alone obese? Furthermore, why does this virus largely afflict the West, despite better technology, living standards, and healthcare? This is likely another instance where the lens of germ theory forcefully imposes itself in an unwarranted attempt to explain diseases. It seems much more likely that environment and social influence are to blame. Specifically, people gain weight when they live in areas abundant in highly refined, nutritionally bereft food, and are prompted to consume it by others who regularly eat this food and gain weight themselves.

Contagious Menstruation

Social contagion takes many unexpected and mysterious forms. For instance, evidence suggests menstruating women living together tend to unintentionally synchronise their cycles. The phenomenon, known as 'menstrual synchrony', occurs when women gradually align on the days they begin their periods. It was first documented by researchers in the 1970s who studied women living together in dormitories.[25] The same effect was replicated in 1980 during an experiment on 18 pairs of close female friends,[26] and then again in 1981 among a group of close friends and roommates living together in a female university dormitory.[27] Some scientists discount menstrual synchrony because not all studies have been able to reliably demonstrate it.[28] Part of the reason for their scepticism is that they cannot account for how such a physiological response communicates from person-to-person.

Other scientists suggest menstrual synchrony may be mediated by pheromones. To test this, researchers in 1980 sampled the underarm perspiration of a healthy female donor, who had a 'normal' menstrual cycle and asked five women to rub this sweat onto their upper lip at regular intervals over four months. During this time, the recipients' menstrual cycles began to conform to that of the donors. In the month before the treatment commenced, recipients' menstrual cycles started an average of nine days after the donors. By the end of the trial, this difference decreased to an average of just three days. Meanwhile, a control group of six women did not show any signs of menstrual synchrony.[29] These results were replicated in a similar experiment conducted a few years later in 1986.[30]

Overall, these various observations and experiments—along with anecdotal evidence—seem to indicate menstruating women can align their physiology and biology. Though menstruation appears to be 'contagious', no one in their right mind would argue menstrual synchrony is caused by a virus. While it is yet unclear why menstrual synchrony occurs, it is unlikely to be an accident. Instead, this phenomenon probably evolved because it granted numerous reproductive and societal benefits, such as reducing internal competition for mates within a specific group, deterring philandery, and synchronising ovulation.[31] This reasoning accords with the broader social contagion account, which suggests there are good reasons to mimic other group members, even if they aren't apparent. While the exact how and why of menstrual synchrony are still open for debate, the fact menstrual synchrony *can* occur is enough to support a social contagion argument for now. At least half the population can detect and convey subtle cues in their social environment, which can alter systems in the body.

Contagious Pain

Social contagion is not always subtle or implicit. Take, for instance, a professor of neuroscience at a university in Turin who, in 2014, offered to take 121 of his students to a research facility located high in the Italian Alps. Before the trip, the professor presented *one* of his students with a flyer and a movie on high-altitude headaches (a symptom of altitude sickness). He also informed this student that a specific aspirin dosage was required to resolve this type of headache. The student was advised to contact the professor a few days before the trip to find out the precise dose of aspirin to take. In the interim, however, 36 students heard the rumour about high-altitude headaches and so they too contacted the professor asking for more information about aspirin and headache prevention.[32] Ironically, during the trip, these 36 students went on to experience *the worst* headaches out of the entire student cohort, despite their preparation. This wasn't simply a figment of their imagination, either. They also produced the highest levels of inflammatory mediators in their saliva compared to other students with headaches.

The results of this study are particularly noteworthy for a few reasons. First, no other study had ever shown that the nocebo effect can increase the synthesis and release of pro-inflammatory chemicals.[32] Second, the study demonstrated that priming a single person with an idea was enough for it to spread within a community. This idea—communicated *explicitly* by the professor—caused the students to manifest and magnify a health condition. Together, these two points indicate that social contagion can travel via everyday communication channels and can exaggerate physiological threat responses. In comparison, the experience of headaches was otherwise trivial or non-existent for other 'uninfected' participants.

What Isn't Contagious?

In addition to these representative examples of yawning, obesity, menstruation, and pain, there are countless other ways social contagion can occur. Depressed people who repeatedly come into contact with those without depression will start to 'transmit' their symptoms over time. Depression isn't called the 'common cold of mental illness' for nothing![33] Likewise, anxiety has also been shown to be contagious and is thought to alert other people in a group about potential threats or to signal a need for emotional support.[34] Emotional contagion occurs when human beings can 'catch' each other's emotional states, spreading things like outrage, fear, or anger just like they would a cold or flu.[35] Beyond these, studies have found many other physical and psychological responses to be contagious, including itching,[36] crying,[37] rudeness,[35] happiness,[38] laughing,[39] smiling,[40] and loneliness.[41] None of these are communicated between people by a pathogen, which would make colds and flu the exception to an otherwise general rule.

More generally, and quite importantly, good health has even been shown to be contagious. Of course, no one thinks this is caused by being infected with 'good bacteria' or a 'health-promoting virus'.[42] There isn't a single case reported anywhere in the literature of a sick person being cured from exposure to another person's 'good' germs. In fact, this is one key limitation of the biological contagion model. It cannot account for *positive* forms of transmission because germs only cause harm. This is worth pointing out because the best scientific theories are simple and generalisable—they rely on fewer assumptions to explain more outcomes. So, compared to contagious germs, which can only account for negative forms of transmission, some kind of 'universal contagion system' would offer a better explanation. The specifics are still up for debate, of course, but the overall effect is clear: humans have a broad, in-built capacity for contagion. The examples listed in this chapter show they are capable of transmitting various aspects of themselves—both good and bad—to one another. Although this 'contagion apparatus' is generally adaptive, it can also be hijacked or misappropriated, resulting in negative outcomes.

Infecting the Airwaves

For this reason, the human capacity to internalise others' thoughts, feelings, words, actions, and appearance is both a blessing and a curse. As a culture, we must be mindful of the information and norms we permit, disseminate, and amplify. This applies especially to mainstream news and media. It is well established that sensationalised media reports about certain diseases can lead people to develop symptoms even though there is no objective reason for doing so.[43-45] It is also well known that sensationalised media reports can increase levels of anxiety, fear, and panic among the general public.[46,47] These are all heightened emotional states that are not only contagious but likely to increase people's reactivity to subsequent events or ideas. Undoubtedly, the media plays an important role in managing population health and well-being. But unfortunately, its track record is not very good. There are many recorded instances where the media has 'infected' large swaths of people with harmful and contagious messaging.

In 2017, a cohort of 45,000 patients in New Zealand were switched from a brand-name anti-depressant drug to a generic one. Several months after the switch, news outlets began reporting that the generic drug was less effective and caused more side effects. Almost immediately, adverse event reports increased for the generic drug. Prior to the news stories airing, consumers reported an average of six adverse events per month for the brand-name drug. After the news stories aired, this increased to an average of 25 adverse effects per month. What was essentially the same drug somehow produced a four-fold increase in adverse events. Another fascinating detail was that this significant increase in side effects only occurred for those mentioned in news stories. This meant there was no increase in the many other known side effects omitted from news reports. Based on this pattern, the researchers studying this cohort concluded that a 'social transmission' mechanism had produced the widespread nocebo response.[43,44,47]

In another study, healthy participants were shown a television report produced by a major media outlet warning them of the adverse health effects of Wi-Fi. After watching the report, the participants were 'exposed' to a non-existent Wi-Fi signal. Of the 147 people who watched the report, 82 (54%) developed symptoms that they attributed to Wi-Fi exposure, despite the fact there was no signal at all.[48] Several other placebo-controlled trials have yielded similar results. They too found that healthy people began experiencing negative effects after watching alarmist media reports on the harms of Wi-Fi, despite being exposed to 'sham' (i.e. non-existent) signals.[49,50]

While these may seem like quirky 'tin-foil-hat' kinds of cases, the influence of the media also affects matters as serious as suicide. A 2021 review found growing support for a 'copycat' effect, whereby suicide rates often spike after news outlets report on them.[51] Now, although this highlights the potential power of the media, there is an important nuance to outline here. It's not simply reporting that is the issue, so mere exposure isn't killing people. This is clear because the copycat effect does not occur in all countries and in all cases. There are even many instances where media portrayals have had helpful effects and reduced suicide rates.[51] What matters is the *nature* of the message and the meaning it conveys. Copycat spikes tend to occur when the media portrays suicide positively, frequently, extensively, and for prominent cases like celebrities. Crafting a message in a particular way can make a morbid act seem viable and normal in the minds of consumers.

But speaking about media in this way implies they can freely manipulate the masses without anyone having a say in the matter. However, there is much more to the story. Many factors determine whether a consumer is more or less psychologically 'ready' to heed a message. To cut a long story short, people respond most strongly to information they see as 'self-relevant'. In other words, they will pay attention to and act on ideas they believe *make sense* in their situation. So, what is often labelled as 'suggestibility' is actually a combination of personality, knowledge, skills (e.g. critical thinking), current circumstances, and life experience. Another example of the copycat effect is crime reporting, where a specific crime will be committed more frequently after it has been reported on the news.[52-54] But media portrayals aren't turning ordinary citizens into crooks, nor are they driving everyday folks to an early grave. The world isn't full of 'sleeper agents' getting triggered by the evening news. Instead, it is select people who face specific conditions and who are inclined to see sensational ideas as feasible solutions. They resort to such drastic means when they are financially destitute, mentally or physically suffering, socially isolated, impressionable, impulsive, and otherwise out of options (at least, in their mind). Remember, desperate people in desperate times are suggestible to desperate measures. This is all to say that most people are trying to move through life as best they can and will use whatever tools and resources are available to them. So, to the extent they view media reports as applicable to their life, they will respond to them. If they don't, then they won't.

Another point that underpins all of this is social context. Other people play a major role in determining whether the media's attempts to influence will 'land'. This is because when a person attempts to make sense of messages, they don't always think for themselves. They often look to relevant others to validate or verify what they hear. Social endorsement can come from 'local' sources like friends, family, or peers. It can also come from 'distant' sources like governments, experts, or famous people. Also, this sense-checking process can happen *explicitly* (e.g. by asking questions) or *implicitly* (e.g. by observing behaviour). In essence, though, the more media content seems to align with the words and actions of people you trust, the more likely it will be to sway you. Of course, this can run into issues when those same people get their information from the news, or when the ideas claimed cannot be verified by simply 'looking out your window', but the general trend remains regardless.[55,56]

This detour into human psychology highlights a few important takeaways for social contagion. The first is *the message* matters. Media wields a double-edged sword in influencing society. They have the power to move the populace in a positive or negative direction. Which will they choose? Well, this very much depends on what *motivates* them (e.g. sources of funding) and what *constrains* them (e.g. ethical principles and regulatory guidelines). If either of these is misguided or corrupted, then the media can easily turn from hero to villain in the battle for population health and wellbeing. It is all too easy for them to engineer media campaigns that prey on basic human emotions and motives in order to satisfy some financial, political, or ideological agenda.

The second takeaway is that *the consumer* counts too. People aren't mindless automatons that blindly follow whatever they are exposed to. Rather, they are constantly trying to find the best way to navigate through life and will pay closest attention to whichever messages they believe will help them do this. Without question, there are better ways to find answers, but for the majority, mainstream media is quick, easy, and accessible.

Not everyone has the time, motivation, or ability to critically evaluate messages. In the absence of better options, consumers should reduce their susceptibility to media by simply discounting it as a reliable source of information.

The third takeaway is *the network* knows best. Despite what the television, radio, or newspapers say, people often look to their social environment to double-check how to respond. If the news says you should stay inside your home, you will be much more likely to follow along if everyone you know (or look up to) agrees and does the same. Humans are very sensitive to social cues like consensus, norms, and status. We evolved a strong tendency to align ourselves with other people like or better than us because, historically, our tribe kept us alive.

The fourth and final takeaway is that all of these levels can interact powerfully to create *the perfect storm*. A persuasive message, a suggestible consumer, and an enthusiastic network—all moving in the same direction. When this happens, it is exceedingly difficult to resist and dissent. This kind of synergy was exemplified during the recent pandemic. Evocative threat-based messages were broadcast extensively and repeatedly. The information seemed personally relevant and made sense for people to follow because it was in the service of safety. Authorities also validated and reinforced the message, while the general populace followed orders and rallied on social media. In all of this, it would be miraculous if social contagion and nocebo *didn't* occur. A similar story occurred during the 2009 swine flu epidemic. The media was accused of *"going over the top"* because they consistently exaggerated the seriousness and severity of the pandemic.[57] The general public viewed the media as a 'fear mongerer' or a 'puppet serving powerful interests'.[58] Some epidemiologists even called it an *"iatrogenic pandemic of panic"*—the consequence of a problem created by health officials and the media.[59] One wonders what role this overdramatisation by the media played in the prevalence and severity of the disease. Rather than speculate, however, it is possible to point to other instances in history where, even with fewer pre-conditions met, social contagion and nocebo came to a head in extreme and widespread ways.

Mass Psychogenic Illness

Although the exact aetiology is unknown, mass psychogenic illnesses are thought to be triggered by sudden exposure to aggravating stimuli like bad odours, loud or peculiar sounds, suspicious-looking substances, or social prompts like rumours, hearsay, and news reports.[4,60,61] It occurs when people believe they have been exposed to a poison, toxin, or a germ,[62] and *spreads* from person-to-person readily via audiovisual cues or by observing behaviour directly.[4]

The signs and symptoms of mass psychogenic illness can last for days, weeks, or even months. They are wide and varied, including dizziness, drowsiness, light-headedness, hyperventilation, shaking, twitching, trouble walking, fainting, heart palpitations, anxiety, itching, communication difficulties, uncontrollable laughter, and trance-like states. Of course, mass psychogenic illness is also associated with flu-like symptoms, including headache, nausea, abdominal cramps, pain, body aches, coughing, fatigue, difficulty breathing, sore throat, sweating, watery eyes, and a long list of other symptoms. Critically, an exaggerated emergency or media response to a particular event is also associated with symptom severity.[60,61] More than 80 recorded instances of mass psychogenic illness have occurred throughout history.[63] To indicate its potential breadth and power, this section briefly describes some of the more notable cases below.

The Dancing Plague of 1518

In the French city of Strasbourg in 1518, a plague broke out among the citizens, causing widespread injury and death. However, this wasn't the kind of plague you might read about in history books. This plague involved a contagious and frenzied form of *uncontrollable dancing*. It began in the middle of July when a lone woman, by the name of Frau Troffea, started dancing in the street for six days straight. Within a few days, 34 others had joined her. By the end of August, more than 400 people were involved in the madness. At one point, over a dozen people per day were allegedly dying of exhaustion as they danced uncontrollably in the searing summer heat. The dancing plague lasted for at least six months. As is the case with many psycho-physiological disorders, the cause remains a mystery. But it is safe to say it was *not* caused by a microscopic, infectious particle.[64,65]

The Lancashire Cotton Mill Prank

In 1787, a young woman working at a Lancashire cotton mill brought a mouse to work with the hope of scaring her co-workers. The woman decided to put the mouse down the shirt neck of a co-worker known to have a phobia of mice. The woman became so terrified she began fitting uncontrollably for 24 hours. The following day, three other workers had fits, and by the fourth day, 24 people working at the mill had been affected. For lack of a better explanation, people believed the fits were being caused not by a mouse, but by a poisonous contaminant in the cotton. Then, when people in the local community heard about these events, the word began to spread, resulting in employees at other cotton mills in the local area suffering the same illness.[66] To this day, the cause of this fit-inducing phenomenon remains unknown.

The June Bug Epidemic

In 1962, workers at a mill in Montana began complaining of a mysterious illness characterised by pain, nausea, fainting, headache, weakness, disorientation, and skin rashes. The illness spread rapidly. Within one week, 62 of the 965 employees (6.5%) at the mill had developed the disease. Those who fell ill believed they had been bitten by an insect hiding amongst a shipment of cloth that had arrived from England. However, no insect was ever found, and the cause of the epidemic could not be explained.[67]

The Tanganyika Laughter Epidemic

An extraordinary example of mass psychogenic illness occurred in the East African country of Tanganyika (now Tanzania) in 1962. The illness was characterised by sudden bouts of uncontrollable laughter and crying, lasting from minutes to hours. Patients also complained of feeling like someone was chasing them. Some people completely recovered after just a few hours, whereas others remained unwell for over two weeks. Three female students at an all-girls middle school began displaying symptoms towards the end of January. Within six weeks, 95 of the 159 students (58%) were affected, forcing the school to close in the middle of March.[66]

When the school reopened in the middle of May, another 57 students were immediately struck down, forcing the school to close once again. Ten days later, the illness broke out in a village where some of the girls lived, approximately 90 kilometres West of the school. Over 200 people in the village developed the illness. A few days later, another school on the outskirts of the village was affected, with 48 out of 158 students (30%) falling ill. When students from this school were sent home to their village, 30 kilometres away, their family members and other people in the village began experiencing the same condition. The laughing epidemic lasted for a total of 18 months, spreading to countless villages across the country, and affecting more than 1,000 people.[66]

The Kosovo Student Poisoning

In 1990, a mass hysteria outbreak occurred in the Serbian province of Kosovo amongst thousands of young adolescents.[68] Between March 24th and March 30th, more than four thousand people requested medical attention for a mysterious illness. More than 1,000 individuals were admitted to hospitals across eight different towns. The outbreak started after students and teachers noticed an unusual smell in the air. A short time later, they began experiencing headaches, dizziness, elevated blood pressure and heart rate, impaired respiration, weakness, burning sensations of the respiratory tract, muscle cramps, conjunctivitis, chest pain, dry mouth, and nausea. Teachers initially thought the illness was influenza. Then, when the most gravely ill students were admitted to the hospital, they were treated as cases of influenza. After receiving medical attention, however, patients recovered rapidly within 15 minutes to two hours. An international team of investigators failed to find any underlying cause for the illness and believed it was a case of mass hysteria.[68]

The Cola Crisis

On the 8th of June 1999, 26 children attending a secondary school in Belgium became acutely unwell, complaining of nausea, vomiting, abdominal pain, dizziness, heart palpitations, malaise, and headache.[69,70]

They were rushed to hospital by ambulance, where 18 of them remained for several days for observation. The students stated they became unwell after drinking bottles of a popular cola-flavoured soft drink. The next evening, the news reported that the cola company would recall its products.

Over the next week, students at four other secondary schools developed the same symptoms. Between the 8th and 20th of June, the Belgian poisons information hotline received more than 1,400 telephone calls for assistance. On the 15th of June, the cola company announced that very low concentrations of hydrogen sulfide were identified on the inside of some bottles, and a fungicide that is sprayed on transport pallets had been detected on the outside of some bottles. A chemical analysis showed that concentrations were too low to cause any toxic effects, though. The company recalled 15 million crates of its products across Europe and temporarily closed three of its factories.[69,70]

On the 23rd of June, the Belgian Ministry of Health commenced an investigation into the matter. They concluded the cause was either due to cola contamination or mass psychogenic illness. However, the investigators drew no definitive conclusion. Though the outbreak in the first school may well have been caused by toxic exposure, it seemed likely the so-called 'spread' of symptoms to other schools in the days that followed was due to mass psychogenic illness. Investigators attributed this to the arrival of ambulances and other emergency personnel at schools, which triggered considerable anxiety and fear. They believed person-to-person transmission of symptoms occurred when students congregated during break periods. They also proposed that extensive media coverage of the event at the first school led to the transmission of the disease to other schools.[70]

Mass psychogenic illness epidemics are nothing more than exceptional nocebo cases caused by socially contagious beliefs, rumours, assumptions, hearsay, anxiety, and fear. They are *not* caused by pathogenic microorganisms, even though they can present in precisely the same way. These examples help to close the earlier discussion on media influence. If such remarkable effects can occur without much assistance, imagine the psychogenic potential of every single government, peak health body, and media outlet on earth sounding the alarm about a highly contagious and deadly threat capable of endangering all of humanity.

A New Mind-Body Model of Contagion

This chapter builds on the previous one by taking the concept of nocebo and explaining how social contagion can cause it to spread and escalate into mass psychogenic outbreaks. Together, these three related concepts provide a reasonable alternative explanation for how colds and flus might spread. Compared to the germ model, this view:

1. Contains the same core features. It specifies an invisible mechanism that is contagious and causes symptoms.

2. Is simple, yet more widely applicable because a generic capacity for contagion also accounts for positive occurrences, like improved health.

3. Accounts for a broader *variety* of symptoms that can be neutral (e.g. yawning, menstruation), negative (e.g. obesity, pain, depression, anxiety, loneliness), or positive (e.g. good health, smiling, laughter).

4. Accounts for a wider range of symptom *severity* that spans from fleeting and harmless, through to enduring and lethal.

5. Emphasises the risks and benefits of social influence and encourages people to pay careful attention to how they contribute and respond to it.

6. Empowers individuals to take personal responsibility and social accountability for health and well-being, rather than off-loading the bulk of this to external entities like germs, authorities, and medical intervention.

This mind-body model of contagion reiterates a key idea mentioned repeatedly throughout this book. Namely, if humans can manifest colds and flu psychologically and spread them socially, then this *confounds* most, if not all, common cold and influenza research. Wherever experimental methods do not adequately control for this phenomenon (with methods like blinding and comparison groups), researchers simply cannot rule out this alternative explanation. Whether or not a 'socially contagious nocebo' replaces germs remains to be seen. But, at the very least, it is a *competing theory* that must be evaluated based on evidence. Until this happens, we cannot place complete certainty in a germ-based account. Instead, we need to remain open to the possibility of a mind-body contagion model.

Chapter 18

Environmental Phenomena

V ery little research looks at alternative causes of the common cold and influenza. There are *three* primary reasons why other possibilities have never been properly investigated. *First*, and foremost, the prevailing paradigm dominates. Germ theory has now secured over a century of purchase in society. It permeates the very fabric of modern life to such an extent that it is hard to find an industry that operates independently of germ principles. But, people are fully immersed in a worldview, it becomes increasingly difficult to see the forest for the trees. More to the point, convincing someone their question is answered will generally end their search. So, with everyone saturated in and satisfied by germs, is it any wonder alternative theories receive minimal attention? No other cause of the cold and flu has been seriously investigated for more than 100 years. This is the definition of *tunnel vision*. Adopting a single-minded view is inherently risky because problems rarely have one solution, and there's always a chance we are mistaken—especially given the fact that other options have not been genuinely considered to the same degree.

The *second* reason for this state of affairs is that the fields of virology and bacteriology receive extraordinary support. Any medical research that 'tips its hat' to germ theory seems to benefit financially. In contrast, scientists exploring alternative theories receive virtually no funding. Adding to this, scholars who publish work aligned with germ theory will enjoy higher rates of journal publication and citation. Meanwhile, anyone looking to explore and offer alternative viewpoints, or even to challenge germ theory, would be lucky to get published in a low-impact journal, if at all. Therefore, without funding and exposure, not to mention the risk of being ostracised, scientists have minimal incentive to venture out into uncharted or adversarial territory.

Third, the growing societal and scientific currents continue to re-circulate into each new generation. For more than 120 years now, universities and schools have taught germ theory as fact to naïve and compliant pupils. In the face of authority, and in the absence of alternative viewpoints, students rarely question the validity of scientific evidence for themselves. Innocent learners don't know any better, so they rely on their teachers and educational institutions to guide them appropriately. The impetus to explore alternative theories rarely crosses the minds of students because course curricula do not make them aware of alternatives, nor do they award grades on this basis. Everyone risks something by 'rocking the boat', so there is no reason to actively endorse views counter to the orthodoxy. Though higher education defended free thinking once upon a time, such values are fast becoming relics of the past. In the end, when students become academics, teachers, health practitioners, or just ordinary members of society, they will uphold and pass on what they are taught.

Because of these three factors, alternative theories tend to be scarce, less sophisticated, and supported by fewer data points. Critics of this book would be rightly justified in pointing out these deficiencies. Nevertheless, it is crucial to discuss other viable viewpoints because, if germs are the only option people know about, it's hard for them not to assume germs cause disease. While alternative models are not necessary to falsify a theory, it's often the case that people need one before they are willing to dismiss what they currently know. Competing hypotheses are also valuable for the process of evaluating evidence. Testing ideas head-to-head means whichever explains the results best will eventually win out. This is particularly relevant to progressing science because there are many instances where committed researchers have refused to see null or contradictory findings as disproving their pet theory.[1-3] They are motivated to downplay or explain away fatal issues rather than admit defeat and move on. With all of this in mind, adequate alternative models are needed to mount a proper challenge to germ theory. To this end, the current and following chapter will offer some *environmental possibilities* to supplement the social and psychological ones provided thus far.

A Primer on the Human Respiratory Tract

To fully appreciate these alternative theories, it helps to have a basic understanding of some of the anatomy and physiology of the human respiratory tract. With a surface area comparable to the size of a tennis court (85 - 200 m^2) and lined by alveolar tissue arranged in a continuous sheet, just one cell thick, the lungs act as an interface between the blood and the outside world.[4-6] The role of the respiratory tract is multi-faceted. It regulates the temperature and humidity of inhaled air and filters out foreign particles. These processes allow for a steady flow of fresh, clean, conditioned air to be absorbed by the lungs, diffused into the bloodstream, and carried around the body to supply the tissues with oxygen.[7]

When air is inhaled, it travels through tubes called bronchi, which divide into smaller and smaller branches, terminating at tiny balloon-shaped air sacs called alveoli. The respiratory tract is highly vascularised, meaning it contains a large amount of blood vessels.[7] When inspired air flows over these vascularised surfaces, it is warmed or cooled to a temperature of 37°C. The respiratory tract is also lined by goblet cells which produce over 100 mL of mucus in the lungs and two litres of mucus in the nasal cavity daily.[7-10] The mucus is called airway surface liquid (ASL) and the tissues it covers are known as mucus membranes. When inspired air flows over the mucous membranes, it is saturated with water vapour, becoming humidified to 100%.[8,10]

In addition to being warmed and humidified, inspired air must also be cleaned before oxygen can be absorbed by the lungs. As inspired air flows over the mucous membranes, any particulate matter or debris suspended within it becomes trapped in the mucus. Once trapped, the debris can be swept up and out of the respiratory tract by cilia—small, hair-like projections that stick out of the epithelial cells lining the respiratory tract. An adult human lung contains more than three trillion (3 x 10^{12}) microscopic cilia. Each cilium is 6 - 7 μm long and 0.1 μm in diameter,[11] orders of magnitude shorter and thinner than a human hair.[12] Cilia function much like a broom, 'sweeping' up to 1,000 times per minute. Cilia help to clear debris out of the respiratory tract and into the mouth, where it is then swallowed or expelled.[13,14] This process is known as mucociliary clearance and can be assisted by coughing and sneezing.[11]

Mucociliary clearance is considered one of, if not the most, important defence systems of the respiratory tract. Impairment of this mechanism is well known to cause several chronic and debilitating airway diseases.[6,11] Any debris the lung cannot clear, via mucociliary clearance, is broken down and removed by white blood cells called alveolar macrophages, which are native to the respiratory tract.[15] During the winter months, when the air becomes cold and dry, the mucous membranes of the respiratory tract can become cooler and dehydrated. This impairs mucociliary clearance, which, in turn, reduces the amount of inhaled particulate matter and pollutants the lungs can remove.[16,17] To compensate, an increased number of macrophages migrate into the respiratory tract.[9] Upon arrival, macrophages secrete *exosomes*, which allow them to collect and process particulate matter.[18]

A useful analogy is to think of the airway as a network of highways, roads, streets, alleyways, and cul-de-sacs. The highways are the primary bronchi, which branch off into narrower secondary bronchi (roads), tertiary bronchi (streets), bronchioles (alleyways), and alveoli (cul-de-sacs). These roadways are full of street sweepers (epithelial cells), water trucks (goblet cells), and rubbish trucks (macrophages). To keep the roadways clean, the street sweepers and water trucks spray water (airway surface fluid) to trap and moisten dirt and grime. Dirt and grime are then swept up and removed by the brooms (cilia) on the street sweepers. Finally, the rubbish trucks (macrophages) collect and remove any larger debris or smaller bits of rubbish missed by the street sweepers. This is an incredibly efficient and highly coordinated process, keeping the roadways (airways) clean and functional. Knowing this process helps to appreciate what is going on when some external or internal factor impacts respiratory tract function.

The Role of Humidity

For hundreds of years, physicians have known a relationship exists between absolute humidity, relative humidity, and respiratory tract infections. To better understand this relationship, it is important to first define absolute and relative humidity. *Absolute humidity* is the total mass of water suspended in the air. It represents the ratio of water vapour mass (in grams) in a given volume of air (per cubic metre).[19] *Relative humidity* is the percentage of water vapour in the air compared to the total amount the air can hold, at a given temperature.[20] For the sake of simplification, consider the following analogies. Think of absolute humidity like the number of litres of petrol in a vehicle's fuel tank, or the number of people sitting in a theatre. Think of relative humidity like a vehicle's fuel gauge, or the percentage of seats in the theatre that are filled. As the temperature increases or decreases, so does the volume of the tank, or the number of seats. Absolute humidity is *lowest* during the winter months because cold air cannot hold as much water vapour. Relative humidity, on the other hand, is at its *highest* during the wintertime because it takes much less water vapour to fully saturate cold air than it does warm air.[21,22] Absolute humidity has a strong seasonal cycle, whereas relative humidity only has a moderate seasonal cycle.[22-24]

Temperate Climates

The reason this information is relevant is because a considerable body of evidence shows that changes in temperature and humidity are significantly associated with influenza activity, specifically in temperate climates (i.e. places with four definite seasons). In these climactic zones, winter air is typically cold and dry. The absolute humidity is low, whereas the relative humidity is high. A drop in temperature and absolute humidity usually precedes the onset of seasonal and epidemic influenza.[25-31] Conversely, an increase in temperature and absolute humidity usually signals the end of the influenza season or an epidemic.[31] These meteorological changes are thought to be one reason why there is a pronounced seasonality of respiratory illnesses like influenza.[32]

The relationship between meteorological changes and influenza activity in temperate climates is so significant that government agencies can predict with great certainty when an influenza outbreak is imminent, simply by monitoring changes in absolute humidity.[19,33] When the absolute humidity falls below a threshold of 8-12 g/m^3, there is a significant chance an outbreak will occur within one month after reaching its nadir (lowest point).[34] For every 0.5 g/m^3 decrease in absolute humidity below this threshold, the risk of influenza increases by a staggering 58%.[35] It is important to note that the *change* (i.e. the relative drop) supposedly heightens flu risk, rather than any specific temperature or humidity level being to blame.[35,36] This may be why, in some experiments, exposing healthy people to consistently low temperatures or humidity levels failed to yield positive cold and flu cases.

Changes in temperature and humidity undoubtedly correlate with influenza activity, but their causal role is not yet verified. Some scholars suspect there is much more to this link. In 2016, a team of scientists and epidemiologists published a paper analysing the effect of environmental variables on influenza activity. They proposed that changes in temperature and absolute humidity are not simply associated with influenza activity, but are *causative*, either directly or indirectly.[37] Naturally, some scientists disagree with this assertion because the specific mechanisms are still hazy despite considerable research in this area.[38-40]

At present, several theories describe how temperature and humidity fluctuations might trigger the onset of seasonal influenza. According to mainstream virology, during the winter months, cold temperatures and low absolute humidity increase the risk of influenza via three different mechanisms:[19]

1. As humidity decreases, viruses can survive longer in the atmosphere.

2. As humidity decreases, respiratory droplets remain suspended in the air longer and travel further due to their smaller size.

3. As humidity and temperature decreases, inhaling air cools and dries the respiratory mucosa, reducing barrier defences and increasing susceptibility to infection.

Virologists believe these three factors increase the risk of being infected by a virus present in the environment,[41,42] and encourage asymptomatic sub-clinical infections to progress into symptomatic ones.[43] At face value, these mechanisms seem to explain why there is a greater prevalence of influenza during the winter months in temperate climates. However, they do not hold water when trying to explain influenza activity in *tropical climates*.[39]

Tropical Climates

While temperate climates have a definite cold and flu season, this is not necessarily the case in tropical and subtropical climates. In these regions, the weather is warmer and more humid for most of the year. Consequently, no strict cold and flu season exists, and people can fall ill year-round.[44-46] There is, however, an increased prevalence of influenza during the rainy season, which is why some consider it to also be the influenza season.[47-51] The incidence of influenza markedly increases when the average monthly rainfall exceeds 150 mm,[34] and the absolute humidity is greater than ~17 g/m^3.[46] There are exceptions to this rule, though. For example, countries like Thailand, Singapore, and Hong Kong have not one, but two distinct influenza seasons per year. One occurs during the rainy summer months (June-August) and the other in the dry winter months (December-February). This is despite a lack of distinct seasonal fluctuations in temperature and humidity.[45,52-54]

Tropical climates pose quite the conundrum as no one knows why the common cold and influenza are prevalent in humid, rainy conditions.[38,39,55] Mainstream virology believes water vapour droplets bind more readily to virus particles. This supposedly increases their concentration in the air, especially within the vicinity of 'infected' individuals who are shedding viral particles.[56] But such an explanation is difficult to accept because virologists also claim high humidity rapidly inactivates viruses.[57] Indeed, this directly contradicts the first two mechanisms mentioned previously (i.e. that viruses survive and stay suspended longer in low humidity). Furthermore, this explanation is purely hypothetical—it is not based on any direct evidence. No one has ever objectively observed or measured a virus particle adhering to water vapour suspended in the atmosphere, let alone shown that this infects humans more readily. Others argue cloud cover in the rainy season blocks ultraviolet radiation (UV) from the sun, mitigating the protective effects of vitamin D against so-called pathogens.[58,59] Furthermore, UV is claimed to inactivate 'respiratory viruses' on surfaces and in aerosols, a process that would be theoretically hindered by cloud cover.[60-62] But if the sun kills airborne viruses so easily, then they should not be able to float around freely in the atmosphere—which drastically limits their spread. Others suggest the greater prevalence of respiratory illnesses during the summer months might be due to the increased amount of air pollution,[56] or from the airways becoming supersaturated with moisture.[63] But these are correlations, not explanations about causal relationships.

The field of infectious disease *cannot* reconcile the common cold and influenza peak during 'dry-cold' conditions in temperate climates and during 'humid-rainy' conditions in tropical climates. The explanations for these different patterns of spread are not only unsatisfactory but are *incompatible with one another.*[64] According to the contagion model, viruses somehow spread optimally in two completely opposite climatic conditions. By this logic, shouldn't outbreaks frequently occur during the hot and humid summer months in temperate regions too? Some might argue that, in both seasons, people stay indoors more, increasing the risk of transmission. But, if that is the case, how do they initially acquire and then pass on an infection readily enough for it to break out across the population? The infectious disease model is yet to resolve this seasonal paradox.

The Role of Temperature

For centuries, society commonly accepted the notion that exposure to cold temperatures caused the cold and flu.[65,66] This concept was acknowledged by countless doctors throughout history, including Dr William Farr,[67] Sir Peter Eade,[68] Dr James Townsend,[69] Dr J. van Loghem,[70] and Dr Andrew Semple.[71] Most people have heard the old wives' tale about cold weather causing influenza, but it is given very little credence because this pet theory was disproven decades ago—or was it? The field of virology dismisses any possible cause-and-effect relationship between meteorological changes, like cold weather and respiratory infections, as mere folklore and misconception.[72] They argue that, while the transmission of respiratory viruses depends on cold temperature,[73] the *only* way to catch a cold or flu is to be infected by a virus. Virologists often refer to a particular set of human experiments as proof that no causal relationship exists between exposure to cold temperature and the development of respiratory illness. However, upon careful review of these studies, it becomes clear that those relationships were never investigated.

Instead of exposing healthy volunteers to cold temperatures and observing whether they develop a cold or flu, these experiments inoculated a group of healthy participants with a common cold virus grown in a cell culture. Some participants were then exposed to cold temperatures, while others were exposed to warm temperatures. Analysis of the results revealed that those participants exposed to cold temperatures were *no more likely* to become sick than those exposed to warm temperatures.[74,75] Somehow, virologists rely on this evidence to support the claim that cold temperatures can only ever be a contributing factor, not a causal one.[76] As it turns out, scientists did not rule out cold temperatures based on rigorous and extensive scientific investigation. So, is it possible then, that an obvious yet discounted answer has been staring us right in the face the entire time?

What the Temperature Science Says

Epidemiological evidence indicates that cold and influenza outbreaks occur in temperate climates following a drop in air temperature. When the temperature falls below 22°C, there is a modest increase in the likelihood of an outbreak. For every 1°C decrease in air temperature below this threshold, the risk of an individual developing influenza increases by 11%, with three-quarters of influenza cases occurring when the temperature is between -10 and 5°C.[35] Not only that but the influenza death rate peaks when the temperature reaches its lowest point—a fact that has been known for over a century.[77] More recent evidence has shown that mortality rates increase 1-2 days after a drop in temperature, before peaking approximately 6-7 days later. This increased risk persists for up to 28 days.[78] The combined effect of air pollution and cold temperatures have also been shown to increase the severity of disease and mortality rates of influenza.[79]

In addition to the epidemiological data, several human experiments have shown cold temperature exposure can cause a common cold, and produce flu-like symptoms, including a runny nose, nasal congestion, nasal itching, post-nasal drip, and sneezing.[72,80-84] In one experiment, 90 healthy people had their feet chilled in icy cold water. After four to five days, 13 (14.4%) people developed colds, whereas only five out of 90 people (5.5%) in the control group became unwell—over *two and a half times fewer*.[43] In a similar experiment, a group of volunteers placed their bare feet in cold water and had electric fans blow cold air onto their exposed skin. Several of the volunteers developed sore throats and common colds the next day.[80]

In another experiment, researchers induced severe chilling in a healthy volunteer to the point of shivering. The morning after the experiment, the volunteer had developed a typical cold. Several other experiments involved healthy volunteers sitting in a cold room wrapped in a blanket. When the blanket was removed, a fan blew a cold stream of air directly onto their bare skin. In the days after the experiment, some of the volunteers developed a sore throat and cold-like symptoms.[80,85]

During World War I, two experiments were conducted involving 8,000 soldiers. In the first experiment, 2,700 men were sent outside into the elements. They lived and slept in the cold, wet trenches for three days and nights. A control group of 5,300 soldiers lived in warm, and dry conditions inside a barracks. The incidence of colds amongst the 2,700 men outside was *four times* greater than the controls. In a second experiment, 4,500 men were once again sent out into the elements for three days and nights. They were exposed to cold (-9° to -12°C), and bitter winds, while another 3,500 men remained warm in the barracks. Once again, the incidence of colds was *four times* greater in those exposed to the elements. Across both experiments, a total of 160 men (2%) exposed to the elements became sick compared to 41 (0.5%) who stayed indoors.[86,87] Although far from definitive, these results are more compelling than those used to debunk cold temperatures.

If exposure to cold temperatures does indeed cause colds, this then raises the question: *how*? To find the answer, Dr van Loghem studied 7,000 Dutch people between September 1925 and June 1926. He found the incidence of common colds followed in parallel with the rise and fall in air temperature. To explore this phenomenon further, Dr van Loghem monitored the core body temperature of 30 children to see how they responded to different ambient room temperatures. He discovered that their core body temperature decreased significantly when the ambient air temperature decreased and vice-versa—a finding that has since been confirmed by several other scholars.[88–90] This led van Loghem to propose that humans are somewhat *poikilothermic*, meaning their internal body temperature varies in response to changes in air temperature. On this basis, he theorised that the common cold occurs when a substantial and sustained change in ambient temperature disturbs the body's capacity to thermo-regulate.[70]

More generally, scientists know that a decrease in ambient temperature of 2-3°C causes several adverse effects on the respiratory tract. This effect is even more pronounced when the temperature drops by 5°C or more.[9] Breathing air at 20°C for short periods of time and chilling the surface of the body can significantly reduce nasal mucosa temperatures by up to 6°C.[9,80,85,91,92] This leads to the mucous membranes drying out, resulting in a panoply of issues including: direct injury to—and shedding of—respiratory epithelial cells,[9,93] nasal irritation,[94,95] broncho-constriction,[95] reactive hyperaemia, vascular leakage, swelling,[10,96,97] greater mucus production and viscosity, increased migration of leukocytes (e.g. macrophages) to the airways,[98] reduced phagocytic activity of leukocytes, and acute cold-like symptoms including sneezing, nasal congestion, and a runny nose.[84,94,95] These symptoms have been proposed as a compensatory mechanism by the body to restore mucosal homeostasis.[99] Furthermore, mucociliary clearance is also hindered by lower ambient temperatures, so it cannot clear pollutants and debris (i.e. particulate matter, sloughed epithelial cells, etc.) from the airway as effectively.[100] To offset the loss of mucociliary clearance, coughing, sneezing, and nose blowing become important mechanisms for clearing the airways.[101–103]

As discussed earlier, these physiological responses are mediated by inflammatory substances including kinins and tachykinins—substances that have been shown to increase in the airways of animals after cold air inhalation.[104] The concentrations of these same inflammatory mediators within the respiratory tract increase 30x during the common cold and influenza.[105,106] In fact, these substances are *responsible* for the symptoms of a common cold or flu, and their concentrations within the respiratory tract are directly proportional to the severity of symptoms experienced during these respiratory illnesses.[105–109] As such, this mechanism might explain why people 'catch colds' after exposure to cold weather.

The Role of the Atmosphere

In 1874, one of the world's leading medical associations established a special committee and asked it to investigate the relationship between meteorological conditions and the prevalence of acute diseases. The committee gathered detailed information on the atmospheric concentrations of a range of substances, including ammonia and ozone. They also examined the relationship between these substances and respiratory illnesses like influenza.[110] Into the late 1880s, various scientific investigators presented official reports to the committee, summarizing their recent findings.

Atmospheric Ammonia

One report described how atmospheric concentrations of *free* and *albuminoid* ammonia would shift across the year. Both forms of ammonia are released as natural by-products when animal matter and human waste are putrefied. When this happens in the presence of moisture, it releases larger amounts of free ammonia into the atmosphere. Meanwhile, when conditions are dry, they release more albuminoid ammonia. Both forms of ammonia can be carried great distances from their source by air currents.[110]

In a controlled experiment, researchers exposed human volunteers to aerosolised ammonia for three hours. They found that relative to the control group, those dosed with airborne ammonia experienced significantly more irritation of the eyes, lacrimation, nasal irritation, rhinorrhoea, throat discomfort, breathing difficulty, headache, fatigue, nausea, and dizziness.[111] More broadly, ammonia impairs mucociliary clearance,[112] in much the same way as other naturally occurring atmospheric compounds, including ozone,[113] nitrogen dioxide,[114] and sulfur dioxide.[115] Ammonia, like other gasses, appears capable of causing an influenza-like illness.[116–118] Therefore, seasonal fluctuations in the atmospheric concentrations of ammonia and other compounds could be responsible for, or at least contribute towards, influenza and the common cold.

The official report also found that certain meteorological conditions encouraged these nitrogen-based substances to undergo microbial decomposition. This releases toxic compounds into the atmosphere, such as toxalbumins and ptomaines.[110,119] Toxalbumins are complex plant-derived proteins that are harmful to humans when ingested or inhaled.[120] Ptomaines are the plant alkaloids responsible for the foul taste or odour associated with putrefying organic matter and are also toxic to humans.[121] The investigators proposed that these toxic substances could damage healthy tissue, stimulate an inflammatory response, and promote the growth of microorganisms in the human body.[119] Ptomaines were often found in the urine of influenza patients. As such, the idea that ptomaine's were a potential cause of respiratory illnesses like influenza gained traction towards the end of the 19th century.[122–124] Unfortunately, this line of research fell out of favour with the inception of germ theory.[125]

Atmospheric Ozone

In the late 1800s, Kline proposed that influenza was caused by sudden and extreme changes in barometric pressure, temperature, and atmospheric electrical activity. These meteorological changes increased the atmospheric concentrations of naturally occurring gasses like ozone, which was purported to trigger influenza epidemics.[126] This perspective was shared by Victor Schönbein, the German chemist who discovered ozone, and by his contemporaries, Dr Frank William Bartlett,[127] Dr Cornelius Fox, Dr Geo Fell,[128] and many others. In 1890, Dr Augustus Harvey published a paper in a leading scientific journal documenting his visit to Victor Schönbein in Germany during the influenza pandemic of 1847. While there, he saw Schönbein's self-experiment which involved inhaling ozone to see if it caused influenza. Harvey was surprised to find that Schönbein had indeed been successful in his attempt—ozone inhalation did induce the disease.[129]

Building on this initial work, scientists conducted a considerable amount of human and animal experiments during the late 1800s and early 1900s to uncover the physiological effects of ozone inhalation. They discovered that when a person inhaled high levels of ozone (i.e. 2 – 3 parts per million), it got absorbed by the mucosal surface of their respiratory tract and caused the tissue to become irritated and swollen. The scientists found that even concentrations as small as one part per million would irritate the respiratory tract and impair mucociliary clearance,[130–132] findings which have been confirmed in more recent times.[133] Other evidence suggests influenza-related hospitalisations and mortality increase significantly when there is a rise in atmospheric ozone concentrations.[130–132]

Even with all of this research, the effect of atmospheric ozone on influenza is not clear-cut. The epidemiological literature contains conflicting findings that complicate the story. For example, some say increased ozone levels *hinder* influenza transmissibility by inactivating airborne viruses, which should reduce hospitalisation and mortality.[134] To confuse things even more, some data show an increased influenza risk at both high (240 – 310 $\mu g/m^3$) and low (0 – 50 $\mu g/m^3$) ozone concentrations.[135] Given these inconsistencies, it is difficult to make any firm conclusions about the relationship between ozone and influenza until more research has been undertaken. Nonetheless, it is important to account for the role of ozone when attempting to explain influenza outbreaks.

Something in the Air

Though the research on alternative theories for the cold and flu is limited, some natural meteorological conditions are commonly associated with symptoms. Changes in relative *humidity* are so tightly linked to colds and flu that they reliably predict outbreaks. In temperate climates, people typically fall ill when the air becomes cold and dry, yet in tropical climates, people tend to fall ill when the air gets warm and wet. Accounting for this pattern with viruses is tricky because they are maximally contagious during opposite conditions. Another environmental factor is cold *temperature*, which is an age-old culprit. Even though many believe the idea of 'catching a cold from the cold' to be disproven, the grounds for dismissing it rest on flimsy evidence. Instead, the data seem to indicate that people are much more likely to fall ill below certain temperature thresholds. This is supported both by epidemiological observations and controlled experiments. Some studies show a four-fold increase in sickness risk when exposed to cold. Low temperatures disrupt the body's thermo-regulatory ability and interfere with normal respiratory tract functions. Last of all, compounds in the *atmosphere* appear to play a role in making people sick. Many airborne substances like ammonia and ozone appear capable of producing flu-like symptoms. Their exact role is less clear-cut, so much more research is needed here. At the very least, the fact that certain ammonia and ozone concentrations harm the respiratory tract means studies should account for these gaseous compounds. With each of these three environmental phenomena contributing to cold and flu symptoms in some way, scientists should dig into them more deeply. Of course, there are many barriers to doing so, but perhaps focused research efforts will find whatever is in the air that's making people ill.

Chapter 19

A Toxic Tale

Natural phenomena aren't the only possible causal factors of environmental illness. There are also many toxic substances suspended in the air that can cause harm to human beings. In the same way that naturally occurring atmospheric compounds can lead to a range of symptoms typically associated with the cold and flu, inhalation of toxins can do the same. What can appear as an infectious disease may simply be a natural adaptive response to foreign material entering the body.

Sick Air Makes People Sick

Every year, commercial and residential activities around the globe release enormous quantities of waste products and pollutants into the atmosphere. Air pollution is a significant threat to human health and well-being, killing ~10.2 million people annually.[1] This number is so large it even exceeds the 9.6 million deaths caused by cancer each year.[2] Equating air quality with cigarette consumption is a helpful way of comprehending the extent of the problem.[3] Spending a day walking around New York City is like smoking 6 cigarettes,[4] living alongside a busy highway in Amsterdam is the same as sucking back 10 cigarettes per day,[5] breathing normally for 24 hours in Beijing is comparable to inhaling 40 cigarettes,[6] whilst doing the same in Delhi is equivalent to 50 cigarettes.[7] Smokers and people living in cities with high levels of air pollution have a much greater incidence of respiratory infections (e.g. influenza) compared to non-smokers and people living in areas with better air quality.[8–10] This is attributed to 'impaired immunity' against 'respiratory viruses',[11,12] however, could it simply be a direct consequence of breathing toxic air?

Particulate matter, the most harmful of all atmospheric pollutants, refers to the cocktail of ultrafine solid and liquid matter suspended in the air. It is measured in two sizes: *fine* (PM diameter ≤ 2.5 μm) and *coarse* (≤ 10 μm).[13] The smaller the particulate matter, the worse its effect on human health. There is also an association between particulate matter concentrations and influenza incidence.[14] Virologists argue this is because airborne particles increase the transmissibility of the influenza virus, but there might be another explanation for why air pollution makes people sick.

Under normal atmospheric conditions, air temperature becomes warmest near the ground when heat from the sun is absorbed by the earth. Given that warm air is lighter than cold air, it then rises into the atmosphere, taking particulate matter away with it. During the winter months, the combination of increased barometric pressure and cooler ground temperature can result in a temperature inversion. Temperature inversions occur when a layer of cold air gets trapped underneath an overlying blanket of warm air, effectively acting as a lid. One consequence of this phenomenon is a gradual buildup of particulate matter in the layer of cold, trapped, stagnant air. Consequently, people living anywhere 'under the lid' will breathe in the highly polluted air.[15-18]

The air quality guidelines developed by peak health bodies suggest that people should not be exposed to air pollution above a certain threshold (i.e. the average annual PM 2.5 recommendation is ≤ 5 μg/m^{-3} with a daily limit of ≤ 15 μg/m^{-3}). Incredibly, not a single country in the world achieved this air quality standard as of 2021.[19] To further expand upon the magnitude of this problem, as of 2023, only 0.18% of all land on the Earth, and just 0.001% of the world's population were exposed to a PM 2.5 of ≤ 5 μg/m^{-3}.[20] For every increment of 50-150 μg/m^{-3} above this limit, the risk of respiratory tract infections *doubles*,[21] and the risk of developing an influenza-like illness increases substantially for up to four weeks after concentrations have peaked.[21] Often, temperature inversions cause particulate matter to exceed safe air quality limits, which subsequently makes people ill.

In one temperature inversion over northern China on 8th January 2013, small particulate concentrations rose from 24 to 84 μg/m^{-3} within a day. Three days later, the concentrations had skyrocketed to 222 μg/m^{-3}, before peaking at 375 μg/m^{-3} on the fourth day. These quantities were merely averages across the North China region, so some localised areas recorded hourly concentrations of over 700 $\mu g/m^{-3}$.[22] This is more than 45 times the recommended daily limit of ≤ 15 $\mu g/m^{-3}$ and could have hypothetically doubled the risk of respiratory tract infections four-fold. Though the temperature inversion subsided a few days later, an influenza epidemic swept across China within a matter of weeks. Experts were quick to point their finger at the novel avian influenza virus H7N9 while overlooking the recent exposure to astronomical air pollution levels.[23,24]

A similar sequence of events occurred seven years later in January of 2020. Major cities across China were shrouded in air pollution from frequent temperature inversions and stagnant air currents. Average daily air pollution levels exceeded 200 $\mu g/m^{-3}$ across many regions. To put this figure into context, for every 1 $\mu g/m^{-3}$ rise in small particulates, SARS-CoV-2 mortality rates increased by 8%.[25] In this way, the severity of the pandemic that broke out at that time was tightly linked to air pollution. Just as they did years earlier, people fell ill shortly after exposure to atmospheric conditions *known* to cause respiratory tract infections and produce flu-like illness. This raises an obvious question: to what extent are people falling ill from a virus or reacting to polluted air?

The Air Can Alter pH

It seems there are many ways humans are affected by particles in the air. For instance, Dr Volney Cheney believed a change in respiratory tract pH ('acid-alkaline balance') caused colds and flu.[26] This idea spawned from a body of research he presented to the American Public Health Association in 1927. In his report, Cheney detailed a series of human experiments conducted over an 11-year period, where he tried to infect thousands of healthy people with common colds by inoculating them with the bodily fluids of sick people.[26] Despite his best efforts, every one of his contagion attempts failed to transmit the common cold. What never failed, however, was inoculating people with ammonium or calcium chloride. This reliably produced colds and flu in healthy people.

As it turns out, this intervention was so reliable that Cheney was also able to reverse engineer it to produce something the medical profession had been in search of for decades—a possible cure. He was able to *reverse* experimentally induced colds and flu by administering a high dose of sodium bicarbonate, every two hours, for six hours. Cheney mixed the sodium bicarbonate with warm water and administered it orally as a drink, or rectally as an enema.[26] Several other scientists have since published similar results, effectively treating the common cold and flu by administering sodium bicarbonate orally, rectally,[27] or nasally.[28]

It was based on these experimental findings that Cheney formulated a hypothesis. Namely, climactic conditions could disturb the electrolyte balance in the blood, which, in turn, diminishes the body's reserves of alkaline substances like calcium, magnesium, potassium, and bicarbonate. This creates a pH imbalance, resulting in mild *acidosis* in the form of acidic urine and nasal secretions. Cheney noted that the body acidifies and excretes bodily fluids as a way of clearing excess acidic substances. It does this in the hope of re-establishing an optimal acid-base balance.[26] While sceptics often dismiss health claims based on pH levels, there is some evidence supporting this line of thinking about respiratory illnesses like the common cold.[29]

The pH Hypothesis

The term 'pH' refers to 'potential hydrogen' (H^+) and is a quantitative measure of how acidic or basic a solution is. A pH of 1 is acidic, 7 is neutral, and 14 is alkaline. The epithelium of the respiratory tract is covered in a thin layer of fluid known as airway surface liquid (ASL). Normally, the pH of ASL sits in a tight range between 6.9 and 7.1. This liquid acts as a physical barrier, protecting the respiratory epithelium from the external environment.[30] ASL contains glycoproteins ('mucins'), which form a mesh-like network, entangling inhaled particulate matter within it. Particulate-laden mucus is constantly removed from the airway by mucociliary clearance and replaced with fresh mucus secreted by goblet cells.[30,31] When the pH of the ASL is close to neutral, epithelial cells stay protected, mucus remains thin, and mucociliary clearance works smoothly. The respiratory tract can remove particulate matter efficiently,[32] though some particles can accumulate in the lung tissue and remain there permanently.[33]

However, when the pH of the ASL becomes too acidic (pH <6.9), it damages epithelial cells, makes mucus more viscous,[34,35] and inhibits mucociliary clearance.[32] With these three acidic impairments, particulate matter starts to accumulate in the respiratory tract. If epithelial cells are exposed to an acidic pH (<6.7) for 24 hours or longer, they begin to die and are sloughed off from the airway.[36,37] This sloughing, along with hindered mucociliary clearance, are considered hallmarks of viral infections like the cold and flu.[38-40] As such, acidic respiratory pH is supposedly a *prerequisite* for viral respiratory infections to occur.[41] During a bout of the cold or flu, the respiratory tract pH decreases significantly, falling as low as 5.2—almost as acidic as a cup of black coffee.[42] To assist with the clearance of unwanted debris from the airway, the body secretes inflammatory chemicals. These force mucociliary clearance by inducing a cough, making mucus extremely runny, secreting larger amounts of mucus into the respiratory tract, and directly stimulating mucociliary motility.[43] These physiological responses are crucial for the removal of inhaled particulate matter and sloughed cells from the airway, especially when normal mucociliary function is impaired.[44,45] This may explain why inflammatory chemical concentrations increase dramatically in the respiratory tracts of people with a cold or flu.[46]

Broadly, there are three non-viral causes of ASL acidification:

1. Particulate matter: When people exhale, the condensation from their breath is a valid pH marker of their ASL and nasal lavage fluid.[47] Research shows these bodily fluids both acidify after inhaling particulate matter.[48] One study found the pH of condensate exhaled by traffic controllers was significantly less alkaline (7.3 – 7.8) than that exhaled by office workers (8.0 – 8.1). The researchers attributed this difference to the relative particulate matter on the streets versus in office buildings.[48] Given the lower baseline in traffic controllers, they may be more prone to developing a respiratory illnesses if further reductions in ASL pH occur. Particulate matter acidifies ASL directly, as well as indirectly by increasing the production of mucin required to clear it.[49] Particulate matter can also set off an acidifying 'loop' because it inhibits the capacity of respiratory macrophages—the very things that clean the respiratory tract.[50]

2. Air temperature and humidity: Changes in air temperature and humidity are known to impact the pH of exhaled breath condensate by *at least* 0.5 points.[29,32] This effect may be mediated by changes in naturally occurring atmospheric compounds like *sulfuric acid* (H_2SO_4) and *sulfur dioxide* (SO_2). Sulfuric acid is one of the strongest naturally occurring acids suspended in the air. Though inhaling sulfuric acid can acidify and damage the respiratory tract,[51] atmospheric concentrations only peak during the spring and summer months.[52,53] Therefore, sulfuric acid may not play a significant role in the development of influenza during wintertime.

Sulfur dioxide is another abundant atmospheric pollutant. While it can be released from natural sources like volcanoes and geothermal springs, the most common source is the combustion of fossil fuels.[54] When the temperature decreases during the wintertime and more fossil fuels are used for heating purposes, sulfur dioxide emissions increase significantly. It is not uncommon for atmospheric sulfur dioxide levels to be 4-6 times higher in wintertime than in the summertime.[55,56] Sulfur dioxide is also a known respiratory irritant. At low concentrations, inhalation of the gas can cause a cough, sore throat, chest tightness, mucus production, and irritation of the airway.[57] At higher concentrations, sulfur dioxide can react with water vapour in the respiratory tract, producing sulfurous acid (H_2SO_3). Like sulfuric acid, this has the potential to acidify the ASL.[58] Sulfurous acid is a far more potent respiratory irritant than sulfur dioxide, causing significant damage and erosion to the mucous membranes.[59] Research has shown that inhaling sulfur dioxide impairs mucociliary clearance by 56%. It also causes epithelial sloughing, intracellular oedema, and various other structural alterations, which are hallmarks of respiratory tract 'infections'.[60]

Exposure to atmospheric sulfur dioxide causes respiratory symptoms in healthy people, and short-term exposure correlates with in-patient hospital visits.[61,62] As atmospheric concentrations of sulfur dioxide increase, so does the incidence of influenza-like illnesses.[63,64] Furthermore, there is a significant relationship between atmospheric sulfur dioxide concentrations and the prevalence of influenza. The mainstream perspective is that sulfur dioxide simply increases the transmissibility of influenza,[14] but this is not supported by any direct evidence. Could it be that sulfur dioxide alone or combined with PM 2.5 directly causes influenza-like illness by acting as a chemical irritant?

3. Acid-Alkaline Balance: The body constantly works to maintain a stable acid-alkaline balance. Various metabolic processes in the body produce acids that must be eliminated by organs like the kidneys, gastrointestinal tract, and lungs.[65] Dietary intake of processed and refined foods—particularly meat and grain-based products—also contributes to the acid load of the body because they contain acid-forming precursors.[66] The capacity of a person's kidneys to neutralise and excrete acids relies on them eating enough fresh fruits and vegetables, which are sources of base-forming precursors.[66,67] When the dietary intake of acid-forming precursors *exceeds* that of alkaline-forming precursors, the body compensates by drawing upon its alkaline reserves to maintain an acid-base equilibrium.[66–70]

The kidneys' capacity to buffer acid is impaired if the body's alkaline reserves become too depleted to meet demands.[66,71,72] This triggers a compensatory mechanism whereby, instead of being dumped into the bloodstream to be buffered by the kidneys, acids are sequestered within the cells and the interstitium (i.e. the fluid surrounding the cells of the body). This conservative process is known as 'low-grade metabolic acidosis' or 'latent acidosis'.[67–69,73] Factors like smoking, drug use, alcohol consumption, a sedentary lifestyle, stress,[74] obesity,[75] and some pharmaceutical drugs[76] can further impair the buffering capacity of the kidneys, exacerbating latent acidosis.[77]

As the pH of the cells and interstitium becomes more acidic, so does the ASL.[30] This may cause abnormal acidification of the airway, leading to inflammation, tissue damage,[78] and respiratory diseases like asthma, chronic obstructive pulmonary disease, cystic fibrosis,[79,80] chronic rhinosinusitis,[81] bronchiectasis,[82] and possibly the common cold.[29] Some evidence suggests an alkaline diet can protect against the cold and flu by alkalizing the pH of respiratory tissue.[83,84] The authors of these papers claim that an alkaline pH denatures the proteins in virus particles and improves host immunity. But could it be that these mechanisms operate independently of viruses?

With these non-viral causes of ASL acidification in mind, the following steps outline how an acidic respiratory pH might trigger influenza or a common cold:

1. Under normal conditions, the airway clears inhaled particulate matter via mucociliary clearance.

2. A change in temperature and humidity increases the amount of particulate matter in the air.

3. The change in temperature and humidity also impairs mucociliary clearance by reducing respiratory tract pH.

4. Inhaled particulate matter begins to accumulate in the respiratory tract, further reducing pH and mucociliary clearance.

5. People with lower baseline pH levels (e.g. traffic controllers) are particularly susceptible to externally induced pH drops.

6. Macrophage concentrations in the respiratory tract increase to deal with the buildup of particulate matter, releasing exosomes to assist with phagocytosis.

7. Mucin production increases to trap and remove particulate matter, further acidifying the ASL in the process.

8. If the acidic pH persists for prolonged periods of time (>24 hours), respiratory epithelial cells slough off.

9. The body releases inflammatory mediators to promote the removal of particulate matter and sloughed cells.

10. This initiates symptoms such as coughing, sneezing, mucus production, and a runny nose to promote clearance of debris from the respiratory tract.

Acting together, accumulated particulate matter, changes in temperature and humidity, as well as pre-existing pH imbalances, can trigger a cascade of physiological responses. Damage to the body, along with its attempts to return to normal, produces symptoms identical to the common cold and influenza. To help ground this abstract sequence of events, let's apply the steps to a real-world situation.

Imagine two people of identical age and gender are exposed to the same atmospheric conditions. Person A is a traffic controller who inhales particulates and eats a junk food diet, causing their lung fluid pH to become more acidic. They can't clear the gunk from their airways, so particulate matter accumulates and drops the pH further. Meanwhile, person B works in an office, breathes cleaner air and has a fresh, whole-food diet, allowing their lung fluid to stay more alkaline. As a result, they have a normal mucociliary clearance, so no foreign debris builds up in their respiratory tract.

When winter arrives, the atmospheric changes reduce both individuals' lung fluid pH. Person A develops a cold or flu because their already low respiratory pH falls below 'the point of no return'. This damages the lungs, creates inflammation, and sets off a range of compensatory processes in the body that appear as symptoms. The severity of this person's cold or flu is determined by the amount of accumulated particulate matter in their lungs. In comparison, person B remains unaffected because their pH does not fall below the same threshold. But, even if it did, they still may not develop a cold or flu because their lungs are relatively free of particulate matter.

From a mainstream perspective, it could be argued that both people were exposed to a virus in the atmosphere. Person A became unwell because their immune system function was impaired due to an unhealthy diet. The severity of their cold or flu was determined by viral load. Person B, on the other hand, had a comparatively strong immune system. They did not develop the flu because they were impervious to the pathogen's effects. Is this really what is going on, or have we confused infection and immunity for internal changes and responses to pH? The differences between person A and B can explain why some people and others don't develop a cold or flu despite being in close proximity to each other.

Respiratory Infection or Desperate Detoxification?

The word 'virus' derives from the Latin word meaning toxin or poison.[85] For centuries, viruses were defined in English dictionaries as *"a poisonous substance produced in the body as the result of some disease"*.[86,87] It was only more recently, after 'scientific advancements' in the mid-1900s, that the definition changed to *"a small, non-cellular obligate parasites carrying non-host genetic information"*.[86] What if there is some truth to the original Latin definition? That is, 'infectious diseases' are caused by toxins and poisons entering the body, rather than invisible parasites. While society obsessed over infectious germs, it turned a blind eye to the obscene amounts of manmade pollution dumped into the environment over the last century. While people have become extremely fearful of and protective against germs in their daily lives, they are indifferent to the toxic substances that permeate almost every product they use and consume.

They are in *everything*—in our air, water, food, fabrics, medications, toiletries, devices, furniture, and building materials. Never in the history of mankind have humans been exposed to as many harmful chemicals as we are today. There are currently more than 350,000 different man-made chemicals in use,[88] and more than 2.5 billion tons of these chemicals are produced each year as a direct consequence of rapid industrialisation.[89-92] This equates to approximately 300 kg of chemicals for every single man, woman, and child.[92] At least 225 million tonnes of microplastic makes its way into the food supply every year.[93,94] This results in the average person consuming about five grams of plastic per week, which is equivalent to a credit card.[94] Many of these chemicals are known as persistent organic pollutants. They are called 'persistent' because they accumulate not only in the environment but also inside human beings.[95] Most people remain breathtakingly ignorant of the harmful environmental and health effects caused by these chemicals, which kill more than 12 million people per year.[96] Compare this to influenza, which allegedly causes between 290,000 and 650,000 yearly deaths.[97]

Toxic substances are also *everywhere*, from the deepest ocean to the highest mountain peak. Estimates suggest over 1,000 metric tons of microplastic rain down onto protected lands every single year in the western United States, which is the equivalent of 132 small pieces of plastic per square meter, per day.[98] As these microplastics fall from the sky, they are inhaled deep into the respiratory tract and absorbed into the bloodstream,[99] which unsurprisingly increases the risk of becoming infected with an 'influenza virus'.[100] Both acute and chronic exposure to toxic and poisonous substances like pesticides,[101] persistent organic pollutants,[102] heavy metals,[103] and pharmaceutical drugs,[104] can cause an influenza-like illness. The symptoms are so similar that, in many cases, patients have been misdiagnosed with influenza when they are actually suffering from the effects of poisoning or toxicity.[105-108]

Influenza and the common cold *may* be detoxification processes initiated by the body to cleanse itself of accumulated toxins. *If* this is the case, then a cure for influenza and the common cold is not required, because...they *are* the cure. The body regularly excretes countless toxic substances every day, in fluids like saliva,[109–113] sweat,[114–116] cervical mucus, [117,118] semen,[119,120] breast milk,[121,122] and urine.[123,124] If the toxic load becomes too high, however, the body *might* need to take a more drastic approach—the initiation of a detoxification response that looks and feels like a cold or flu. The body responds in any way it can to detoxify—sloughing off respiratory cells,[125–127] ramping up respiratory mucus production,[128] and expelling unwanted materials through urine, saliva, tears, and sweat.[129,130] This *could* be why sick people experience fevers and sweat profusely—to excrete more waste through the skin. In this way, a cold or flu is not some foe to fend off. Instead, it might just be the body's way of 'cleaning house', desperately trying to free itself from harmful substances and restore homeostasis.

This perspective rings true when examining the toxins and poisons that cause influenza-like illness.

Toxic & Poisonous Causes of Influenza-like Illness	
Air pollution[59]	Paraquat poisoning[103]
Botox therapy[126]	Persistent organic pollutants[97]
Carbon monoxide poisoning[127]	Pesticide exposure[96,134]
Dippers' flu[128,129]	Phenol poisoning[135]
Electromagnetic radiation[130]	Polymer fume fever[136]
Metal fume fever[98,131]	Ricin poisoning[137]
Organophosphate toxicity[132]	Silo-fillers disease[138]
Organic dust inhalation[133]	Vaping illness[139,140]

Table 4 – Toxic & Poisonous causes of Influenza-like Illness

A range of drugs (and withdrawal from them) are also known to produce flu-like illness.

Drug Associated Influenza-like Illness	
Antibiotics[142-144]	Chemotherapy[149]
Anticonvulsant medication withdrawal[145]	Diuretic drugs[150]
	Opiate withdrawal[151]
Anti-depressant overdose[146]	Oral contraceptives[152]
Anti-depressant withdrawal[147]	Methoxsalen[100]
Caffeine withdrawal[148]	Smoking cessation[153]

Table 5 – Drug-associated Influenza-like Illness.

Cleaning House

The metaphor of 'cleaning house' helps illustrate what happens when the body induces a cold or flu. Imagine two families of four living next door to each other. Both families rent their houses and buy the same amount of groceries each week. Family One, however, is health conscious and tries to minimise the amount of plastic they use. They buy fresh produce from the local farmer's market and use their own shopping bags. They recycle some of their rubbish and have a compost pile for food scraps. The total rubbish they produce weekly amounts to *five* garbage bags. Being good, clean, respectful tenants, family one dispose of their garbage bags weekly. No garbage bags accumulate week by week.

Family Two, on the other hand, buys groceries from the supermarket. Nearly all their food is processed and refined, so it all comes in plastic packaging, which they carry home in plastic bags. They don't recycle anything, nor do they compost food scraps. The total amount of garbage they produce is equivalent to *ten* weekly bags. Unlike Family One, though, Family Two does not take pride in their home, and they are generally lazy. They aren't good tenants and often forget to take out the rubbish. They only take out two garbage bags per week. Consequently, Family Two accumulates eight garbage bags weekly.

Every three months, both families have a rental house inspection. Family One doesn't have to do much in preparation for the inspection because they have maintained the property and haven't accumulated any rubbish bags. In contrast, Family Two must do a lot of cleaning if they want to pass the inspection. Over three months, they have accumulated 96 rubbish bags. There is a lot to clean all at once, so they must rally together and ramp up their cleaning efforts. They rent a skip and hire some professional cleaners to help them clean the house. It's unpleasant and chaotic, but they get there in the end.

Could a similar thing be happening with a cold or flu? The body accrues various waste products and needs to spring-clean them periodically. Cleaning house needs to be undertaken to prevent 'eviction'—which, for the body, might mean serious disease or dysfunction. So, if someone takes care of their body by eating whole food, drinking filtered water, exercising, abstaining from alcohol and cigarettes, and managing their stress levels, their body won't accumulate much garbage over time. There isn't ever much mess to clean up, so once a year they might feel briefly run down while their body does a quick clean up. Compare this to someone who eats junk food, lives a sedentary lifestyle, drinks, smokes, and is chronically stressed. Their body will accumulate much more garbage, which piles up quickly and gets out of hand. Consequently, their body needs to do a giant spring clean every few months, which manifests as half a dozen moderate-to-severe colds and flu each year. This cleaning metaphor helps indicate how a detoxification response can appear as a cold or flu. It also accounts for why environment and lifestyle make some people more prone to colds and flu than others. Of course, it might be that their immune system is 'run down' and more prone to a 'viral infection', but the same set of events can occur from a *toxic* overload as the body's way of taking care of business.

A Disease in the Trees

Every autumn, tree leaves turn yellow and fall off. This is a natural, cyclical process necessary for trees to survive winter. But imagine if this was mistaken for 'yellow leaf disease'. Each year, groups of arborists would gather around trees, trying to understand what causes the disease and why it seems to spread so quickly over the season. They suspect an infectious agent that jumps to other trees when the wind blows falling yellow leaves around. Though they admit the change in season is related to yellow-leaf disease, the scientists are convinced environmental changes merely render the trees more susceptible to the yellow-leaf pathogen. The arborists collect leaf samples from green trees—which somehow remained uninfected—to make a 'green leaf vaccine' for the others. The following year, the arborists return to fields and parks before autumn to inject the deciduous trees with their new green leaf vaccine. They know this doesn't stop the spread of disease, but claim it reduces the likelihood of trees dying—something they admit was already rare. The arborists also state that trees will need this intervention indefinitely, otherwise, they will suffer even more from the dreaded yellow leaf disease. In this scenario, the arborists completely ignore and actively interfere with the natural, cyclical process of leaf shedding, which helps trees survive the winter. They produce an intervention that not only fails to stop yellow leaf disease but can cause separate issues by interfering with naturally occurring processes and by introducing foreign material into a living organism.

It's essential to consider and respect *why* trees shed their leaves. Every leaf on a tree serves two main purposes: *photosynthesis* and *respiration*.[1268] As a leaf ages, it loses its ability to perform these metabolic functions.[131,132] Therefore, it makes sense for trees to shed old leaves and grow new ones to optimise leaf efficiency for the following season. But there is more to shedding than simply leaves. In the autumn months, deciduous trees limit a hormone called auxin, which results in their leaves, fruits, flowers, seed pods, and branches falling away. This cleanse helps trees to survive the winter by reducing evaporative water loss and conserving energy expenditure. Shedding these 'organs' also prevents the heavy build-up of snow and ice which minimises the risk of structural damage. If any of these processes is artificially inhibited, the dead matter would remain attached to the tree. This would (1) undermine the tree's metabolism long-term, (2) make it susceptible to acute injury, and (3) cause disease as it decomposes while attached to the tree.[133]

Just like a deciduous tree sheds its breathing apparatus (leaves) in autumn,[134] could the human body shed a part of its breathing apparatus (respiratory tract cells) in winter, to achieve some functional benefit? Humans, like trees, possess remarkable innate intelligence and a range of automatic responses and instincts. These allow them to exist harmoniously in their natural environment and convey some kind of survival benefit. As another example of this, contemporary mental health models increasingly frame aversive states like depression and anxiety as *adaptive responses*. The mind and body try their best to protect people and return them to a better state, albeit primitively. Yet, traditionally, people view these as mental health disorders that need to be fixed or eliminated.[135] Likewise, the germ model sees cold and flu only as infectious diseases that must be combatted and eradicated. But what if at least some portion of colds and flu were natural and adaptive processes, like a tree shedding its leaves each season, or a person reacting to life stressors? If this were the case, it would cause people to rethink why they attempt to suppress or eliminate natural responses using extreme countermeasures, especially where these cause more issues than they resolve. It would also cause society to carefully consider what colds and flu arise in response *to*. Before waging war on symptoms, it seems prudent to address the toxic tidal wave they might be trying to shield us from.

Let's Clear the Air

Airborne particulate matter is harmful to human health. Concentrations can rise when cold air gets trapped near the earth's surface. The higher the concentration, the greater the risk of respiratory tract infections and influenza-like illness, even weeks later. One of the ways air pollution makes people sick is by messing with their pH balance—something doctors like Volney Cheney have shown can experimentally induce and reverse colds and flu. Normally, airway surface liquid (ASL) captures particulate matter and clears it from the lungs. However, accumulated air pollution, air temperature and humidity, as well as lifestyle can cause ASL to acidify. When this happens, the respiratory cleansing process completely derails. Acid damages the lungs, thickens mucus, and hinders its clearance. When this goes on for too long, cells in the respiratory tract start to slough off too, adding more debris to be cleaned up. To force the material out, the body shifts into overdrive by releasing inflammatory chemicals that bring about a variety of symptoms. In this way, what appears as a cold or flu may simply be the body engaging in a natural detoxification process. This response is reminiscent of trees shedding their leaves each fall season, which is ultimately adaptive. Given that modern humans are frequently exposed to toxins, drugs, and poisons, it is fortunate that the body evolved a defence mechanism to periodically clear itself out. Instead of viewing colds and flu simply as diseases to fight, then, it is wise to consider how they might be primitive attempts by the body to remain healthy in an increasingly toxic environment.

Chapter 20

Bringing It All Together

C an you catch a cold? What may have seemed like a silly or strange question now holds much more weight and meaning. As you now know, challenging germ theory and the contagion model is neither new nor fringe. When these ideas first arrived on the scene, mainstream doctors and scientists found them unappealing and inadequate. The weather doctors, for instance, argued that contagious germs could not account for the pace, scope, timing, or direction of seasonal outbreaks. Also, prominent thinkers like Antoinne Béchamp fervently opposed Louis Pasteur's ideas and findings. Though Béchamp had shown them to be inferior and deficient in many ways, germs eventually won the battle and came to be revered by modern science. This was also in spite of the fact that Pasteur was unoriginal and dishonest in his academic work.

Experts at the time took sides in the Pasteur vs. Béchamp debate, forming contagionist and anti-contagionist camps, respectively. In their opposition to germs, anti-contagionists championed concepts like the terrain and zymotic theories to argue that environmental conditions and toxins were the real cause of disease. They also rallied around the principle of spontaneous generation. This emerged from experiments that detected microscopic 'base units' (i.e. microzyma) in sterile media which would supposedly transform into specific germs as a *response* to environmental stimuli. From this perspective, germs couldn't cause disease because they followed rather than preceded it. Pasteur himself remained open to these opposing arguments—acknowledging their importance on his deathbed. Nevertheless, contemporary science disregarded them and led us down the path we remain on to this day.

This current path, however, is a particularly puzzling one. Many of germ theory's foundations, like Koch's and Rivers' postulates, crumble under scrutiny. These criteria were crafted specifically so that scientists could prove bacteria and viruses cause disease. Yet, despite erecting these central pillars of germ theory themselves, neither Koch nor Rivers could satisfy the postulates. Others failed to fulfil them, too. Rather than follow the data, men like Koch shifted the goalposts and invented convenient 'rescue devices' (e.g. asymptomatic infections) to explain away contradictory findings.

The path continued to veer even further away from reason in the many attempts to isolate viruses. Ideally, scientists should be able to purify and directly observe cold and flu viruses as a prerequisite for proving they exist and cause disease. However, virologists cannot convincingly achieve either of these two feats, even with sophisticated methods like cell cultures, plaque assays, electron microscopy, density gradient centrifugation, and genomic sequencing. In fact, when virologists find a particle they believe is a virus, they can't reliably tell it apart from other alleged viruses, or from non-viral particles like 'exosomes'. Instead, what virologists tend to do is *infer* a virus is present by observing a separate phenomenon: cell death. Virologists assume viruses kill cells, so when cultured cells die, a virus must therefore be present. The logic here is fatally flawed, especially considering it relies on a method specifically designed to produce a cytopathic effect. What's more, this same effect occurs even when no virus could hypothetically be present. Such fraudulent scientific reasoning is exemplified by Enders and Peebles' landmark study supposedly 'isolating' the measles virus. They took cell death as indicating that the measles virus was present, despite culture cells also dying in their control procedure—which did not contain any viral material.

These fundamental issues aren't merely exceptions or outliers. Rather, they reflect a broader crisis in science. Though the scientific method ought to be our most valuable tool, its widespread misuse in modern medical research is particularly troubling. Given such a questionable context, it is perhaps unsurprising that contemporary virology finds it acceptable to: (1) assume rather than observe, (2) lack a true independent variable, (3) misinterpret the dependent variable, (4) draw simple conclusions from overly complicated methods, and (5) fail to control for confounding variables. Altogether, the various shortcomings that plague this discipline make it difficult to trust their story.

What's more, the issues extend beyond the laboratory and out into the real world. Using contagious germs as a 'lens' to view disease has led doctors and scientists into all sorts of strife. There are many historical incidents where authorities and experts mistook non-communicable ailments (like scurvy, pellagra, and Minimata disease) for contagious ones. They were so invested in their germ-based worldview that it was all they could see. Such errors of judgement caused much unnecessary suffering. But the confusion and its consequences didn't stop there.

Those subscribing to germ theory also struggled to make sense of major influenza pandemics. During the Russian flu, for example, doctors weren't even sure it *was* a flu. Cases presented with so many different symptoms that they found them difficult to properly categorise or diagnose. Many other anomalous cases were also inconsistent with how a contagious germ should spread. At the time, germ theorists were so desperate to point the finger at a pathogenic agent, that they became wrongly convinced that a specific bacteria caused the flu. This misled everyone and sent the field of medicine on a wild goose chase for over thirty years. In much the same way, the Spanish flu pandemic proved to be just as mysterious from a germ perspective. Scientists found it difficult to account for its point of origin, its pattern of spread, its wave-like recurrence, and its targeting of young men. Again, the symptoms varied so wildly in form and severity as to bewilder healthcare practitioners. Not only was Spanish flu hard to pin down as 'one disease', but its symptom profile closely resembled that of battle gas and aspirin poisoning. This further muddied the waters of understanding.

If these natural events weren't baffling enough, germ theorists continued to hit brick walls when deliberately attempting to transmit diseases from the sick to the well. This started with the self-inoculation experiments of Napoleon during the bubonic plague and persisted through to 20th-century experimental efforts encompassing more than 50 failed self-inoculation attempts with so-called disease-causing germs. Innovative methods to filter out bacteria ended one wild goose chase but started another. Though filtration allowed experts to rule out bacteria, they simply presumed an even smaller culprit was to blame. Scientists assumed that the only substances capable of causing disease in filtered bodily fluids were viruses, remaining oblivious to the fact that inflammatory mediators, which are known to cause cold and flu symptoms, could also pass through.

Nevertheless, this suspicion inspired wave after wave of human transmission experiments attempting to unlock the secrets of influenza. The U.S. military's dedicated and diligent efforts came up empty-handed, even after performing 25 of the most elaborate contagion studies that have ever been conducted in the history of medicine. Other researchers followed suit, finding little to no evidence of viral spread. Some scientific efforts, like Yamanouchi's and Schmidt's, actually did a disservice to the germ narrative. Yamanouchi achieved one of the highest transmission rates using dubious patient sampling and experimental methods. Meanwhile, Schmidt managed to produce his highest positive case rate using saline—an *inert* substance. By and large, the studies conducted during this period are some of the best available attempts to transmit the flu, even to this day. Regardless, they were unable to spread the cold and flu convincingly and consistently.

The same fruitless pursuit was true for cold transmission as well. After almost two decades of trying, the purpose-built Common Cold Research Unity (CCRU) was, by its own admission, largely unsuccessful in spreading the common cold. When this facility was threatened to be shut down, the CCRU was overhauled by Tyrrell and the newly developed cell culture method. Though this approach was much more successful, it still led to lower-than-expected case rates, notwithstanding the major flaws inherent to cell cultures. In the same vein, other scientific efforts challenged contagion further by failing to transmit colds and flu via droplets, aerosols, or fomites. Reviewing the cold and flu literature reveals a double bind: under-represented null findings and problematic positive findings. It also uncovers various real-world cases like oceanic voyages and Antarctic expeditions that a germ account cannot explain without contradicting other virological principles.

In the face of all these woes, there are also other viable explanations for cold and flu outbreaks. Though these may or may not replace germ theory, they at least present competing hypotheses that scientists need to rule out before they can be sure that pathogenic germs cause cold and flu outbreaks. This includes processes like nocebo and social contagion. Many studies show how expectation and suggestion alone can cause all sorts of illnesses—even as serious as cancer. Funnily enough, just the *idea* of germs is sufficient to make people sick when lifelong conditioning piques in critical moments. Without a doubt, the contagion story is psychologically toxic. It causes people to be fearful and avoidant. It is also physically unhealthy because protecting oneself from germs often interferes with the actions people normally take to look after their health. On the flip side, processes like placebo hint at the untapped positive potential of the mind. If society were to change its guiding narrative, people would be in a much better position to take control of their lives and cultivate more constructive patterns that are conducive to health.

In addition to social and psychological factors, there are also environmental factors that influence the risk, onset, spread, and severity of colds and flu. This includes natural phenomena like humidity, temperature, and atmospheric compounds. It also includes man-made phenomena like environmental toxins suspended in polluted air. Furthermore, both natural and man-made phenomena can interact with one another and may even trigger social contagion to create a 'perfect storm'.

Revisiting Our Aims

Having covered all of this content, it makes sense to return to the original goals of this book. In satisfying aim #1, you now have the information you need to understand a complex and unwieldy topic. Although it's impossible to cover everything, there is enough detail and guidance to start connecting the dots and forming your own picture. If you would like more information still, there is a detailed appendix at the end of this book summarising the results of more than 200 contagion studies—many of which are not mentioned in-text. After parsing through this additional data, you will be in an even better position to formulate your own answer to the book's titular question.

In satisfying aim #2, you now have an example of how to ask difficult questions and confront sacred topics more generally in your life. If there is so much uncertainty around something as 'settled' as germs, then what other deeply held beliefs might be worth interrogating? The overall stance of this book is not a definitive one. Instead, it queries whether germs make people sick, and cites legitimate sources to show why this is a reasonable and worthwhile question to ask. In the same way, you should cast a critical eye over any area of your life that is impacted by 'big ideas'. Examine the available evidence and follow where it leads, even if it's uncomfortable.

In satisfying aim #3, you now have a myriad of new possibilities to consider. The book asked many questions and ideally prompted even more. Are germs the answer? If not, then what is? As example answers, the book proposed alternative viewpoints to bring concepts to the fore that people often underestimate or ignore. Remember, these are only a sample of possible pathways and processes. They may be completely wrong or only reflect a subset of all the forces that determine our health. So, keep that mind of yours open. No one knows what humans are truly capable of.

What Does All This Mean?

With all this said, how might uprooting our current understanding of colds and flu impact the way we live our lives? Well, let's suppose the current model of pathogenic and contagious germs is indeed *wrong*. The implications of this would be numerous and far-reaching. Shattering the illusion of disease-causing germs could make the world a much better place to live, both on an individual and societal level. To put this into context, consider the following positives.

Individual Benefits

1. Your appreciation for the human body grows because you realise the symptoms of 'so-called' infectious diseases are not the problem, but the remedy to the problem.

2. Your relationships with other people solidify because you no longer fear catching something *from* or passing something *to* fellow humans.

3. Your connection with nature deepens because you realise it's not out to get you. Potentially, germs signal help rather than hindrance.

4. Your beliefs about the cause of disease change. Instead of disease being something you *catch* randomly and innocently, it is

something you *cultivate* much more reliably and deliberately. If you adopt improper dietary and lifestyle practices or continually expose yourself to harmful environmental materials (e.g. poisons, toxins, pollutants, chemicals), you will get sick.

5. Your perspective towards health also transforms. Just like disease, health is not caught but cultivated through proper dietary and lifestyle practices as well as minimising your exposure to harmful environmental materials. With this view, you feel engaged and empowered because you come to appreciate the amount of control you have over your own health.

Societal Benefits

1. We reallocate the precious time, money, and energy we normally dedicate to things like research, technology, and education. Our resources go towards grappling with the actual cause(s) of disease instead.

2. We offer a better standard of healthcare because our systems address the true underlying cause(s) of disease. Perhaps they bring nutrition, lifestyle, sanitation, toxins, poisons, and even psychological trauma into focus.

3. We call a ceasefire to the war against germs and lay down 'arms' in the form of invasive pharmaceutical interventions like vaccines, antiviral medication, and antibiotics.

4. We reject the need for heavy-handed public health mandates like lockdowns, quarantines, injections, social distancing, and face masks. Governments and institutions can no longer exert power over people by using fear of germs as a justification.

5. We become less tolerant of grotesque industries that install infrastructure, manufacture products, and provide services which rely on harmful and destructive substances. No more pharmaceuticals in the water supply, no more pesticides in the soil, no more micro-plastics in the air, and no more heavy metals and artificial byproducts accumulating in the ecosystem.

A Certain Contradiction

It is widely accepted, as a fact, that influenza and the common cold are caused by transmissible viruses. Most of the population embraces this belief because it aligns with their lived experience. Healthy individuals *seem* to fall ill after close contact with sick individuals. However, drawing firm conclusions from an observation is problematic because it doesn't necessarily provide any meaningful insight into how or why. So, simply witnessing groups of people becoming sick at the same time, with the same symptoms, one after another, does not necessarily mean some common agent passed between them, nor does it prove a 'virus' was present. To establish claims like these and demonstrate a cause-and-effect relationship, rigorously controlled scientific experiments are essential. As this book highlights, however, many such trials attempted to do just this over the last century and a half. Time and again, researchers exposed healthy recipients directly to sick donors and their bodily fluids. Time and again, those same researchers struggled to make people ill. Although some participants did become sick, these positive results are difficult to interpret with high levels of confidence. There are too many methodological flaws that undermine the strength of these conclusions.

This core critique is important to reiterate because it reveals a massive contradiction and 'meta' problem in society. As we've established, people cling unquestioningly to the model of contagious germs—a concept they cannot adequately explain nor sufficiently justify. But this is merely a secondary symptom of a deeper and more concerning dilemma. Namely, we live in a world where the most powerful and widespread ideas are at odds with the available evidence. To make matters worse, people willingly attack or dismiss anyone who challenges 'accepted' beliefs, despite their questionable validity. Cold and flu contagion is just one of many instances where this intellectual contradiction has occurred. Faulty ideas with flimsy support are flaunted about and fiercely protected. Thinking in this way is antithetical to a functioning and flourishing society. Collectively, we need to do better. So, what's the solution?

One option is for each person to 'flip the script' on how they build and maintain their belief system. That is, don't start at 100% certainty. Not only does this make you complacent, but you'll tend to perceive anything other than agreement as a threat. Instead, take a leap of humility and start at 0% certainty. Earn your knowledge and beliefs from the ground up, don't mindlessly inherit them. Regard your knowledge as provisional and subject to change. Realise that what you know is just a hunch until proven otherwise. This means tentatively extending trust in ideas and only increasing your confidence and conviction when you have quality data available. This sounds nice in theory, but there's an unpleasant downside. You need to get used to saying, "I don't know" and accept that, for many things, you will never know for sure. It's not as much fun to admit you might be wrong—it's a fragile ego's worst nightmare. But, ultimately, this tougher road to travel is the right one to take.

All of this is similar to the principle of 'innocent until proven guilty'. Just like in the criminal justice system, claims need to be substantiated before a verdict can be given. This resembles true scientific thinking. Unfortunately, however, many scientists don't think like this. They over-invest in 'pet' ideas and become unwilling or unable to see beyond them. There's an adage, "*science progresses one funeral at a time*" precisely for this reason. We only leave behind outdated ideas when those who derive power from them are no longer around to prop them up. It usually takes a fresh generation of thinkers to move a field forward. Bringing this back to colds and flus, experts and lay people alike need to take stock of the state of 'the science' and adjust their confidence level accordingly. It's definitely not 100 percent, so is it 90, 80, 70, or even less? Where exactly would *you* place your certainty in cold and flu contagion, given there are so many studies that do not support it? Acknowledging we have an imperfect understanding is a pre-requisite for giving others the space to engage in dialogue and debate. Even if you still think others are wrong about colds and flu, appreciate that the state and betterment of society relies on people thinking openly and flexibly. How we arrive at ideas is just as valuable as the ideas themselves.

The World's at Stake

As a final thought exercise, this book will describe two 'end game' scenarios. The first will be of a world that continues to align itself with the doctrine of contagion. The second will reject it. Now, a world ruled by contagious germs is not that difficult to imagine because everyone already knows it well. Just like in recent memory, the freedoms and liberties we enjoyed for decades have been insidiously whittled away by bureaucrats who proclaim themselves as the only ones capable of protecting humanity against an invisible enemy. Our bodily autonomy, freedom of movement, freedom of association, freedom of speech, and other inalienable human rights have become nothing more than distant memories. Governments and institutions have appointed themselves as unquestionable arbiters of truth and decreed that the science of germs is *settled*. Anyone who disagrees or dissents is deemed a threat to public safety and dealt with accordingly. Those citizens who have opted to acquiesce not only live in constant fear of the state, but of their germ-ridden family, friends, pets, surfaces, neighbours, and the very air they breathe. In ongoing efforts to thwart future pandemics, infection control measures return in force. Quarantines, entry-point screenings, lockdowns, curfews, face masks, social distancing, tracking and tracing, vaccine passports, non-essential business closures, and travel restrictions have been mandated permanently. But, remember, these protective measures didn't achieve the desired result the first time, so they only grow in form and intensity. People with a cold or flu are viewed as lepers and shunned by society. Sometimes just an innocent cough or sneeze in public is enough to get you in hot water. Germs are used as a scapegoat for diseases that are caused by some concoction of toxic man-made chemicals, processed and refined food, polluted air and water supplies, mass medication, and a dash of chronic fear. As the control state tightens its grip, memories of a free world slowly fade into oblivion, and humanity is left shackled by germ theory into perpetuity.

In contrast, a world that has untethered itself from the doctrine of contagion sees fear of sick-to-well transmission as a thing of the past. Medical, scientific, educational, and government institutions have changed course and made a concerted effort to uncover the true cause of infectious diseases. As a result, they have discovered some of the important mechanisms that keep us well versus ill. Society has shifted its focus away from killing germs and towards abolishing toxic man-made chemicals, environmental pollution, and ultra-processed foods. This has allowed them to implement targeted public health initiatives that address the things that really make people sick. Consequently, the human race has become happier, healthier, and wealthier. Such a move coincides with a deeper understanding of the relationships between health and environmental phenomena, too. Individuals in this world are more motivated and inspired to take responsibility for their own health because they have realised disease is cultivated, not caught. Natural reactions like the cold and flu are treated the way they have always been, with a box of tissues, chicken soup, and plenty of bed rest. People have also felt moved to co-exist in harmony with Mother Nature because they understand human health is inextricably linked to that of the environment.

Now, ask yourself, which of these two worlds do you want to live in? The choice is yours.

Appendix

The appendix details human experiments attempting to infect volunteers with a cold or flu.

656	417 of 4054 (10%)	2629 of 8165 (32%)
Sick donor(s)	Control recipient(s) became sick	Healthy recipient(s) became sick

Direct Exposure

Of the 203 experiments, 26 directly exposed healthy people to sick people. A total of 172 sick donors were exposed to 252 healthy recipients in every way imaginable. They lived in the same houses, slept in the same beds, drank from the same cups, kissed each other, used one another's handkerchiefs, and coughed and sneezed in each other's faces. Despite these efforts, a mere 21 recipients (12%) came down with a cold or flu. None of the studies used participant blinding, or controls.

Exposure to Bodily Fluids

Of 6,522 healthy people exposed directly (i.e., aerosols, droplets, injections) or indirectly (i.e., fomites) to the bodily fluids of sick people across 117 experiments, approximately one-third (2,125 people) developed a cold or flu. Only one-quarter of these experiments used some form of control group. Of the 1,585 control participants exposed to an inert placebo, 157 (10%) developed a cold or flu, which implies that inert substances and the nocebo effect can cause respiratory illnesses. Just one-third of the experiments used blinding, and no studies used positive controls.

Cell Culture Experiments

Across 42 experiments inoculating healthy people with cell culture fluid, 381 out of 1215 (31%) recipients contracted a cold or flu. Interestingly, 81 (7%) developed illnesses other than a cold or flu. It is debatable whether a single experiment utilized an independent variable (i.e., a purified virus sample). Less than half of the studies used negative controls or participant blinding, and none used a positive control. Of the 2,427 control recipients inoculated with an inert placebo, 252 (10%) fell ill with a cold or flu.

Exposure to Bacteria

A total of 26 experiments exposed 107 participants to cultures of bacteria (e.g. Pfeiffer's bacillus). Of these, 24 (22%) developed a cold or flu. These results are peculiar because viruses, not Pfeiffer's bacillus, are claimed to be the cause of influenza and the common cold.

Key Takeaways

Across 203 experiments, 417 of 4,054 controls (10%) became sick after exposure to an inert substance, while 2,629 of 8,165 healthy people (32%) became sick after being exposed to sick people, their bodily fluids, or cell culture fluid. A 32% positive rate is dismally low considering participants were inoculated with massive doses of so-called virus material, or exposed to sick people under conditions specifically designed to maximise disease transmission. After accounting for 'false positives' and the nocebo effect, this number drops even further to 28%. Of the 203 experiments, four of them (2%) accounted for almost half of the 2,629 positive cases. Removing these 'outliers' reduces the case rate to a woeful 22%. Meanwhile, a total of 73 experiments (36%) failed to make a single person ill. So, whilst the mean contagion rate is 32% at best, the *modal* contagion rate is 0%. In other words, the most frequently occurring experimental outcome, by far, is *no contagion.*

At face value, a 32% contagion rate might seem like evidence for viral contagion, but this conclusion is unjustified for two main reasons. *First*, the experiments lack external validity because direct inoculation methods do not reflect the natural modes of transmission. This means that, even if the contagion rate were higher, the results of these studies cannot be extrapolated to the real world. *Second*, the experiments lack internal validity because they did not implement positive controls, random sampling, or sufficient blinding. Without these measures, there is no way to know what made people sick. Participants' symptoms could have been caused by a so-called 'virus', a mechanical or chemical irritation, an allergic or inflammatory response, a nocebo effect, natural acquisition, or some other unknown factor. With so many possibilities, any conclusion drawn from these trials about the cause of the participants' symptoms is purely speculative. Ultimately, the number of high-quality scientific experiments that unambiguously demonstrate contagion is *zero*.

The next section of the appendix presents (in tables and text) the results of all 203 experiments that have been conducted over the last century attempting to demonstrate sick-to-well transmission of the cold and flu.

Appendix (Experiments 1.1 - 10.8)

1. The Bacteriology of Whooping Cough

Author(s): Davis, D.[1] **Year:** 1906

Experiment 1.1

1	0 of 0 (0%)	1 of 1 (100%)
Sick donor(s)	Control recipient(s) became sick	Healthy recipient(s) became sick

Method: Respiratory mucus was obtained from one person with whooping cough and used to culture Pfeiffer's bacillus. The cultured bacteria were mixed with saline and smeared over the throat, tonsils, and nasal mucosa of one healthy male recipient.

Result: The healthy recipient complained of a mild productive cough, headache, and fever for two days. The cough persisted for four weeks.

Notes: The recipient developed an illness different to the sick donor. No controls were used. Participants were not blinded.

2. The Causative Agents of Cough and Common Cold

Author(s): Kruse, W.[2]   **Year:** 1914

Experiment 2.1

1	0 of 0	4 of 12
	(0%)	(33%)
Sick donor(s)	Control recipient(s) became sick	Healthy recipient(s) became sick

Method: Nasal secretions from one person with a cold were mixed with saline, filtered, and dropped into the nasal cavities of 12 healthy recipients.
Result: Four healthy recipients developed symptoms of a common cold.
Notes: The causative agent was not identified. No controls were used. Participants were not blinded.

Experiment 2.2

1	0 of 0	15 of 36
	(0%)	(42%)
Sick donor(s)	Control recipient(s) became sick	Healthy recipient(s) became sick

Method: Respiratory mucus from one person with a cold was mixed with saline, filtered, and dropped into the nasal cavities of 36 healthy volunteers.
Result: Fifteen recipients developed symptoms of a common cold.
Notes: The causative agent was not identified. No controls were used. Participants were not blinded.

3. The Etiology of Common Colds

Author(s): Foster, G.[3]   **Year:** 1916

Experiment 3.1

3	0 of 0	9 of 10
	(0%)	(90%)
Sick donor(s)	Control recipient(s) became sick	Healthy recipient(s) became sick

Method: Respiratory mucus from three people with colds was mixed with saline, filtered, and dropped into the noses of 10 healthy soldiers.
Result: Nine soldiers developed common cold symptoms.
Notes: The causative agent was not identified. No controls were used. Participants were not blinded.

Experiment 3.2

3	0 of 0	11 of 11
	(0%)	(100%)
Sick donor(s)	Control recipient(s) became sick	Healthy recipient(s) became sick

Method: Respiratory mucus was obtained from three people with colds, and mixed with ascitic fluid, rabbit kidney, petroleum jelly, and saline. The solution was filtered and dropped into the noses of 11 healthy soldiers.
Result: All soldiers developed symptoms of a common cold. One soldier recovered within 8 hours and the others recovered in under a week.
Notes: The causative agent was not identified. No controls were used. Participants were not blinded.

4. Contributions to the Etiology of Colds

Author(s): Dold, V.[4]   **Year:** 1917

Experiment 4.1

1	0 of 15 (0%)	7 of 17 (41%)
Sick donor(s)	Control recipient(s) became sick	Healthy recipient(s) became sick

Method: Respiratory mucus was obtained from an individual with a cold, mixed with saline, filtered, and inoculated into 17 healthy recipients. Fifteen healthy participants served as controls and worked, ate, and slept, in the same quarters as the inoculated group.
Result: Seven of the inoculated participants developed colds.
Notes: No transmission occurred between the inoculated and control group. The causative agent was not identified. No mention of blinding.

Experiment 4.2

1	0 of 0 (0%)	1 of 40 (3%)
Sick donor(s)	Control recipient(s) became sick	Healthy recipient(s) became sick

Method: Forty patients in surgical wards were inoculated with the filtered nasal secretions obtained from an individual with a cold.
Result: One of the 40 healthy patients contracted a cold.
Notes: No mention of blinding.

Experiment 4.3

1	0 of 0 (0%)	2 of 3 (67%)
Sick donor(s)	Control recipient(s) became sick	Healthy recipient(s) became sick

Method: Respiratory mucus was obtained from a person with a cold, mixed with saline, and inoculated into three healthy volunteers.
Result: Two recipients experienced sneezing, nasal discharge, and irritation of the conjunctiva.
Notes: The causative agent was not identified. No controls were used. Participants were not blinded.

5. Pandemic Influenza & Pneumonia in a Large Civil Hospital

Author(s): Nuzum, J. & Bonar, B.[5] **Year:** 1918

Experiment 5.1

1	0 of 0 (0%)	1 of 4 (25%)
Sick donor(s)	Control recipient(s) became sick	Healthy recipient(s) became sick

Method: Mucus was obtained from a person with influenza, mixed with saline, filtered and dropped into the noses of four healthy volunteers.
Result: One recipient developed a headache, a slight temperature, and conjunctivitis. These symptoms 'rapidly disappeared'.
Notes: The authors concluded pandemic influenza was not caused by a virus. No controls were used. Participants were not blinded.

Experiment 5.2

2	0 of 0	1 of 4
	(0%)	(25%)
Sick donor(s)	Control recipient(s) became sick	Healthy recipient(s) became sick

Method: Respiratory mucus was collected from two participants, filtered, and inoculated intranasally into four healthy recipients.
Result: One recipient developed a headache, nasal discharge, conjunctivitis, and teary eyes. The symptoms resolved within 24 hours. The other recipients remained well.
Notes: The causative agent was not identified. No controls were used. Participants were not blinded.

Experiment 5.3

1	0 of 0	0 of 1
	(0%)	(0%)
Sick donor(s)	Control recipient(s) became sick	Healthy recipient(s) became sick

Method: Tracheal and bronchial tissue was obtained from a man who had died from influenza, ground up into a paste, mixed with sterile saline, centrifuged, and filtered. This solution was inoculated into the nasal cavity and injected intravenously into a rhesus monkey.
Result: The monkey remained perfectly well.
Notes: No controls were used.

Experiment 5.4

4	0 of 0	0 of 1
	(0%)	(0%)
Sick donor(s)	Control recipient(s) became sick	Healthy recipient(s) became sick

Method: Respiratory mucus was obtained from four people with influenza. Approximately 2 mL of the mixed washings were inoculated into the monkey used in experiment 5.3.
Result: The monkey remained perfectly well.
Notes: No controls were used.

6. On the Etiology of Influenza

Author(s): Selter, H.[6]   **Year:** 1918

Experiment 6.1

5	0 of 0	2 of 2
	(0%)	(100%)
Sick donor(s)	Control recipient(s) became sick	Healthy recipient(s) became sick

Method: Respiratory mucus was collected from five influenza patients, filtered, put in an atomizer, and sprayed into the nasal cavities of the author and his assistant.
Result: The author developed a headache and coryza which resolved within 12 hours. The assistant developed mild joint pain, chills, and coryza. These symptoms lasted for two days.
Notes: It is doubtful whether either recipient developed influenza. The causative agent was not identified. No controls were used. The participants were not blinded.

7. Some Experimental Notions on the Influenza Virus

Author(s): Nicolle, C. & Lebailly, C.[7] **Year:** 1918

Experiment 7.1

?	0 of 0	2 of 3
	(0%)	(66%)
Sick donor(s)	Control recipient(s) became sick	Healthy recipient(s) became sick

Method: Respiratory mucus was collected from patients with influenza and inoculated into a monkey. The mucus was then mixed with saline, filtered, and injected subcutaneously into two healthy men.
Result: The monkey developed a fever. One man developed a headache, fatigue, and a mild fever. The other man remained completely healthy.
Notes: Injection of a foreign substance directly into the body does not reflect the natural routes of transmission. It is doubtful whether the recipient developed influenza. The causative agent was not identified. No controls were used. Participants were not blinded.

Experiment 7.2

1	0 of 0	0 of 1
	(0%)	(0%)
Sick donor(s)	Control recipient(s) became sick	Healthy recipient(s) became sick

Method: A blood sample was collected from the monkey in experiment 7.1. and injected subcutaneously into one healthy volunteer.
Result: The healthy recipient remained completely well.
Notes: No controls were used. The participant was not blinded.

Experiment 7.3

1	0 of 0 (0%)	0 of 1 (0%)
Sick donor(s)	Control recipient(s) became sick	Healthy recipient(s) became sick

Method: A blood sample was collected from the monkey in experiment 7.1. and injected subcutaneously into one healthy volunteer.
Result: The healthy recipient remained completely well.
Notes: No controls were used. The participant was not blinded.

Experiment 7.4

1	0 of ? (0%)	2 of 3 (66%)
Sick donor(s)	Control recipient(s) became sick	Healthy recipient(s) became sick

Method: Lung fluid from an influenza patient was inoculated into a monkey. The lung fluid was also filtered and injected intravenously into one healthy man and subcutaneously into another.
Result: The monkey developed a fever. The man injected intravenously remained well. The man injected subcutaneously developed mild flu-like symptoms. He shared quarters with several healthy people (control group), none of whom developed influenza.
Notes: The injection of a foreign substance does not reflect a natural transmission route. Participants were not blinded.

8. Is Influenza a Filterable Virus Disease?

Author(s): Dujarric de la Rivière, R.[8]   **Year:** 1918

Experiment 8.1

4	0 of 0 (0%)	1 of 1 (100%)
Sick donor(s)	Control recipient(s) became sick	Healthy recipient(s) became sick

Method: Blood from four influenza patients was pooled together, and filtered. The author injected himself with 4 mL of the blood.
Result: The author developed a headache, muscle pain, chills, and a slight temperature. He recovered within 24 hours.
Notes: It is unlikely that the author developed influenza. The causative agent was not identified. No controls were used. The participant was not blinded.

9. Experiments Upon Volunteers to Determine the Cause and Mode of Spread of Influenza (Boston)

Author(s): Rosenau, M., Keegan, W. & Goldberger, G.[9]   **Year:** 1918

Introduction: The following experiments were undertaken by the United States Navy and the United States Public Health Service in the city of Boston in November and December of 1918. This is the first of three series of experiments. They are arguably the most comprehensive human contagion experiments ever undertaken in the history of medicine. These experiments were conducted at the height of the Spanish Influenza epidemic to determine the cause and mode of spread of the disease.

The men subjected to these experiments were all volunteers from the United States Naval Training Station located in Deer Island, Boston. There were 62 men in total ranging in age from 15 – 34 years, with 54 of them aged between 18 – 21 years. All men were in excellent physical condition.

Of the 62 subjects, 39 reported they had never previously contracted influenza at any point during their lives. Eight of the 62 men had been ill the previous flu season with non-specific symptoms that may or may not have been influenza.

At the time of these experiments, an epidemic of influenza had broken out at the naval base on Deer Island and the sick men at the local naval hospital and surrounding military hospitals were used as a source of infectious material (i.e., body fluids). As the participants were all sailors stationed at naval hospitals, they could be carefully monitored to observe any response following each experiment.

Experiment 9.1

1	0 of 0 (0%)	0 of 6 (0%)
Sick donor(s)	Control recipient(s) became sick	Healthy recipient(s) became sick

Method: Pfeiffer's bacillus was isolated from the sputum of a sailor with influenza and cultured. The cultured bacteria were mixed with saline, and 0.5 mL was instilled into the nostrils of six healthy sailors.
Result: None of the sailors became sick.
Notes: No controls were used. The participants were not blinded.

Experiment 9.2

16	0 of 0 (0%)	0 of 20 (0%)
Sick donor(s)	Control recipient(s) became sick	Healthy recipient(s) became sick

Method: Respiratory mucus was collected from 16 sailors with influenza and mixed with saline. Approximately 6 mL of the solution was sprayed into the noses and throats of 10 healthy sailors. Some of the solution was swallowed. The unfiltered secretions were then filtered and exposed to a different group of 10 healthy men.
Result: None of the 20 men became unwell.
Notes: No controls were used. The participants were not blinded.

Experiment 9.3

4	0 of 0 (0%)	0 of 10 (0%)
Sick donor(s)	Control recipient(s) became sick	Healthy recipient(s) became sick

Method: Respiratory mucus samples were obtained from four influenza patients. The secretions were pooled together, and 6 mL was instilled into the eyes and noses of each of the 10 healthy sailors.
Result: None of the 10 healthy recipients became sick.
Notes: No controls were used. The participants were not blinded.

Experiment 9.4

10	0 of 0 (0%)	0 of 19 (0%)
Sick donor(s)	Control recipient(s) became sick	Healthy recipient(s) became sick

Method: Using a swab, respiratory mucus was transferred directly from 10 sailors with influenza into the noses and throats of 19 healthy sailors.
Result: None of the 19 healthy participants became unwell.
Notes: No controls were used. The participants were not blinded.

Experiment 9.5

3	0 of 0 (0%)	0 of 10 (0%)
Sick donor(s)	Control recipient(s) became sick	Healthy recipient(s) became sick

Method: Respiratory mucus from three people with influenza was mixed with saline and filtered. Approximately 2 mL of the mucus was injected subcutaneously into each of the 10 healthy recipients.
Result: None of the healthy recipients became sick.
Notes: No controls were used. The participants were not blinded.

Experiment 9.6

5	0 of 0 (0%)	0 of 10 (0%)
Sick donor(s)	Control recipient(s) became sick	Healthy recipient(s) became sick

Method: Approximately 20 mL of blood was drawn from five influenza patients and mixed with saline. The blood samples were pooled together, and 1 mL was injected subcutaneously into each of the 10 healthy recipients.

Result: None of the men became ill.

Notes: No controls were used. The participants were not blinded.

Experiment 9.7

30	0 of 0 (0%)	0 of 10 (0%)
Sick donor(s)	Control recipient(s) became sick	Healthy recipient(s) became sick

Method: Ten healthy sailors were taken to a quarantine ward where 30 men were being treated for influenza. Each of the sailors sat next to the bed of a sick man and spoke with each other face-to-face for two to three minutes. The sick man was directed to breathe five times and cough five times into the face of a sailor, whilst the sailor breathed in. The sailor repeated the process with another 10 patients. The total exposure time was between 30 - 50 minutes.

Result: None of the healthy men became ill.

Notes: No controls were used. The participants were not blinded.

Experiment 9.8

13	0 of 0	2 of 19
	(0%)	(11%)
Sick donor(s)	Control recipient(s) became sick	Healthy recipient(s) became sick

Method: Pfeiffer's bacillus was isolated from 13 different cases of influenza, cultured, mixed with saline and sprayed into the nasal cavities and throats of 19 healthy men.

Results: One man vomited and complained of malaise, but was ill before the experiment. Another man experienced a headache, sore throat, and a mild temperature. Both men recovered within 24 hours.

Notes: The two instances of illness were not cases of Spanish flu and cannot be considered proof of transmission. No controls were used. The participants were not blinded.

10. Experiments Upon Volunteers to Determine the Cause and Mode of Spread of Influenza (San Francisco)

Author(s): McCoy, G. & Richey, D.[10]   **Year:** 1918

Introduction: The following experiments were undertaken by the United States Navy and the United States Public Health Service in the city of San Francisco in November and December of 1918. This is the second of three experiments. These experiments were conducted at the United States Quarantine Station on Angel Island, San Francisco.

The men subjected to these experiments were all volunteers from the United States Naval Training Station, Yerba Buena. There were 50 men in total, all of whom had been quarantined for one month before the experiments. Of the 50 men, only five had fallen ill with influenza in the previous season and 46 had suffered from influenza at some point in their lives. The age of the men ranged from 18 – 23 and they were all in very good physical condition. As per the previous set of experiments, the sailors who volunteered were carefully monitored by naval doctors to observe any response following each experiment.

Experiment 10.1

1	0 of 4 (0%)	0 of 6 (0%)
Sick donor(s)	Control recipient(s) became sick	Healthy recipient(s) became sick

Method: Respiratory mucus from a girl with influenza was mixed with sterile beef broth and dropped into the noses and throats of three men. Filtered secretions were dropped into the nasopharynx of another three men. Four men served as controls and received sterile water.
Result: None of the volunteers in the active or control groups became ill.
Notes: The participants were not blinded.

Experiment 10.2

1	0 of 2 (0%)	1 of 8 (13%)
Sick donor(s)	Control recipient(s) became sick	Healthy recipient(s) became sick

Method: Mucus from the respiratory tract of an infant with influenza was mixed with sterile beef broth and instilled into the nasal cavities of four men. Another four men were inoculated with the *filtered* secretions. Two men served as controls.
Result: One recipient developed tonsilitis, a headache, and constipation. His symptoms resolved within four days.
Notes: The participant who developed tonsilitis had a history of recurrent tonsilitis. This was not a case of influenza and therefore cannot be considered a positive case of influenza transmission. No controls were used. The participants were not blinded.

Experiment 10.3

1	0 of 2 (0%)	0 of 8 (0%)
Sick donor(s)	Control recipient(s) became sick	Healthy recipient(s) became sick

Method: Lung fluid samples were collected from a man with influenza and used to culture Pfeiffer's bacillus. The bacteria were mixed with beef bouillon, filtered, and sprayed into the mouth and nose of four healthy men. An additional man acted as a control and received no intervention. The *unfiltered* solution was also exposed to another group of four men. An additional man acted as a control and received no intervention.
Result: All participants remained perfectly well.
Notes: The participants were not blinded.

Experiment 10.4

1	0 of 0 (0%)	2 of 10 (20%)
Sick donor(s)	Control recipient(s) became sick	Healthy recipient(s) became sick

Method: Respiratory mucus was collected from a man with influenza, put in an atomiser and sprayed into the noses and throats of 10 healthy sailors.
Result: Two men developed tonsilitis which lasted four days. The other eight men remained completely healthy despite being in close contact with the two cases of tonsilitis.
Notes: The supervising doctors remarked that they had no reason to believe that these positive cases were attacks of influenza. No controls were used. The participants were not blinded.

Experiment 10.5

1	0 of 2 (0%)	0 of 4 (0%)
Sick donor(s)	Control recipient(s) became sick	Healthy recipient(s) became sick

Method: Respiratory mucus was obtained from a female nurse with influenza and mixed with saline. The *unfiltered* solution was sprayed into the nose and throat of two men. The solution was then *filtered* and sprayed into the noses and throats of two healthy men. Two other men remained as controls and received no intervention.
Result: None of the participants became unwell.
Notes: The participants were not blinded.

Experiment 10.6

1	0 of 0 (0%)	0 of 2 (0%)
Sick donor(s)	Control recipient(s) became sick	Healthy recipient(s) became sick

Method: Filtered mucus from experiment 10.5 was dropped into the conjunctiva of two healthy men.
Result: Neither man became sick.
Notes: No controls were used. The participants were not blinded.

Experiment 10.7

1	0 of 0 (0%)	0 of 1 (0%)
Sick donor(s)	Control recipient(s) became sick	Healthy recipient(s) became sick

Method: The mucus from experiment 10.5 was taken up into a syringe. Precisely 2 mL of the filtered mucus solution was injected subcutaneously into the deltoid muscle of the left arm of one healthy volunteer.
Result: The man did not develop any symptoms.
Notes: No controls were used. The participants were not blinded.

Experiment 10.8

1	0 of 0 (0%)	0 of 1 (0%)
Sick donor(s)	Control recipient(s) became sick	Healthy recipient(s) became sick

Method: A female nurse with influenza had 10 mL of blood collected from her left arm. The blood was mixed with one per cent sodium citrate solution and injected into the left arm of a healthy sailor.
Result: The male recipient remained completely healthy.
Notes: No controls were used. The participants were not blinded. The doctors undertaking these experiments stated their disbelief that not a single man fell ill with influenza despite their most desperate attempts.

Appendix (Experiments 11.1 - 20.3)

11. Experiments Upon Volunteers to Determine the Cause and Mode of Spread of Influenza (Boston)

Author(s): Rosenau, M., Keegan, W. & Richey, D.[11]   **Year:** 1919

Introduction: The following experiments were conducted at the United States Quarantine Station on Gallups Island, Boston, in February and March of 1919. The volunteers, 49 in total, came from the United States Naval Detention Training Camp located on Deer Island, Massachusetts. They ranged in age from 19 – 36 years of age and were in very good physical condition. Two of the men had contracted influenza in the previous flu season. The rest of the 47 men had not suffered from influenza in the previous season, suggesting that they were unlikely to be immune.

Experiment 11.1

?	0 of 0	0 of 10
	(0%)	(0%)
Sick donor(s)	Control recipient(s) became sick	Healthy recipient(s) became sick

Method: Bacteria isolated from cases of influenza were cultured and added to sterile broth. A thick solution totaling 1.5 mL was sprayed and dropped into the nasal cavities and throats of 10 healthy sailors.
Result: All 10 men remained completely healthy.
Notes: No controls were used. The participants were not blinded.

Experiment 11.2

1	0 of 0 (0%)	2 of 10 (20%)
Sick donor(s)	Control recipient(s) became sick	Healthy recipient(s) became sick

Method: Respiratory mucus was obtained from a naval doctor who developed influenza, mixed with saline, inoculated into the nasal cavities and throats of 10 healthy men.

Result: One man developed tonsilitis, and another developed an influenza-like illness. The other eight men remained well.

Notes: The man with tonsilitis had a history of the condition for several years. The man who developed the influenza-like illness was diagnosed with a "a syndrome somewhere between influenza and a sore throat". No controls were used. The participants were not blinded.

Experiment 11.3

?	0 of 0 (0%)	1 of 10 (10%)
Sick donor(s)	Control recipient(s) became sick	Healthy recipient(s) became sick

Method: Bacterial cultures of Pfeiffer's bacillus and *Staphylococcus aureus*, were mixed with 30 mL of beef broth. Ten healthy men each had 3 mL (approximately 5 billion bacteria) of the solution sprayed and dropped into their noses and throats. Three of the men gargled a two per cent sodium bicarbonate solution before inoculation whilst another three gargled with 0.5 per cent acetic acid.

Result: One man developed acute tonsilitis.

Notes: No controls were used. The participants were not blinded.

Experiment 11.4

1	0 of 0 (0%)	0 of 10 (0%)
Sick donor(s)	Control recipient(s) became sick	Healthy recipient(s) became sick

Method: Respiratory mucus was collected from a patient with influenza. Approximately 3 mL of the mucus was instilled into the nasal cavities and throats of 10 healthy men. Three men also had capsicum oleoresin sprayed into their nasal cavities, whilst another received adrenaline.
Result: None of the men became ill.
Notes: No controls were used. The participants were not blinded.

Experiment 11.5

10	0 of 0 (0%)	2 of 4 (50%)
Sick donor(s)	Control recipient(s) became sick	Healthy recipient(s) became sick

Method: Respiratory mucus was collected from four influenza patients and sprayed and dropped into the nose and throat of four healthy participants. Mucus was also collected from six other influenza patients and mixed with fresh milk. Each of the four healthy men drank 250 mL of the milk which contained 2.5 mL of the mucus.
Result: Two of the men developed tonsilitis and recovered completely within 48 hours.
Notes: No controls were used. The participants were not blinded.

Experiment 11.6

10	0 of 0 (0%)	0 of 4 (0%)
Sick donor(s)	Control recipient(s) became sick	Healthy recipient(s) became sick

Method: Ten healthy men recently exposed to people with influenza had their nasal cavities and throats washed out with saline. This was done in the hope that the infectious agent might only be present (and therefore transmissible) in the respiratory tract before the onset of symptoms. Approximately 10 mL of the washings were sprayed and dropped into the nose and throat of four healthy volunteers.

Result: All of the recipients remained healthy.

Notes: No controls were used. The participants were not blinded.

Experiment 11.7

1	0 of 0 (0%)	5 of 10 (50%)
Sick donor(s)	Control recipient(s) became sick	Healthy recipient(s) became sick

Method: Respiratory mucus was collected from one of the men in experiment 11.5 who developed tonsilitis. The mucus was mixed with saline and inoculated into the noses and throats of each of the 10 healthy volunteers.

Result: Four of the men developed tonsilitis. One man developed influenza-like symptoms. All men recovered completely within one week. The other five men remained well.

Notes: The causative agent was not identified. No controls were used. The participants were not blinded.

Experiment 11.8

3	0 of 0 (0%)	1 of 9 (11%)
Sick donor(s)	Control recipient(s) became sick	Healthy recipient(s) became sick

Method: Respiratory mucus was obtained from three men with influenza, and inoculated into the noses and throats of nine healthy men.

Result: One man developed symptoms of influenza (a cough, general body pain, temperature, and light sensitivity). He recovered within a week. The other eight men remained completely well.

Notes: The causative agent was not identified. The authors stated the case of influenza might have been naturally acquired. No control group was used. The participants were not blinded.

Experiment 11.9

1	0 of 1 (0%)	3 of 14 (21%)
Sick donor(s)	Control recipient(s) became sick	Healthy recipient(s) became sick

Method: Mucus secretions from a patient were mixed with saline and inoculated into the noses and throats of 14 healthy recipients. One man served as a control.

Result: Three men developed tonsilitis.

Notes: The participants were not blinded.

12. The Infecting Agent of Influenza

Author(s): Yamanouchi, T., Sakakami, K. et al.[12]   **Year:** 1919

Experiment 12.1

43	0 of 0	18 of 24
	(0%)	(75%)
Sick donor(s)	Control recipient(s) became sick	Healthy recipient(s) became sick

Method: The lung fluid of 43 patients with influenza was mixed with Ringer's solution and inoculated into the noses and throats of 12 people. The solution was *filtered* and inoculated into another 12 people.
Result: Eighteen recipients developed influenza. Six recipients remained well, however, they had recently recovered from influenza and were considered immune.
Notes: The causative agent was not identified. No adequate controls were used. Participants were not blinded.

Experiment 12.2

?	0 of 0	6 of 6
	(0%)	(100%)
Sick donor(s)	Control recipient(s) became sick	Healthy recipient(s) became sick

Method: Blood was collected from people with influenza and inoculated into the noses and throats of six healthy people.
Result: All recipients developed influenza.
Notes: The causative agent was not identified. No adequate controls were used. Participants were not blinded.

Experiment 12.3

43	0 of 0 (0%)	7 of 8 (88%)
Sick donor(s)	Control recipient(s) became sick	Healthy recipient(s) became sick

Method: The *filtered* sputum from experiment 12.1 was injected subcutaneously into four healthy participants. The *unfiltered* sputum was also injected into another four healthy participants.
Result: Seven of the eight recipients developed influenza. The participant who did not fall ill reported recovering from influenza previously.
Notes: The causative agent was not identified. No adequate controls were used. Participants were not blinded.

Experiment 12.4

?	0 of 0 (0%)	0 of 14 (0%)
Sick donor(s)	Control recipient(s) became sick	Healthy recipient(s) became sick

Method: Pfeiffer's bacillus was mixed with pneumococci, streptococci, staphylococci, and diplococci and inoculated into the nose and throat of 14 participants.
Result: All recipients remained well.
Notes: Pathogenic bacteria did not induce illness in healthy people. No controls were used. The participants were not blinded.

13. On the Etiological Problem of Today's Influenza Pandemic

Author(s): Michelli, F. & Satta, G.[13]   **Year:** 1919

Experiment 13.1

5	0 of 0 (0%)	0 of 12 (0%)
Sick donor(s)	Control recipient(s) became sick	Healthy recipient(s) became sick

Method: Respiratory mucus was obtained from five people with influenza, mixed with saline, whey, and filtered. Twelve healthy men were injected subcutaneously with the solution.
Result: None of the men became ill.
Notes: The authors concluded influenza cannot be transmitted through exposure to mucus secretions injected into the body. No controls were used. The participants were not blinded.

Experiment 13.2

1	0 of 0 (0%)	0 of 6 (0%)
Sick donor(s)	Control recipient(s) became sick	Healthy recipient(s) became sick

Method: Blood was drawn from a sick patient with influenza, left unfiltered, defibrinated, and injected subcutaneously into six healthy men.
Result: None of the healthy participants became sick.
Notes: The authors concluded that influenza cannot be transmitted via exposure to infected blood. No controls were used. Participants were not blinded.

14. Research on the Etiology of Influenza

Author(s): Paraf, J. & Goubalt, A.[14]   **Year:** 1919

Experiment 14.1

?	0 of 0 (0%)	0 of 8 (0%)
Sick donor(s)	Control recipient(s) became sick	Healthy recipient(s) became sick

Method: Respiratory mucus was filtered, sprayed into the noses of four men, and injected subcutaneously into four others.
Result: All eight participants remained completely healthy.
Notes: No controls were used. Participants were not blinded.

15. Pandemic Influenza in Korea

Author(s): Schofield, F. & Cynn, H.[15]   **Year:** 1919

Experiment 15.1

2	0 of 0 (0%)	2 of 3 (67%)
Sick donor(s)	Control recipient(s) became sick	Healthy recipient(s) became sick

Method: *Unfiltered* blood from influenza patients was injected intravenously into two men. *Filtered* blood was injected into one man.
Result: One man developed flu-like symptoms, and one developed a mild flu. The other man remained well.
Notes: The causative agent was not identified. No controls were used. Participants were not blinded.

Experiment 15.2

1	0 of 0 (0%)	0 of 2 (0%)
Sick donor(s)	Control recipient(s) became sick	Healthy recipient(s) became sick

Method: Blood was drawn from one person with influenza and filtered. Two healthy participants were injected with 2 mL of the blood.
Result: Both participants remained well.
Notes: No controls were used. Participants were not blinded.

Experiment 15.3

1	0 of 0 (0%)	2 of 2 (100%)
Sick donor(s)	Control recipient(s) became sick	Healthy recipient(s) became sick

Method: Lung fluid was obtained from a case of influenza, mixed with saline, centrifuged, and filtered. Two healthy recipients were then injected with 2 mL of the solution.
Result: Both healthy participants became acutely ill with chills, vomiting, rapid pulse, headache, and muscle pains for six hours.
Notes: The authors concluded that the participants had become ill with acute toxaemia. This result highlights that a flu-like illness can be produced in response to a toxin. No controls were used. Participants were not blinded.

Experiment 15.4

1	0 of 0	0 of 1
	(0%)	(0%)
Sick donor(s)	Control recipient(s) became sick	Healthy recipient(s) became sick

Method: The lung fluid from a case of influenza was prepared in the same manner as Exp. 15.3 Precisely 2 mL of the filtered lung fluid was injected intravenously into a healthy man.
Result: The man remained completely healthy.
Notes: No controls were used. Participants were not blinded.

16. Experimental Investigation of Epidemic Influenza at Durban

Authors(s): Lister, F & Taylor, E.[16] **Year:** 1919

Experiment 16.1

?	0 of 0	1 of 9
	(0%)	(11%)
Sick donor(s)	Control recipient(s) became sick	Healthy recipient(s) became sick

Method: Pfeiffer's bacillus and two other strains of cocci bacteria were inoculated into the noses and throats of nine healthy men.
Result: One of the men developed influenza.
Notes: The authors concluded that the bacteria did not cause the case of influenza. No controls were used. The participants were not blinded.

Experiment 16.2

?	0 of 0	0 of 11
	(0%)	(0%)
Sick donor(s)	Control recipient(s) became sick	Healthy recipient(s) became sick

Method: Healthy volunteers were taken by boat, to a remote island 500 miles from their hometown, where influenza had not yet occurred. Respiratory mucus was collected from people with influenza, mixed with saline, filtered, and inoculated into the noses of 11 healthy men.
Result: None of the men became unwell.
Notes: No controls were used. The participants were not blinded.

Experiment 16.3

?	0 of 0	2 of 5
	(0%)	(40%)
Sick donor(s)	Control recipient(s) became sick	Healthy recipient(s) became sick

Method: Mucus from experiment 16.1 was left unfiltered and then inoculated into the nasal cavities of 5 healthy men.
Result: Two of the men developed symptoms of influenza.
Notes: Specific details about the methodology and results (i.e. symptoms) were not available. No firm conclusions can be deduced from this experiment. No controls were used. The participants were not blinded.

17. Some experiments on the Transmission of Influenza

Author(s): Wahl, H., White, G. & Lyall, H.[17]   **Year:** 1919

Experiment 17.1

2	0 of 0	0 of 2
	(0%)	(0%)
Sick donor(s)	Control recipient(s) became sick	Healthy recipient(s) became sick

Method: Lung tissue was removed from a person who had died from influenza and another person who was suffering from influenza. Ten grams of the lung tissue was finely chopped, ground up with saline and sterile sand in a mortar, centrifuged, and filtered. The solution was sprayed into the nostrils and throats of two healthy volunteers.
Result: Both healthy recipients remained well.
Notes: No controls were used. The participants were not blinded.

Experiment 17.2

1	0 of 0	0 of 5
	(0%)	(0%)
Sick donor(s)	Control recipient(s) became sick	Healthy recipient(s) became sick

Method: Pfeiffer's bacillus was isolated from a person with influenza and cultured. The bacteria were mixed with saline and inoculated into five healthy volunteers.
Result: The recipients remained well.
Notes: No controls were used. The participants were not blinded.

Experiment 17.3

1	0 of 0 (0%)	0 of 5 (0%)
Sick donor(s)	Control recipient(s) became sick	Healthy recipient(s) became sick

Method: Pfeiffer's bacillus was isolated from a person who had died from influenza. The bacteria were mixed with a saline solution and "massive doses" were inoculated into five healthy recipients.
Result: One man had a slight local reaction that resolved rapidly. The other recipients remained well.
Notes: No controls were used. The participants were not blinded.

18. The Occurrence of the Pfeiffer Bacillus in Measles

Author(s): Sellards, A. & Strum, E.[18]   **Year:** 1919

Experiment 18.1

5	0 of 0 (0%)	0 of 4 (0%)
Sick donor(s)	Control recipient(s) became sick	Healthy recipient(s) became sick

Method: Pfeiffer's bacillus isolated from measles patients were mixed with saline, and inoculated into four healthy recipients.
Result: All four recipients remained completely well.
Notes: No controls were used. The participants were not blinded.

19. The Fate of Influenza Bacilli

Author(s): Bloomfield, A.[19] **Year:** 1920

Experiment 19.1

?	0 of 0 (0%)	0 of 14 (0%)
Sick donor(s)	Control recipient(s) became sick	Healthy recipient(s) became sick

Method: Three strains of Pfeiffer's bacillus were isolated from influenza patients. The bacteria were cultured and then swabbed onto the tongue, nasal septum, nasopharynx, and tonsils of 14 volunteers.
Result: All recipients remained completely healthy.
Notes: No controls were used. The participants were not blinded.

20. On the Etiology of Colds and Influenza

Author(s): Schmidt, P.[20] **Year:** 1920

Experiment 20.1

16	0 of 0 (0%)	24 of 196 (12%)
Sick donor(s)	Control recipient(s) became sick	Healthy recipient(s) became sick

Method: Respiratory mucus was obtained from 16 people with common colds and filtered. One drop of the solution was inoculated into the conjunctiva of both eyes of 196 healthy participants.
Result: Three recipients developed flu and 21 developed colds.
Notes: Some participants developed an illness different from the one being studied. Participants were not blinded.

Experiment 20.2

12	0 of 0 (0%)	9 of 84 (11%)
Sick donor(s)	Control recipient(s) became sick	Healthy recipient(s) became sick

Method: Respiratory mucus was obtained from 12 people with influenza. The secretions were filtered and dropped into the conjunctiva of 84 healthy recipients. Both nostrils were also swabbed with the mucus.
Result: Five recipients developed influenza and four developed colds.
Notes: Some of the participants developed an illness different from the one being studied. Participants were not blinded.

Experiment 20.3

0	8 of 43 (19%)	0 of 0 (0%)
Sick donor(s)	Control recipient(s) became sick	Healthy recipient(s) became sick

Method: Saline solution was inoculated into 43 healthy volunteers.
Result: Eight healthy volunteers developed a common cold.
Notes: A higher percentage of people who received physiological saline solution developed a common cold compared to those being exposed to the mucus secretions of people with colds and flu (Exp. 20.1 & 20.2). The author concluded that the results do not support the assumption that influenza and the common cold are caused by viruses.

Appendix (Experiments 21.1 - 30.1)

21. Acute Respiratory Infection in Man

Author(s): Cecil, R. & Steffen, G.[21]   **Year:** 1921

Experiment 21.1

2	0 of 0 (0%)	2 of 2 (100%)
Sick donor(s)	Control recipient(s) became sick	Healthy recipient(s) became sick

Method: Pfeiffer's bacillus was mixed with sterile broth and inoculated into the noses and throats of two healthy volunteers.
Result: Both participants developed a mild influenza-like illness including headache, sore throat, rhinitis, malaise, and nasal obstruction.
Notes: Pfeiffer's bacillus induced an influenza-like illness despite not being the cause of influenza. The participants were not blinded.

Experiment 21.2

1	0 of 0 (0%)	2 of 2 (100%)
Sick donor(s)	Control recipient(s) became sick	Healthy recipient(s) became sick

Method: Pfeiffer's bacillus were injected directly into the abdominal cavity of a monkey. Within 24 hours the monkey had died. Fluid from the monkey's abdomen was inoculated into the nostrils of two healthy volunteers. A cotton swab soaked in the abdominal fluid was also swabbed over the throats of both volunteers.

Result: Both volunteers developed symptoms of an influenza-like illness including a headache, rhinitis, cough, malaise, pharyngitis, sore throat, backache, and conjunctivitis.

Notes: The methods do not reflect the natural route of transmission. The causative agent was never identified. The participants were not blinded.

Experiment 21.3

1	0 of 0 (0%)	2 of 2 (100%)
Sick donor(s)	Control recipient(s) became sick	Healthy recipient(s) became sick

Method: Pfeiffer's bacillus was isolated from a patient with influenza and cultured in a blood broth. Approximately 0.5 mL was inoculated into the nostrils of two healthy recipients.

Result: Both recipients fell ill with an influenza-like illness. They experienced headaches, rhinitis, malaise, pharyngitis, tracheitis, conjunctivitis, backache, and a sore chest.

Notes: Pfeiffer's bacillus induced an influenza-like illness despite not being the cause of influenza. The participants were not blinded.

Experiment 21.4

1	0 of 0 (0%)	0 of 2 (0%)
Sick donor(s)	Control recipient(s) became sick	Healthy recipient(s) became sick

Method: Pfeiffer's bacillus was isolated from a patient with influenza and cultured in a blood broth. The broth was filtered and then inoculated into the nose of two recipients.
Result: Both participants remained completely well.
Notes: The participants were not blinded.

Experiment 21.5

1	0 of 0 (0%)	1 of 2 (50%)
Sick donor(s)	Control recipient(s) became sick	Healthy recipient(s) became sick

Method: *Streptococcus hemolyticus* was isolated from a patient with acute tonsilitis and inoculated intranasally into two healthy recipients. Their throats were also swabbed with the bacteria.
Result: One volunteer developed an inflamed sore throat which lasted a few hours whilst the other patient remained completely well.
Notes: Neither volunteer was seriously adversely affected after being directly exposed to a pathogenic bacterium that allegedly causes pharyngitis, tonsilitis, and pneumonia. No mention of blinding.

Experiment 21.6

2	0 of 0 (0%)	0 of 2 (0%)
Sick donor(s)	Control recipient(s) became sick	Healthy recipient(s) became sick

Method: A 'highly virulent' pneumococcus bacteria strain was isolated from a sick patient with pneumonia, and a patient with acute tonsilitis. Two healthy recipients were inoculated intranasally with 0.5 mL of a blood broth culture containing the bacteria. Their throats were also swabbed with the bacteria.

Result: Both healthy recipients remained well.

Notes: Neither volunteer fell ill after being directly exposed to a pathogenic bacterium that allegedly causes pharyngitis, tonsilitis, and pneumonia. No mention of blinding.

22. Studies on Acute Respiratory Infections

Author(s): Williams, A., Nevin, M. & Gurley, C.[22] **Year:** 1921

Experiment 22.1

7	0 of 0 (0%)	0 of 45 (0%)
Sick donor(s)	Control recipient(s) became sick	Healthy recipient(s) became sick

Method: Respiratory mucus was collected from seven people with influenza, mixed with saline, and filtered. The solution was then dropped into the nasal cavities of 45 healthy recipients.

Result: Every single recipient remained well.

Notes: No controls were used. The participants were not blinded.

23. Experimental Human Inoculations with Filtered Nasal Secretions from Acute Coryza

Author(s): Robertson, R. & Groves, R.[23]   **Year:** 1924

Experiment 23.1

11	0 of 0 (0%)	5 of 100 (5%)
Sick donor(s)	Control recipient(s) became sick	Healthy recipient(s) became sick

Method: Respiratory mucus from people with common colds was mixed with saline, filtered, and sprayed into the nostrils of 100 healthy volunteers.
Result: One volunteer developed bronchitis, one developed a cold, one developed influenza, and two developed laryngitis.
Notes: The authors concluded the positive cases were naturally acquired. No controls were used. The participants were not blinded.

24. Production of Cold with Micrococcus Catarrhalis

Author(s): Walker, J.[24]   **Year:** 1929

Experiment 24.1

0	0 of 0 (0%)	1 of 1 (100%)
Sick donor(s)	Control recipient(s) became sick	Healthy recipient(s) became sick

Method: *Micrococcus catarrhalis* was cultured, diluted in saline, and sprayed into the nostrils of one healthy volunteer.
Result: The recipient developed an acute cold for three days.
Notes: No controls were used. The participants were not blinded.

Experiment 24.2

0	0 of 0 (0%)	0 of 1 (0%)
Sick donor(s)	Control recipient(s) became sick	Healthy recipient(s) became sick

Method: *Micrococcus catarrhalis* was cultured, diluted in saline, and sprayed into the nostrils of one healthy volunteer with an atomizer.
Result: The healthy recipient remained well.
Notes: No controls were used. The participant was not blinded.

Experiment 24.3

0	0 of 0 (0%)	1 of 1 (100%)
Sick donor(s)	Control recipient(s) became sick	Healthy recipient(s) became sick

Method: *Micrococcus catarrhalis* was cultured, diluted in saline, and sprayed into the nostrils of one healthy volunteer with an atomizer.
Result: The recipient developed symptoms of a moderate cold including a headache, nasal congestion, and profuse nasal discharge.
Notes: No controls were used. The participant was not blinded.

25. Studies of the Etiology of the Common Cold

Author(s): Dochez, A., Shibley, G. & Mills, K.[25]   **Year:** 1930

Experiment 25.1

?	0 of 0	4 of 9
	(0%)	(44%)
Sick donor(s)	Control recipient(s) became sick	Healthy recipient(s) became sick

Method: Respiratory mucus was collected from people with influenza, filtered, and inoculated intranasally into nine men.
Result: Four of the nine participants developed colds.
Notes: One participant was told he was inoculated with infected mucus. Later that evening he developed a severe cold. The next day it was revealed he received saline. His symptoms resolved within the hour.

26. Study of the Virus of the Common Cold

Author(s): Dochez, A., Mills, K. & Kneeland, Y.[26]   **Year:** 1931

Experiment 26.1

3	0 of 0	9 of 16
	(0%)	(56%)
Sick donor(s)	Control recipient(s) became sick	Healthy recipient(s) became sick

Method: Respiratory mucus from a person with a cold was cultured in a chicken embryo. The embryo fluid was inoculated into 16 healthy men.
Result: Nine recipients developed colds.
Notes: No controls were used. The participants were not blinded.

27. Cultivation of the Virus of the Common Cold

Author(s): Dochez, A., Mills, K. & Kneeland, Y.[27]   **Year:** 1931

Experiment 27.1

3	0 of 2	2 of 3
	(0%)	(67%)
Sick donor(s)	Control recipient(s) became sick	Healthy recipient(s) became sick

Method: Three recipients were inoculated with chicken embryo fluid as per experiment 26.1. Two controls received 'uninfected' embryo fluid. **Result:** Both recipients developed colds. The controls remained well. **Notes:** A negative control was used.

28. Cultivation of the Virus of Common Cold

Author(s): Powell, H. & Clowes, G.[28]   **Year:** 1931

Experiment 28.1

1	0 of 0	2 of 3
	(0%)	(67%)
Sick donor(s)	Control recipient(s) became sick	Healthy recipient(s) became sick

Method: Respiratory mucus was obtained from a person with a cold, filtered, and added to a chicken embryo. Embryo fluid was instilled into each nostril of three healthy volunteers. **Result:** Two out of three healthy recipients developed colds. **Notes:** No proper controls were used. No mention of blinding.

Experiment 28.2

1	0 of 0 (0%)	3 of 5 (67%)
Sick donor(s)	Control recipient(s) became sick	Healthy recipient(s) became sick

Method: The methodology of this experiment was the same as 28.1. Five healthy recipients were inoculated with chicken embryo fluid.
Result: Three out of five healthy recipients developed colds.
Notes: No proper controls were used. No mention of blinding.

Experiment 28.3

1	71 of 717 (10%)	4 of 5 (80%)
Sick donor(s)	Control recipient(s) became sick	Healthy recipient(s) became sick

Method: The methodology of this experiment was the same as 28.1. Five healthy recipients were inoculated with chicken embryo fluid. A group of 717 people did not receive any intervention and were used as controls to gauge the prevalence of colds amongst the general population.
Result: Four out of five healthy recipients developed colds. Seventy-one people in the control group developed colds.
Notes: No proper controls were used. No mention of blinding.

Experiment 28.4

1	56 of 700 (8%)	4 of 6 (67%)
Sick donor(s)	Control recipient(s) became sick	Healthy recipient(s) became sick

Method: The methodology of this experiment was the same as 28.1. Six healthy recipients were inoculated with chicken embryo fluid. A group of 700 people did not receive any intervention and were used as controls to gauge the prevalence of colds amongst the general population.

Result: Four out of six healthy recipients developed colds. Fifty-six people in the control group developed colds.

Notes: No proper controls were used. No mention of blinding.

Experiment 28.5

1	50 of 496 (10%)	3 of 4 (75%)
Sick donor(s)	Control recipient(s) became sick	Healthy recipient(s) became sick

Method: The methodology of this experiment was the same as 28.1. Four healthy recipients were inoculated with chicken embryo fluid. A group of 496 people did not receive any intervention and were used as controls to gauge the prevalence of colds amongst the general population.

Result: Three out of four healthy recipients developed colds. Fifty people in the control group had colds.

Notes: No proper controls were used. No mention of blinding.

Experiment 28.6

1	16 of 210 (8%)	4 of 5 (80%)
Sick donor(s)	Control recipient(s) became sick	Healthy recipient(s) became sick

Method: The methodology of this experiment was the same as 28.1. Five healthy recipients were inoculated with chicken embryo fluid. A group of 210 people did not receive any intervention and were used as controls to gauge the prevalence of colds amongst the general population.
Result: Four out of five healthy recipients developed colds. Sixteen people in the control group had colds.
Notes: No proper controls were used. No mention of blinding.

Experiment 28.7

1	10 of 200 (5%)	3 of 4 (75%)
Sick donor(s)	Control recipient(s) became sick	Healthy recipient(s) became sick

Method: The methodology of this experiment was the same as 28.1. Four healthy recipients were inoculated with chicken embryo fluid. A group of 200 people did not receive any intervention and were used as controls to gauge the prevalence of colds amongst the general population.
Result: Three out of four healthy recipients developed colds. Ten people in the control group developed colds.
Notes: No proper controls were used. No mention of blinding.

29. Report of Studies of the 1932 Epidemic of Influenza in Puerto Rico

Author(s): Mandry, O., Morales, P. & Suarez, J.[29]   **Year:** 1932

Experiment 29.1

5	0 of 0 (0%)	0 of 10 (0%)
Sick donor(s)	Control recipient(s) became sick	Healthy recipient(s) became sick

Method: Respiratory mucus was collected from five patients with influenza, filtered, and inoculated into 10 healthy participants.
Result: None of the healthy recipients became unwell.
Notes: No controls were used. The participants were not blinded.

Experiment 29.2

5	0 of 0 (0%)	0 of 8 (0%)
Sick donor(s)	Control recipient(s) became sick	Healthy recipient(s) became sick

Method: Respiratory mucus was collected from five patients with influenza, filtered, and inoculated into eight healthy participants.
Result: None of the healthy recipients became unwell.
Notes: No controls were used. The participants were not blinded.

30. Studies of the Etiology of Influenza

Author(s): Dochez, A., Mills, K. & Kneeland, Y.[30]   **Year:** 1933

Experiment 30.1

1	0 of 0	2 of 2
	(0%)	(100%)
Sick donor(s)	Control recipient(s) became sick	Healthy recipient(s) became sick

Method: Respiratory mucus was collected from a person with influenza, filtered and inoculated into a chicken embryo. The chicken embryo fluid was inoculated intranasally into two healthy volunteers.
Result: Both recipients developed symptoms of a severe common cold including nasal obstruction, nasal discharge, sneezing, and a productive cough. They recovered within one week.
Notes: No controls were used. The participants were not blinded.

Appendix (Experiments 31.1 - 40.6)

31. Transmissibility of the Common Cold. Exposure of Susceptible Individuals Under Controlled Conditions

Author(s): Kerr, W. & Lagen, J.[31]   **Year:** 1934

Experiment 31.1

5	0 of 0 (0%)	0 of 19 (0%)
Sick donor(s)	Control recipient(s) became sick	Healthy recipient(s) became sick

Method: Nineteen people were divided into five groups of three to five people. Each group was isolated in an air-locked, climate-controlled, pressure-controlled room with a person with a naturally acquired cold for 48 hours. They ate together, played cards with each other, drank from the same glass, and had the sick person sneeze directly in their faces.
Result: None of the healthy participants developed a cold.
Notes: No controls were used. The participants were not blinded.

Experiment 31.2

1	0 of 0 (0%)	0 of 5 (0%)
Sick donor(s)	Control recipient(s) became sick	Healthy recipient(s) became sick

Method: Oral thermometers were covered in mucus from a person with a cold and used to take the temperatures of five volunteers.
Result: None of the healthy participants developed a cold.
Notes: No controls were used. The participants were not blinded.

Experiment 31.3

1	0 of 1 (0%)	0 of 4 (0%)
Sick donor(s)	Control recipient(s) became sick	Healthy recipient(s) became sick

Method: Respiratory mucus was collected from a person with a cold and dropped into the conjunctiva of four healthy recipients. One person served as a control and received heat-treated mucus.
Result: All participants remained completely well.
Notes: Participants were not blinded.

Experiment 31.4

1	0 of 1 (0%)	0 of 4 (0%)
Sick donor(s)	Control recipient(s) became sick	Healthy recipient(s) became sick

Method: The mucus collected in experiment 31.3 was centrifuged and the clear supernatant was dropped into the conjunctiva of four healthy men. One person served as a control.
Result: All participants remained completely well.
Notes: No controls were used. The participants were not blinded.

Experiment 31.5

1	0 of 1 (0%)	0 of 5 (0%)
Sick donor(s)	Control recipient(s) became sick	Healthy recipient(s) became sick

Method: Mucus was collected from a person with a cold and dropped into the conjunctiva of five healthy recipients. One person served as a control.
Result: All participants remained completely well.
Notes: No controls were used. The participants were not blinded.

32. Observations on the Recovery of Virus from Man

Author(s): Andrewes, C., Smith, W & Laidlaw, P.[32]   **Year:** 1935

Experiment 32.1

1	0 of 0 (0%)	0 of 2 (0%)
Sick donor(s)	Control recipient(s) became sick	Healthy recipient(s) became sick

Method: A mucus sample was collected from a ferret with experimentally induced influenza. Two healthy people had 1 mL of a solution containing the ferret's mucus instilled into each nostril.
Result: Both recipients remained well.
Notes: No controls were used. The participants were not blinded.

33. Investigation of Volunteers Infected with Influenza

Author(s): Smorodintseff, A., Tushinsky, M., et al.[33]   **Year:** 1937

Experiment 33.1

?	0 of 12 (0%)	14 of 72 (19%)
Sick donor(s)	Control recipient(s) became sick	Healthy recipient(s) became sick

Method: Lung tissue from mice with influenza was ground with sand and saline, centrifuged, and sprayed in the noses of 72 recipients. A control group received an aerosol made from the lung tissue of healthy mice.
Result: Fourteen of 72 recipients developed influenza.
All of the controls remained well.
Notes: The causative agent was not identified.

34. The Antibody Response of Human Subjects

Author(s): Francis, T. & Magill, T.[34]   **Year:** 1937

Experiment 34.1

0	0 of 0	0 of 23
	(0%)	(0%)
Sick donor(s)	Control recipient(s) became sick	Healthy recipient(s) became sick

Method: Cell culture fluid allegedly containing influenza virus was inoculated into 23 healthy volunteers as a 'vaccine'.
Result: In no instance was evidence of infection observed.
Notes: No controls were used. The participants were not blinded.

35. Influenza Virus on the Developing Egg VII

Author(s): Burnet, F. & Lush, D.[35]   **Year:** 1938

Experiment 35.1

0	0 of 0	0 of 200
	(0%)	(0%)
Sick donor(s)	Control recipient(s) became sick	Healthy recipient(s) became sick

Method: Melbourne type virus was cultured in chicken embryos. The live virus was then inoculated intranasally into 200 healthy volunteers as a 'vaccine' to afford protection against seasonal influenza.
Result: No recipients developed influenza. No influenza occurred in Melbourne that winter, so no evidence of protection from the 'vaccine' could be obtained.
Notes: No controls were used. The participants were not blinded.

36. Intranasal Inoculation of Human Individuals

Author(s): Francis, T.[36]   **Year:** 1940

Experiment 36.1

0	0 of 0 (0%)	3 of 11 (27%)
Sick donor(s)	Control recipient(s) became sick	Healthy recipient(s) became sick

Method: Cell culture fluid allegedly containing influenza A (PR8 strain) was inoculated intranasally into 11 healthy volunteers.
Result: Three participants became unwell. One participant developed a cold, one developed a temperature, and one experienced a cold sore.
Notes: The illnesses differed to the one being studied. No controls were used. The participants were not blinded.

37. The Common Cold: A Note Regarding Isolation

Author(s): Topping, A. & Atlas, L.[37]   **Year:** 1947

Experiment 37.1

1	0 of 0 (0%)	5 of 5 (100%)
Sick donor(s)	Control recipient(s) became sick	Healthy recipient(s) became sick

Method: Mucus from a person with a common cold was mixed with milk and inoculated intranasally into five healthy volunteers.
Result: All five volunteers developed mild symptoms including fatigue, a headache, nasal obstruction, coughing, and sneezing.
Notes: No controls were used. The participants were blinded.

Experiment 37.2

1	24 of 48 (50%)	57 of 60 (95%)
Sick donor(s)	Control recipient(s) became sick	Healthy recipient(s) became sick

Method: Mucus from people with colds was added to chicken embryos. The embryo fluid was inoculated into 60 participants. A total of 48 volunteers were inoculated with non-infected chicken embryo fluid.
Result: Fifty-seven recipients developed mild colds. Twenty-four controls developed mild cold-like symptoms.
Notes: Uninfected chicken embryo fluid caused flu-like symptoms. The participants were blinded.

38. Experimental Transmission of Minor Respiratory Illness to Human Volunteers by Filter Passing Agents

Author(s): Commission on Acute Respiratory Diseases[38] **Year:** 1947

Experiment 38.1

0	0 of 9 (0%)	0 of 0 (0%)
Sick donor(s)	Control recipient(s) became sick	Healthy recipient(s) became sick

Method: Respiratory mucus was obtained from healthy people. They were inoculated with their own mucus a few days later.
Result: None of the participants became unwell.
Notes: No mention of participant blinding.

Experiment 38.2

1	0 of 0 (0%)	12 of 14 (86%)
Sick donor(s)	Control recipient(s) became sick	Healthy recipient(s) became sick

Method: Respiratory mucus was obtained from one sick donor with an acute respiratory disease, mixed with sterile broth and inoculated with an atomiser into the noses and throats of 14 healthy volunteers.
Result: Twelve of the 14 men became ill and two remained unaffected.
Notes: The symptoms in the inoculated group differed from that of the sick donor. No proper controls were used.

Experiment 38.3

1	0 of 0 (0%)	9 of 14 (64%)
Sick donor(s)	Control recipient(s) became sick	Healthy recipient(s) became sick

Method: Fourteen healthy men were inoculated intranasally with a mucus sample obtained from one sick man with a severe cold.
Result: Nine of the 14 men became unwell.
Notes: The symptoms in the inoculated group differed from that of the sick donor. No proper controls were used.

Experiment 38.4

1	0 of 0 (0%)	6 of 10 (60%)
Sick donor(s)	Control recipient(s) became sick	Healthy recipient(s) became sick

Method: Ten healthy men were inoculated with a mucus sample obtained from one sick man with a common cold.
Result: Six of the 10 men became unwell.
Notes: The symptoms in the inoculated group differed from that of the sick donor. No proper controls were used.

Experiment 38.5

1	0 of 0 (0%)	4 of 10 (40%)
Sick donor(s)	Control recipient(s) became sick	Healthy recipient(s) became sick

Method: Ten healthy men were inoculated with a mucus sample obtained from one sick man with a common cold.
Result: Four of the 10 men became unwell.
Notes: The symptoms in the inoculated group differed from that of the sick donor. No proper controls were used.

39. Experiments at the Common Cold Research Institute

Author(s): Andrews, C.[39,40]   **Year:** 1947-1948

Experiment 39.1

4	0 of 0	1 of 19
	(0%)	(5%)
Sick donor(s)	Control recipient(s) became sick	Healthy recipient(s) became sick

Method: Four people were inoculated with 'common cold germs'. Before developing symptoms, they were exposed to eight healthy people. Once the four inoculated people developed symptoms, they were exposed to 11 healthy people in a room for 10 hours.

Result: Only one of the 19 participants developed a cold.

Notes: No controls were used. No information was available about how the colds were experimentally induced.

Experiment 39.2

?	0 of 0	0 of 4
	(0%)	(0%)
Sick donor(s)	Control recipient(s) became sick	Healthy recipient(s) became sick

Method: People with experimentally induced colds were directly exposed to four healthy people.

Result: None of the healthy people became unwell.

Notes: No mention of blinding or controls.

Experiment 39.3

?	0 of 0	1 of 5
	(0%)	(20%)
Sick donor(s)	Control recipient(s) became sick	Healthy recipient(s) became sick

Method: As per experiment 39.2.
Result: One of the five healthy participants developed a cold.
Notes: No mention of blinding or controls.

Experiment 39.4

1	0 of 0	0 of 5
	(0%)	(0%)
Sick donor(s)	Control recipient(s) became sick	Healthy recipient(s) became sick

Method: As per experiment 39.2.
Result: None of the healthy participants became unwell.
Notes: No mention of blinding or controls.

40. An Experiment on the Transmission of Colds

Author(s): Andrewes, C. & Lovelock, J.[40]   **Year:** 1951

Introduction: Twelve healthy volunteers were sent to a remote island in the Hebrides and isolated from all other contact for ten weeks. The volunteers were separated into three groups of four people (groups A, B and C). No one had lived on the island for 12 years and the volunteers were sent there with enough supplies to last them 3 months so that no person-to-person contact with anyone from the outside world occurred.

Experiment 40.1

6	0 of 0	0 of 4
	(0%)	(0%)
Sick donor(s)	Control recipient(s) became sick	Healthy recipient(s) became sick

Method: Group A (consisting of four healthy people) lived in a house together for 10 weeks. The healthy volunteers vacated the house for several hours whilst six volunteers with colds contaminated playing cards, books, cutlery, cups, chairs, door handles, and tables inside the house by dripping their nasal discharge onto the items. The six sick people then vacated the house and members of group A returned to the house. Neither the sick nor healthy volunteers had any direct contact. Group A then exposed themselves to these objects for 3 hours.

Result: None of the healthy participants became unwell.

Notes: No controls were used. No mention of blinding.

Experiment 40.2

6	0 of 0	0 of 4
	(0%)	(0%)
Sick donor(s)	Control recipient(s) became sick	Healthy recipient(s) became sick

Method: Group B (consisting of four healthy people) lived in a house together for 10 weeks. Six sick participants with experimentally induced colds visited the room with the healthy participants for 3 hours. The sick participants coughed and sneezed and spoke freely in the presence of the healthy participants, whilst they sat quietly.

Result: None of the healthy volunteers became unwell.

Notes: No controls were used. No mention of blinding.

Experiment 40.3

6	0 of 0 (0%)	0 of 4 (0%)
Sick donor(s)	Control recipient(s) became sick	Healthy recipient(s) became sick

Method: Group C (consisting of four healthy people) lived in a house together for 10 weeks. Four sick participants lived and ate in the same house as Group C for four days.

Result: None of the healthy volunteers became unwell.

Notes: No controls were used. No mention of blinding.

Experiment 40.4

4	0 of 0 (0%)	0 of 4 (0%)
Sick donor(s)	Control recipient(s) became sick	Healthy recipient(s) became sick

Method: Another group of four people with experimentally induced colds were brought to the island. They were directly exposed to group A for three hours on the evening of their arrival to the island and for three hours the next morning.

Result: None of the participants in group A developed a cold.

Notes: No controls were used. No mention of blinding.

Experiment 40.5

1	0 of 0 (0%)	3 of 4 (75%)
Sick donor(s)	Control recipient(s) became sick	Healthy recipient(s) became sick

Method: A man on a nearby island who had acquired a natural cold five days prior was brought to the island and exposed to Group B. He interacted with the healthy volunteers inside their house and sat by a fire with each person for a total of 2 hours.
Result: Three of the four healthy people in Group B developed a cold.
Notes: No controls were used. No mention of blinding.

Experiment 40.6

5	0 of 0 (0%)	0 of 4 (0%)
Sick donor(s)	Control recipient(s) became sick	Healthy recipient(s) became sick

Method: The man with the natural cold from exp. 40.5 spent 3.5 hours with the members of group C. When none of the participants became sick, the four sick people with experimentally induced colds then lived with Group C for four days.
Result: None of the participants became unwell.
Notes: No healthy people exposed to people with natural or experimental colds became unwell. No controls were used. No mention of blinding.

Appendix (Experiments 41.1 - 50.2)

41. Further Studies on the Natural Transmission of the Common Cold

Author(s): Lovelock, J., Roden, A. & Porterfield, J.[41]   **Year:** 1952

Experiment 41.1

22	0 of 0	2 of 25
	(0%)	(8%)
Sick donor(s)	Control recipient(s) became sick	Healthy recipient(s) became sick

Method: A room was divided in half with a partition made from a large blanket with a one-foot gap between the blanket and the walls, floor, and ceiling. Air was circulated through the room with a fan. Five to six healthy participants sat quietly reading or knitting on one side of the blanket. A group of people with naturally acquired colds played games, sang, and shouted on the other side of the partition for two hours. The sick participants were also administered sneezing powder (o-dianisidine hydrochloride) to fill the room with respiratory droplets. This experiment was repeated five times on five separate days.
Result: Out of 25 healthy participants exposed to infected droplets in the air, two developed colds.
Notes: No controls were used. No mention of blinding.

Experiment 41.2

22	0 of 0 (0%)	3 of 32 (9%)
Sick donor(s)	Control recipient(s) became sick	Healthy recipient(s) became sick

Method: A group of people with naturally acquired colds spent two hours in a room with a group of healthy volunteers. They ate lunch together, conversed with each other and played card games together. The sick participants were encouraged to sneeze and cough and blow their nose 'violently'. At the end of the experiment, the healthy and sick participants vacated the room. This experiment was repeated five times.

Result: Out of 32 healthy people who had full direct contact with sick people, three developed colds.

Notes: No controls were used. No mention of blinding.

Experiment 41.3

22	0 of 0 (0%)	2 of 25 (9%)
Sick donor(s)	Control recipient(s) became sick	Healthy recipient(s) became sick

Method: A group of healthy people were brought into the vacant room where experiment 41.2 took place. They were encouraged to handle the objects used by the sick participants for two hours. This experiment was repeated five times on five separate days.

Result: Two healthy participants out of 25 developed colds, however, the authors expressed doubt as to whether these colds occurred as a consequence of the experiment.

Notes: No controls were used. No mention of blinding.

Experiment 41.4

5	0 of 0 (0%)	4 of 8 (50%)
Sick donor(s)	Control recipient(s) became sick	Healthy recipient(s) became sick

Method: Five children with colds played games with a group of eight healthy adults for two hours.
Result: Four of the healthy adults developed colds.
Notes: No controls were used. No mention of blinding.

Experiment 41.5

0	0 of 0 (0%)	26 of 89 (29%)
Sick donor(s)	Control recipient(s) became sick	Healthy recipient(s) became sick

Method: Healthy participants wore oxygen masks fitted over their mouths and noses. A 1 mL mixture of cultured cold virus particles mixed with saline and bovine albumin was then administered through the masks. The participants inhaled the mist for five minutes.
Result: Twenty-six out of 89 participants developed cold symptoms.
Notes: No controls were used. No mention of blinding.

Experiment 41.6

0	0 of 0	0 of 7
	(0%)	(0%)
Sick donor(s)	Control recipient(s) became sick	Healthy recipient(s) became sick

Method: Cotton wool swabs were soaked in viral culture material and then painted onto the skin around the nostrils of seven healthy volunteers. Volunteers were instructed not to touch or wipe their nose for an hour.
Result: None of the healthy participants became unwell.
Notes: No controls were used. No mention of blinding.

Experiment 41.7

5	0 of 0	0 of 8
	(0%)	(0%)
Sick donor(s)	Control recipient(s) became sick	Healthy recipient(s) became sick

Method: Five adults with colds blew their noses into plastic handkerchiefs. The mucus was washed off with a saline solution into a container. The fluid was then centrifuged and 1 mL of supernatant was sprayed onto clean handkerchiefs and given to eight healthy volunteers who blew and wiped their noses for 24 hours.
Result: None of the healthy participants became unwell.
Notes: No controls were used. No mention of blinding.

Experiment 41.8

?	0 of 0	0 of 7
	(0%)	(0%)
Sick donor(s)	Control recipient(s) became sick	Healthy recipient(s) became sick

Method: Sterile gauze was soaked in undiluted nasal washings obtained from people with colds. Seven healthy volunteers were instructed to wipe the skin around their nostrils with the gauze several times over an hour.
Result: None of the healthy participants became unwell.
Notes: No controls were used. No mention of blinding.

Experiment 41.9

?	0 of 0	5 of 8
	(0%)	(63%)
Sick donor(s)	Control recipient(s) became sick	Healthy recipient(s) became sick

Method: Mucus secretions from people with colds were diluted in saline and dropped into the nasal passages of eight volunteers.
Result: Five of the eight participants developed colds.
Notes: No controls were used. No mention of blinding.

Experiment 41.10

?	0 of 0	2 of 7
	(0%)	(29%)
Sick donor(s)	Control recipient(s) became sick	Healthy recipient(s) became sick

Method: Sterile gauze was soaked in undiluted nasal washings obtained from people with colds. The gauze was then packed into the nasal cavities of seven healthy volunteers for two hours.
Result: Two of the healthy participants became unwell.
Notes: No controls were used. No mention of blinding.

Experiment 41.11

?	0 of 0	2 of 19
	(0%)	(11%)
Sick donor(s)	Control recipient(s) became sick	Healthy recipient(s) became sick

Method: Gauze was soaked in nasal mucus obtained from people with colds and packed into the nasal cavities of two groups of healthy participants. One group received dry gauze, whilst the other was wet.
Result: Two healthy participants in the wet gauze group developed colds.
Notes: No controls were used. No mention of blinding.

42. Type C Influenza Virus. II. Intranasal Inoculation

Author(s): Quilligan, J., Minuse, E & Francis, T.[42]   **Year:** 1954

Experiment 42.1

0	0 of 5 (0%)	0 of 6 (0%)
Sick donor(s)	Control recipient(s) became sick	Healthy recipient(s) became sick

Method: The JJ strain of influenza C virus was cultured in a chicken embryo. The embryo fluid was inoculated intranasally into six recipients. Five people served as controls and received no intervention.
Result: None of the recipients or controls developed any symptoms.
Notes: No adequate controls were used. No mention of blinding.

43. Artificially Induced Asian Influenza

Author(s): Bell, J., Ward, T & Kapikian, A.[43]   **Year:** 1957

Experiment 43.1

?	18 of 23 (78%)	32 of 58 (58%)
Sick donor(s)	Control recipient(s) became sick	Healthy recipient(s) became sick

Method: Influenza vaccine was given to 58 participants and 23 received a placebo. A few weeks later, both groups were inoculated intranasally with cell culture fluid containing 'influenza virus'.
Result: The flu occurred in 18 controls and 32 vaccinated participants.
Notes: The authors concluded the vaccine provided incomplete protection against the influenza virus. No positive controls were used.

44. Transmission of Experimental Cold in Volunteers. II.

Author(s): Dowling, H., Jackson, G & Inouye, T.[44]   **Year:** 1957

Experiment 44.1

?	0 of 0 (0%)	279 of 836 (33%)
Sick donor(s)	Control recipient(s) became sick	Healthy recipient(s) became sick

Method: The bodily fluids of sick people with colds were inoculated into 143 participants with allergies, and 693 non-allergic participants. A total of 836 people were inoculated.
Result: Colds were induced in 64 (45%) out of 143 allergic participants, compared to 241 (31%) out of 693 non-allergic participants.
Notes: No controls were used.

Experiment 44.2

?	0 of 0 (0%)	271 of 827 (33%)
Sick donor(s)	Control recipient(s) became sick	Healthy recipient(s) became sick

Method: The bodily fluids of sick people with colds were inoculated into 363 participants who had their tonsils previously removed, and 464 people whose tonsils were intact. A total of 827 people were inoculated.
Result: Colds were induced in 123 (34%) out of 363 participants without tonsils, compared to 148 (32%) out of 464 participants with tonsils.
Notes: No controls were used.

Experiment 44.3

?	0 of 0	87 of 249
	(0%)	(35%)
Sick donor(s)	Control recipient(s) became sick	Healthy recipient(s) became sick

Method: The bodily fluids of sick people with colds were inoculated into 249 participants who smoked tobacco and a group of non-smokers.
Result: Colds were induced in 87 (35%) out of 249 smokers, compared to 34% of non-smokers.
Notes: No controls were used.

Experiment 44.4

?	0 of 0	10 of 13
	(0%)	(77%)
Sick donor(s)	Control recipient(s) became sick	Healthy recipient(s) became sick

Method: The bodily fluids of sick people with colds were inoculated into 13 women during the first, middle, and last third of their menstrual cycle. These women were also exposed to cold temperatures.
Result: Colds were induced in 10 (77%) of 13 women inoculated during the middle third of their menstrual cycle, compared to 28% and 30% inoculated during the first and final third of their cycles, respectively.
Notes: No controls were used.

45. Transmission of the Common Cold to Volunteers. I.

Author(s): Jackson, G., Dowling, H. & Dowling, I.[45]   **Year:** 1958

Experiment 45.1

1	6 of 89 (7%)	77 of 217 (58%)
Sick donor(s)	Control recipient(s) became sick	Healthy recipient(s) became sick

Method: Nasal secretions were obtained from a person with a cold, filtered and diluted in saline. Yeast, or human haemoglobin was added as a stabilising protein. Approximately 0.2 mL was instilled into both nostrils of 217 healthy volunteers. A saline solution containing the same amount of yeast or haemoglobin was used as a control in 89 volunteers.
Result: Of the 217 healthy inoculated volunteers, 77 (36%) developed colds, whilst 6 (7%) of the 89 controls developed colds.
Notes: No positive controls were used. Participants were blinded.

Experiment 45.2

1	10 of 85 (12%)	66 of 182 (36%)
Sick donor(s)	Control recipient(s) became sick	Healthy recipient(s) became sick

Method: The methodology was the same as experiment 45.1. A total of 182 healthy volunteers were exposed to the filtered mucus solution and 85 were exposed to the control solution.
Result: Of the 182 healthy volunteers that were inoculated, 66 (36%) developed colds, whilst 10 (12%) of the 85 controls developed colds.
Notes: No positive controls were used. Participants were blinded to the challenge substance.

Experiment 45.3

1	8 of 85	105 of 293
	(9%)	(36%)
Sick donor(s)	Control recipient(s) became sick	Healthy recipient(s) became sick

Method: The methodology was the same as experiment 45.1. A total of 293 healthy volunteers were exposed to the filtered mucus solution and 85 were exposed to the control solution.

Result: Of the 293 healthy volunteers that were inoculated, 105 (36%) developed colds, whilst 8 (9%) of the 85 controls developed colds.

Notes: No positive controls were used. Participants were blinded to the challenge substance.

Experiment 45.4

1	5 of 56	77 of 180
	(9%)	(43%)
Sick donor(s)	Control recipient(s) became sick	Healthy recipient(s) became sick

Method: The methodology was the same as that employed in experiment 45.1. A total of 180 healthy volunteers were exposed to the filtered mucus solution and 56 were exposed to the control solution.

Result: Of the 180 healthy volunteers that were inoculated, 77 (43%) developed colds, whilst 5 (9%) of the 56 controls developed colds.

Notes: No positive controls were used. Participants were blinded to the challenge substance.

46. Transmission of the Common Cold to Volunteers. III.

Author(s): Dowling, H., Jackson, G., Spiesman, I., et al.[46]   **Year:** 1958

Experiment 46.1

?	15 of 96 (16%)	63 of 175 (36%)
Sick donor(s)	Control recipient(s) became sick	Healthy recipient(s) became sick

Method: Mucus secretions from people with colds were filtered, diluted in saline, and instilled into the nostrils of 175 recipients. The recipients were then put in a climate-controlled room. A total of 96 participants were inoculated with a placebo and exposed to the same conditions.
Result: Of the 175 inoculated participants, 63 (36%) developed colds. Of the 96 controls, 15 (16%) developed colds.
Notes: Controls developed colds despite receiving a placebo.

Experiment 46.2

?	5 of 63 (8%)	55 of 168 (32%)
Sick donor(s)	Control recipient(s) became sick	Healthy recipient(s) became sick

Method: A group of 168 healthy recipients were inoculated as per experiment 46.1. The recipients were then put in a climate-controlled room and exposed to 15.5°C and 80% relative humidity for up to four hours. A total of 63 participants were inoculated with a control solution as per experiment 46.1 and exposed to the same conditions.
Result: Of the 168 inoculated participants, 55 (32%) developed colds. Of the 63 controls, 5 (8%) developed colds.
Notes: Controls developed colds despite being inoculated with an inert substance.

Experiment 46.3

?	5 of 74	33 of 85
	(8%)	(39%)
Sick donor(s)	Control recipient(s) became sick	Healthy recipient(s) became sick

Method: A group of 85 healthy recipients were inoculated as per Exp. 46.1. A total of 74 participants were inoculated with a control solution as per experiment 46.1.

Result: Of the 85 inoculated participants, 33 (39%) developed colds. Of the 74 controls, 5 (8%) developed colds.

Notes: Controls developed colds despite being inoculated with an inert substance.

47. Inoculation of Volunteers with J.H Strain of New Respiratory Virus

Author(s): Tyrrell, D. & Bynoe, M.[47]   **Year:** 1958

Experiment 47.1

1	0 of ?	0 of 16
	(0%)	(0%)
Sick donor(s)	Control recipient(s) became sick	Healthy recipient(s) became sick

Method: Mucus secretions allegedly containing rhinovirus (J.H strain) were added to a cell culture. A group of 16 healthy volunteers were inoculated intranasally with cell culture fluid. Saline was inoculated into an unknown number of control recipients.

Result: None of the 16 recipients became sick.

Notes: The recipients were claimed to be asymptomatically infected.

Experiment 47.2

2	0 of 0 (0%)	2 of 11 (18%)
Sick donor(s)	Control recipient(s) became sick	Healthy recipient(s) became sick

Method: Nasal washings were obtained from two volunteers who developed an 'asymptomatic infection' in experiment 47.1 and was used to grow the virus in a cell culture inoculated. Cell culture fluid was inoculated into 11 healthy volunteers. Saline was inoculated into an unknown number of controls.

Result: Two (18%) of the 11 recipients developed mild cold symptoms, and three developed 'asymptomatic infections'.

Notes: The authors claim the illnesses were caused by an agent other than the J.H virus lying dormant in the throat of the recipients.

Experiment 47.3

2	0 of ? (0%)	2 of 21 (10%)
Sick donor(s)	Control recipient(s) became sick	Healthy recipient(s) became sick

Method: Nasal washings were obtained from the two volunteers who developed colds in experiment 47.2 and were added to a cell culture. The cell culture fluid was diluted in saline and inoculated intranasally into 21 healthy volunteers.

Result: Two (10%) of the 21 recipients developed colds. One recipient developed a cold, but it was not considered to be caused by the virus because no 'virus material' was identified in their nasal washings.

Notes: The authors claim the illnesses were caused by an agent other than the J.H virus lying dormant in the throat of the recipients.

Experiment 47.4

1	0 of ? (0%)	1 of 10 (10%)
Sick donor(s)	Control recipient(s) became sick	Healthy recipient(s) became sick

Method: Mucus was obtained from a volunteer with a cold from Exp 47.3 and added to a cell culture. Virus material was inoculated intranasally into 10 healthy volunteers. The control group received saline.
Result: One (10%) of the 10 recipients developed cold-like symptoms, however, the authors concluded this was not caused by the virus because no virus material could be recovered from them.
Notes: N/A.

48. Transmission of the Common Cold to Volunteers. IV.

Author(s): Jackson, G & Dowling, H.[48]   **Year:** 1959

Experiment 48.1

5	70 of 696 (10%)	449 of 1034 (42%)
Sick donor(s)	Control recipient(s) became sick	Healthy recipient(s) became sick

Method: Respiratory mucus from five people with colds was filtered, mixed with saline, haemoglobin, yeast, and instilled into the noses of 1034 recipients. A total of 696 controls received buffered saline.
Result: Of the 1034 recipients, 449 (42%) developed a cold. Of the 696 controls, 70 (10%) developed a cold.
Notes: Buffered saline induced colds.

Experiment 48.2

5	0 of 0	7 of 73
	(0%)	(10%)
Sick donor(s)	Control recipient(s) became sick	Healthy recipient(s) became sick

Method: Seventy-three people who did not develop colds in experiment 48.1 were rechallenged with the same nasal secretions between 3 and 45 weeks later.
Result: Seven (10%) of the 73 recipients developed a cold.
Notes: N/A.

Experiment 48.3

5	0 of 0	6 of 71
	(0%)	(8%)
Sick donor(s)	Control recipient(s) became sick	Healthy recipient(s) became sick

Method: Seventy-one people who developed colds in experiment 48.1 were rechallenged with the same nasal secretion up to 45 weeks later.
Result: Six (8%) of the 71 recipients developed a cold.
Notes: N/A.

Experiment 48.4

5	0 of 0 (0%)	31 of 74 (40%)
Sick donor(s)	Control recipient(s) became sick	Healthy recipient(s) became sick

Method: Seventy-four people who did not develop colds in experiment 48.1 were rechallenged with a different nasal secretion up to 45 weeks later.
Result: Thirty-one (40%) of the 74 recipients developed a cold.
Notes: N/A.

Experiment 48.5

5	0 of 0 (0%)	19 of 41 (46%)
Sick donor(s)	Control recipient(s) became sick	Healthy recipient(s) became sick

Method: Forty-one people who did develop a cold in experiment 48.1 were rechallenged with a different nasal secretion up to 45 weeks later.
Result: Nineteen (46%) of the 41 recipients developed a cold.
Notes: N/A.

49. Inoculation of Volunteers with Parainfluenza Viruses

Author(s): Tyrrell, D., Bynoe, M., Sutton, R., et al.[49]   **Year:** 1959

Experiment 49.1

1	0 of 0	6 of 18
	(0%)	(33%)
Sick donor(s)	Control recipient(s) became sick	Healthy recipient(s) became sick

Method: Parainfluenza 1 virus was 'isolated' from a sick child by adding their mucus to a cell culture. Cell culture fluid was mixed with Hank's saline and dropped into the noses of 18 healthy recipients.
Result: Six out of 18 (33%) healthy recipients developed mild colds.
Notes: No controls were used.

Experiment 49.2

1	0 of 0	5 of 15
	(0%)	(33%)
Sick donor(s)	Control recipient(s) became sick	Healthy recipient(s) became sick

Method: Parainfluenza 3 virus was 'isolated' from a sick child by adding their mucus to a cell culture. Cell culture fluid was then mixed with Hank's saline and dropped into the nasal cavities of 15 healthy recipients.
Result: Five out of 15 (33%) healthy recipients developed mild colds.
Notes: No controls were used.

50. Infectivity and Interrelationships of 2060, and JH Viruses in Volunteers

Author(s): Jackson, G., Dowling, H. & Mogabgab, W.[50]   **Year:** 1960

Experiment 50.1

0	9 of 56 (16%)	25 of 90 (28%)
Sick donor(s)	Control recipient(s) became sick	Healthy recipient(s) became sick

Method: Virus strain 2060 was cultured and inoculated into 90 healthy volunteers. The control group received saline.
Result: Twenty-five (28%) of the 90 recipients developed a common cold. Nine (16%) of the 56 controls developed a common cold.
Notes: The difference between the active and control groups was not statistically significant.

Experiment 50.2

0	8 of 40 (20%)	23 of 69 (34%)
Sick donor(s)	Control recipient(s) became sick	Healthy recipient(s) became sick

Method: Rhinovirus was grown in a cell culture and inoculated intranasally into 69 healthy volunteers. Uninfected culture medium was inoculated into 40 healthy controls.
Result: Twenty-three (34%) of the 69 recipients developed a common cold. Eight (20%) of the 40 controls developed a common cold.
Notes: The difference between the active and control groups was not statistically significant.

Appendix (Experiments 51.1 - 60.3)

51. Some Virus Isolations from Common Colds. I.

Author(s): Tyrrell, D., Bynoe, M., Hitchcock, G., et al.[51]   **Year:** 1960

Experiment 51.1

?	0 of 78 (0%)	22 of 102 (22%)
Sick donor(s)	Control recipient(s) became sick	Healthy recipient(s) became sick

Method: Nasal washings obtained from people with a cold were added to cell cultures. The cell culture fluid was inoculated intranasally into 102 healthy participants. A control group of 78 participants were inoculated with saline, or uninoculated cell culture fluid.
Result: Twenty-two (22%) out of 102 healthy participants developed colds. None of the control group developed colds.
Notes: N/A.

Experiment 51.2

?	0 of 0	0 of 42
	(0%)	(0%)
Sick donor(s)	Control recipient(s) became sick	Healthy recipient(s) became sick

Method: Nasal washings obtained from people with a cold were added to cell cultures using a different cell line to the one in experiment 51.1. The cell culture fluid was inoculated intranasally into 42 healthy participants.
Result: None of the 42 healthy participants developed colds.
Notes: The negative results were explained away by the authors as a failure of the virus to grow in the different cell line.

Experiment 51.3

?	3 of 55	14 of 71
	(5%)	(20%)
Sick donor(s)	Control recipient(s) became sick	Healthy recipient(s) became sick

Method: Nasal washings obtained from people with a cold were added to cell cultures. The cell culture fluid was inoculated intranasally into 71 healthy participants. A group of 55 healthy recipients were used as controls and received uninoculated cell culture fluid.
Result: Fourteen (20%) of the 71 healthy participants developed colds. Three (5%) of the controls developed colds.
Notes: N/A.

52. Inoculation of Human Volunteers with Parainfluenza

Author(s): Kapikian, A., Chanock, R., et al.[1299]   **Year:** 1961

Experiment 52.1

1	1 of 11 (9%)	9 of 17 (53%)
Sick donor(s)	Control recipient(s) became sick	Healthy recipient(s) became sick

Method: Respiratory mucus from an infant with influenza was added to a cell culture. Cell culture fluid was inoculated intranasally into 17 recipients. Eleven controls received a saline placebo.
Result: Nine recipients and one control group developed an acute respiratory illness.
Notes: No positive controls were used. Saline caused a respiratory illness.

53. Inoculation of Human Volunteers with a Strain of Virus Isolated from a Common Cold

Author(s): Bynoe, M., Horner, J., Schild, G., et al.[1300]   **Year:** 1961

Experiment 53.1

?	0 of 0 (0%)	14 of 33 (42%)
Sick donor(s)	Control recipient(s) became sick	Healthy recipient(s) became sick

Method: Nasal washings from people with colds were collected, pooled together, and dropped into the nasal passages of 33 healthy volunteers.
Result: Fourteen people developed colds.
Notes: No controls were used.

Experiment 53.2

?	0 of 7	16 of 54
	(0%)	(30%)
Sick donor(s)	Control recipient(s) became sick	Healthy recipient(s) became sick

Method: Respiratory mucus from people with colds was collected, pooled together, and inoculated into 54 healthy recipients using nasal drops, and conjunctival and throat swabs. Seven people were inoculated with saline.
Result: Of the 54 people inoculated, 16 (30%) developed colds. The controls remained well.
Notes: N/A.

54. Inoculation of Human Volunteers with E.C.H.O Virus Type 20

Author(s): Buckland, F., Bynoe, M., Rosen, L., et al.[54]   **Year:** 1961

Experiment 54.1

2	0 of 0	5 of 8
	(0%)	(63%)
Sick donor(s)	Control recipient(s) became sick	Healthy recipient(s) became sick

Method: Throat swabs were taken from two people with colds, mixed with Hank's saline and dropped into the nasal cavities of eight people.
Result: Five (63%) of eight people became ill, but only one (13%) developed a mild cold.
Notes: The recipients developed an illness different to the sick donors.

Experiment 54.2

1	0 of 0 (0%)	5 of 6 (83%)
Sick donor(s)	Control recipient(s) became sick	Healthy recipient(s) became sick

Method: Respiratory mucus was collected from the participant who developed a cold in Exp. 52.1 and inoculated into six healthy volunteers.
Result: Five (83%) of the six recipients became ill, but only one (17%) developed symptoms of a mild cold.
Notes: The recipients developed an illness different to the sick donors.

Experiment 54.3

1	0 of 0 (0%)	11 of 15 (73%)
Sick donor(s)	Control recipient(s) became sick	Healthy recipient(s) became sick

Method: A throat swab from the sick participant in experiment 54.1 was added to cell cultures. Cell culture fluid was pooled and inoculated into 15 healthy volunteers.
Result: Eleven (73%) of the 15 recipients became ill, but only one (6%) developed a mild cold.
Notes: The inoculation of bodily fluids resulted in an illness different to the sick donors.

Experiment 54.4

0	0 of 0 (0%)	3 of 9 (33%)
Sick donor(s)	Control recipient(s) became sick	Healthy recipient(s) became sick

Method: Antiserum was added to two separate samples of the cell culture fluid from experiment 52.3 to neutralise the 'virus' and inoculated into nine healthy volunteers.

Result: Three (33%) of the nine recipients became ill. None developed colds.

Notes: The inoculation of bodily fluids resulted in an illness different to the sick donors.

Experiment 54.5

0	7 of 33 (21%)	0 of 0 (0%)
Sick donor(s)	Control recipient(s) became sick	Healthy recipient(s) became sick

Method: Hank's saline solution or uninoculated cell culture fluid was inoculated intranasally into 33 healthy volunteers.

Result: Seven (21%) of the 33 control recipients became ill.

Notes: The inoculation of bodily fluids resulted in an illness different to the sick donors.

55. Para-influenza 2 Virus Infections

Author(s): Taylor-Robinson, D. & Bynoe, M.[55]   **Year:** 1963

Experiment 55.1

0	7 of 28 (25%)	12 of 28 (43%)
Sick donor(s)	Control recipient(s) became sick	Healthy recipient(s) became sick

Method: Influenza cell culture fluid was inoculated intranasally into 28 healthy volunteers. Another 28 received a placebo.
Result: Four recipients (14%) developed mild colds and 28 recipients (29%) developed cold-like symptoms. Six (21%) controls developed cold-like symptoms and one (4%) developed a cold.
Notes: No positive controls were used.

56. Inoculation of Volunteers with H Rhinoviruses

Author(s): Taylor-Robinson, D & Bynoe, M.[56]   **Year:** 1964

Experiment 56.1

?	2 of 29 (7%)	6 of ? (?%)
Sick donor(s)	Control recipient(s) became sick	Healthy recipient(s) became sick

Method: Swabs with TH, P, and T viruses were mixed with saline and inoculated into healthy people. Twenty-nine controls received saline.
Result: Two people who became sick were used as donors in Exp. 56.2 – 56.4. Two (7%) controls developed colds.
Notes: No controls were used. No mention of blinding.

Experiment 56.2

2	0 of 0	4 of 14
	(0%)	(29%)
Sick donor(s)	Control recipient(s) became sick	Healthy recipient(s) became sick

Method: Pooled nasal secretions (allegedly containing the 'TH' strain) obtained from the two sick people in experiment 56.1 were filtered and dropped into the noses of 14 healthy volunteers.
Result: Four (29%) of the 14 participants developed colds.
Notes: N/A.

Experiment 56.3

2	0 of 0	11 of 24
	(0%)	(46%)
Sick donor(s)	Control recipient(s) became sick	Healthy recipient(s) became sick

Method: Pooled nasal secretions (allegedly containing the 'T' strain) obtained from the two sick people in experiment 56.1 were filtered and dropped into the noses of 24 healthy recipients.
Result: Eleven (46%) of the 24 participants developed colds.
Notes: N/A.

Experiment 56.4

2	0 of 0 (0%)	4 of 8 (50%)
Sick donor(s)	Control recipient(s) became sick	Healthy recipient(s) became sick

Method: Pooled nasal secretions (allegedly containing the 'P' strain) obtained from the two sick people in experiment 56.1 were filtered and dropped into the noses of 8 healthy recipients.
Result: Four (50%) of the 8 participants developed colds.
Notes: N/A.

57. Studies with Rhinoviruses in Volunteers

Author(s): Cate, T., Couch, R. & Johnson, K.[57]   **Year:** 1964

Experiment 57.1

3	0 of 0 (0%)	38 of 56 (68%)
Sick donor(s)	Control recipient(s) became sick	Healthy recipient(s) became sick

Method: Rhinovirus strains (NIH 353, NIH 1734, and NIH 11757) were isolated from three people in cell cultures. Cell culture fluid was inoculated intranasally into healthy volunteers.
Result: Twenty-nine out of 45 volunteers (54%) inoculated with 1734 became ill, 4 of 6 (67%) inoculated with 353 became ill, and 5 of 5 (100%) inoculated with 11757 became ill. A total of 38 out of 56 (68%) became ill.
Notes: When eight volunteers with low levels of antibodies were rechallenged one month later with the same strain they exhibited resistance to reinoculation. This contrasts to 13 of 25 volunteers who became ill despite having naturally acquired antibodies. This demonstrates resistance against reinfection independent of antibody response.

58. Experiments on the Spread of Colds II: Studies in Volunteers with Coxsackievirus A21

Author(s): Buckland, F., Bynoe, M. & Tyrrell, D[58]   **Year:** 1965

Experiment 58.1

24	0 of 0 (0%)	1 of 20 (5%)
Sick donor(s)	Control recipient(s) became sick	Healthy recipient(s) became sick

Method: Healthy people had a solution of mucus from a sick person, or a 'virus' grown in a tissue culture, dropped into their noses. Twenty-four people in this group developed non-specific symptoms suggestible of a cold. Each of these 'sick' people was housed with one or two healthy volunteers for nine days to see if the cold could be transmitted.
Result: Only one (5%) out of 20 participants developed a mild cold.
Notes: No controls were used. No blinding was used.

Experiment 58.2

6	0 of 0 (0%)	0 of 11 (0%)
Sick donor(s)	Control recipient(s) became sick	Healthy recipient(s) became sick

Method: Six sick participants with experimentally induced colds (as per the methodology of 58.1) sneezed or snorted and spat their snot into a bag three times. Eleven healthy participants inhaled air directly from the bag.
Result: None of the healthy participants became unwell.
Notes: No controls or blinding were used.

Experiment 58.3

6	0 of 0 (0%)	0 of 8 (0%)
Sick donor(s)	Control recipient(s) became sick	Healthy recipient(s) became sick

Method: Six participants with experimental colds attended 'sneeze parties' with eight healthy volunteers. They spent one hour twice per day for three days (6 hours total) playing card games in a room with closed windows and doors. The sick participants snorted and sneezed throughout each session.
Result: None of the healthy participants became unwell.
Notes: No controls were used. No blinding was used.

59. Homologous & Heterologous Resistance to Rhinovirus

Author(s): Fleet, W., Cough, R., Cate, T & Knight, V.[59]   **Year:** 1965

Experiment 59.1

1	0 of 0 (0%)	10 of 32 (31%)
Sick donor(s)	Control recipient(s) became sick	Healthy recipient(s) became sick

Method: Two rhinovirus strains (NIH 1734 and 353) were grown in a cell culture and inoculated into two groups of 16 prisoners.
Result: All 16 prisoners inoculated with NIH 1734 developed symptoms (i.e. malaise, myalgia, temperature). Six (38%) developed 'colds'. Of the 16 volunteers inoculated with 353, 15 (94%) developed symptoms (i.e. malaise, myalgia, temperature). Four (25%) developed 'colds' and one (6%) remained well.
Notes: No controls were used. No blinding was used.

Experiment 59.2

1	0 of 0	10 of 32
	(0%)	(31%)
Sick donor(s)	Control recipient(s) became sick	Healthy recipient(s) became sick

Method: Prisoners from Exp 59.1 were reinoculated with the same (homologous) or different (heterologous) strains at 2, 5, and 16 weeks. Their antibody response was measured before and after inoculation.

Result: At two weeks, none of the seven volunteers reinoculated with the homologous strain became unwell despite having no detectable antibodies. None of the 10 volunteers inoculated with the heterologous strain became unwell despite having no detectable antibodies. At five weeks, nine volunteers were inoculated with the heterologous strain. Five had a marked increase in detectable antibodies before inoculation, and four (44%) became ill. At 16 weeks, 11 volunteers were inoculated with the heterologous strain. A total of seven (64%) became ill. Two individuals failed to exhibit any detectable rise in antibodies.

Notes: The authors concluded the results did not support the notion that antibodies provide protection against reinfection, nor does the lack of antibodies increase susceptibility to infection. They stated that specific antibodies nor any virus-specific factor provides protection against infection. No controls were used. Single blinding was used.

60. Inoculation of a Novel Type of Rhinovirus

Author(s): Hoorn, B., Bynoe, M., Chapple, P., et al.[60]   **Year:** 1965

Experiment 60.1

?	0 of 0 (0%)	3 of 6 (50%)
Sick donor(s)	Control recipient(s) became sick	Healthy recipient(s) became sick

Method: Nasal washings were collected from people with colds and added to a cell culture. Pooled cell culture fluid was mixed with Hank's saline and inoculated into the noses of six healthy people.
Result: Three (50%) of the six recipients developed colds. Two colds were mild, and one was severe.
Notes: N/A.

Experiment 60.2

3	0 of 0 (0%)	2 of 7 (29%)
Sick donor(s)	Control recipient(s) became sick	Healthy recipient(s) became sick

Method: Nasal mucus was collected from three people with colds in Exp. 60.1. The washings were pooled, mixed with saline and inoculated intranasally into seven healthy volunteers.
Result: Two (29%) of the seven recipients developed mild colds.
Notes: N/A.

Experiment 60.3

0	0 of 12 (0%)	0 of 0 (0%)
Sick donor(s)	Control recipient(s) became sick	Healthy recipient(s) became sick

Method: A group of 12 healthy people served as controls. They were inoculated intranasally with cell culture fluid that had not been inoculated with bodily fluids from sick people.

Result: None of the controls became sick.

Notes: No positive controls were used.

Appendix (Experiments 61.1 - 70.1)

61. The Leukocyte Response During Viral Respiratory Illness in Man

Author(s): Douglas, G., Alford, R., Cate, T., et al.[61]   **Year:** 1966

Experiment 61.1

0	0 of 0 (0%)	17 of 32 (53%)
Sick donor(s)	Control recipient(s) became sick	Healthy recipient(s) became sick

Method: Fluid from a cell culture allegedly containing rhinovirus type 1734 was inoculated via intranasal instillation or inhalation into 32 healthy volunteers.

Result: Seventeen (53%) of the 32 participants developed symptoms ranging from mild nasal symptoms to bronchitis.

Notes: No controls were used. Participants were not blinded.

Experiment 61.2

0	0 of 0 (0%)	21 of 32 (66%)
Sick donor(s)	Control recipient(s) became sick	Healthy recipient(s) became sick

Method: Fluid from a cell culture allegedly containing influenza virus type A2 was inoculated via intranasal instillation or inhalation into 38 healthy volunteers.

Result: Twenty-one (66%) of the 32 participants developed upper respiratory symptoms.

Notes: No controls were used. Participants were not blinded.

Experiment 61.3

0	0 of 0 (0%)	20 of 28 (71%)
Sick donor(s)	Control recipient(s) became sick	Healthy recipient(s) became sick

Method: Fluid from a cell culture allegedly containing coxsackie virus A type 21 was inoculated via intranasal instillation or inhalation into 28 healthy volunteers.

Result: Twenty (71%) of the 28 participants developed symptoms ranging from mild nasal symptoms to tracheobronchitis.

Notes: No controls were used. Participants were not blinded.

Experiment 61.4

0	0 of 0 (0%)	9 of 15 (60%)
Sick donor(s)	Control recipient(s) became sick	Healthy recipient(s) became sick

Method: Fluid from a cell culture allegedly containing adenovirus type 4 was inoculated via inhalation into 15 healthy volunteers.
Result: Nine (60%) of the 15 participants developed upper and lower respiratory symptoms including pneumonia.
Notes: No controls were used. Participants were not blinded.

62. Effect of a New Human Respiratory Virus in Volunteers

Author(s): Bradburne, A., Bynoe, M & Tyrrell, D.[62]   **Year:** 1967

Experiment 62.1

0	0 of 0 (0%)	4 of 6 (67%)
Sick donor(s)	Control recipient(s) became sick	Healthy recipient(s) became sick

Method: Tissue culture fluid allegedly containing respiratory virus 2229-E was inoculated via instillation into the noses of six recipients.
Result: Four (67%) of the 6 recipients developed colds.
Notes: No controls were used.

Experiment 62.2

0	0 of 0	4 of 6
	(0%)	(67%)
Sick donor(s)	Control recipient(s) became sick	Healthy recipient(s) became sick

Method: The nasal secretions from one of the sick people in experiment 62.1 were filtered and instilled into the noses of 20 recipients. Twenty healthy controls were inoculated with saline.

Result: Nine (45%) of the 20 recipients developed colds. One cold was graded as serve, two as moderate and the rest as mild. None of the participants in the control group developed a cold.

Notes: No positive controls were used.

Experiment 62.3

?	0 of 0	34 of 75
	(0%)	(45%)
Sick donor(s)	Control recipient(s) became sick	Healthy recipient(s) became sick

Method: Nasal washings obtained from sick people allegedly containing respiratory virus B814 were instilled into the noses of 75 recipients.

Result: Thirty-four (45%) of the 75 recipients developed colds. About 70% of the colds were mild.

Notes: No controls were used.

Experiment 62.4

0	0 of 0 (0%)	78 of 213 (37%)
Sick donor(s)	Control recipient(s) became sick	Healthy recipient(s) became sick

Method: Tissue culture fluid containing respiratory virus 'HGP' or 'PK' was instilled into the noses of 213 healthy recipients.

Result: Seventy-eight (37%) of the 213 recipients developed colds. About 80% of the colds were mild.

Notes: No controls were used.

Experiment 62.5

?	0 of 0 (0%)	77 of 251 (31%)
Sick donor(s)	Control recipient(s) became sick	Healthy recipient(s) became sick

Method: Nasal washings from people allegedly containing respiratory virus 'DC' were instilled into the noses of 251 recipients.

Result: Seventy-seven (31%) of the 251 recipients developed colds.

Notes: No controls were used.

63. Exposure to Cold Environment and Rhinovirus

Author(s): Douglas, R., Lindgren, K & Couch, R.[63]   **Year:** 1968

Experiment 63.1

0	0 of 0 (0%)	24 of 44 (55%)
Sick donor(s)	Control recipient(s) became sick	Healthy recipient(s) became sick

Method: Forty-four healthy prison inmates were inoculated with cell culture fluid containing 'rhinovirus'. Nine men were then exposed to a temperature of 4°C, six were exposed to 10°C, seventeen were exposed to 23°C, and seven were exposed to 32°C for two hours. Five men were exposed to both cold (4°C) and warm (32°C) temperatures.

Result: Of nine exposed to 4°C, four (44%) developed colds. Nine of 17 (29%) exposed to 23°C, and 11 (85%) of 13 exposed to 10°C or 32°C, developed colds. A total of 24 out of 44 (55%) developed colds.

Notes: No controls were used. No blinding was used. The authors concluded that cold temperatures do not affect the common cold.

64. An Outbreak of Common Colds at an Antarctic Base

Author(s): Allen, T., Bradburne, A., Stott, E[64]   **Year:** 1973

Experiment 64.1

8	0 of 0 (0%)	1 of 17 (6%)
Sick donor(s)	Control recipient(s) became sick	Healthy recipient(s) became sick

Method: Twelve Antarctic explorers lived together in huts. After 17 weeks in isolation, one man developed a severe cold, eight developed colds, and two had 'sneezing attacks'. Mucus samples were sent to the CCRU, pooled, and inoculated into 17 healthy volunteers.
Result: One of the 17 recipients developed a 'doubtful' cold.
Notes: No controls were used.

65. Hand-to-hand Transmission of Rhinovirus Colds

Author(s): Gwaltney, J., Moskalski, P. & Hendley, J.[65]   **Year:** 1978

Experiment 65.1

0	0 of 0 (0%)	9 of 11 (82%)
Sick donor(s)	Control recipient(s) became sick	Healthy recipient(s) became sick

Method: The HH 'strain' of rhinovirus was mixed in Hank's balanced salt solution and inoculated intranasally into 11 healthy people.
Result: Nine (82%) of 11 developed cold-like symptoms.
Notes: No controls were used. No blinding was used.

Experiment 65.2

6	0 of 0	9 of 15
	(0%)	(60%)
Sick donor(s)	Control recipient(s) became sick	Healthy recipient(s) became sick

Method: Six participants from Exp. 65.1 with severe symptoms blew their nose into their hands. Fifteen healthy participants touched the sick donor's hands for 10 seconds and then touched their eyes and nose.

Result: Nine (60%) out of 15 recipients developed colds.

Notes: The way in which colds were diagnosed is questionable. No controls were used. No blinding was used.

Experiment 65.3

6	0 of 0	1 of 12
	(0%)	(8%)
Sick donor(s)	Control recipient(s) became sick	Healthy recipient(s) became sick

Method: Six sick participants from Exp. 65.1 sat at a table, with two to four healthy participants for 15 minutes. They were positioned 70 cm away from each other and encouraged to talk loudly, sing, cough, and sneeze at the healthy participants.

Result: One (8%) out of 12 recipients developed colds.

Notes: No controls were used. No blinding was used. The single sick participant acquired a natural cold outside of the experimental setting.

Experiment 65.4

6	0 of 0	0 of 10
	(0%)	(0%)
Sick donor(s)	Control recipient(s) became sick	Healthy recipient(s) became sick

Method: The six sick donors from experiment 65.1 and 10 healthy participants were housed in one large, closed room for three days and nights. They were separated by a double wire mesh barrier preventing any direct physical contact. The donors were allowed to cough and sneeze at will. No fresh air was introduced into the room. Each donor was intentionally exposed to at least one or two healthy recipients.
Result: None of the healthy recipients developed colds.
Notes: No controls were used. No blinding was used.

66. Short Duration Exposure and the Transmission of Rhinoviral Colds

Author(s): D'Alessio, D., Meschievitz, C., Dick, C., et al.[66]   **Year:** 1984

Experiment 66.1

2	0 of 0	0 of 5
	(0%)	(0%)
Sick donor(s)	Control recipient(s) became sick	Healthy recipient(s) became sick

Method: Two people with experimentally induced colds sat at a table in a small unventilated room, 90 cm away from five healthy recipients. They played cards, sang, and conversed freely.
Result: None of the healthy volunteers became unwell.
Notes: No controls were used. No blinding was used.

Experiment 66.2

3	0 of 0 (0%)	0 of 4 (0%)
Sick donor(s)	Control recipient(s) became sick	Healthy recipient(s) became sick

Method: Three sick people with experimentally induced colds sat at a table in a small unventilated room 90 cm away from four healthy recipients. They played cards, sang, and conversed freely.
Result: None of the healthy volunteers became unwell.
Notes: No controls were used. No blinding was used.

Experiment 66.3

11	0 of 0 (0%)	1 of 11 (9%)
Sick donor(s)	Control recipient(s) became sick	Healthy recipient(s) became sick

Method: Eleven participants were experimentally infected with colds. They were divided into five groups and matched with five groups of healthy participants. The groups of healthy and sick people spent 12 hours per day over three consecutive days together in a small room.
Result: One (9%) of the eleven healthy participants developed a 'laboratory confirmed' cold (their bodily fluids induced cytopathic effects in a cell culture and had an increase in the titre of neutralising antibodies).
Notes: No controls were used. No blinding was used.

Experiment 66.4

4	0 of 0 (0%)	0 of 4 (0%)
Sick donor(s)	Control recipient(s) became sick	Healthy recipient(s) became sick

Method: Four people were experimentally infected with colds. They kissed five healthy recipients for one minute each.
Result: None of the healthy participants became ill.
Notes: No controls were used. No blinding was used.

Experiment 66.5

4	0 of 0 (0%)	1 of 11 (9%)
Sick donor(s)	Control recipient(s) became sick	Healthy recipient(s) became sick

Method: Six participants with experimentally induced colds kissed 11 healthy people (two 45-second contacts).
Result: Only one case of a 'laboratory confirmed' cold occurred (their bodily fluids induced cytopathic effects in a cell culture, and an increase in the titre of neutralising antibodies).
Notes: No controls were used. No blinding was used.

67. Experimental Rhinovirus Infection in Volunteers

Author(s): Bardin, P., Sanderson, G., et al.[67]   **Year:** 1996

Experiment 67.1

0	0 of 0 (0%)	20 of 25 (80%)
Sick donor(s)	Control recipient(s) became sick	Healthy recipient(s) became sick

Method: Twenty-five volunteers were experimentally infected with rhinovirus (HRV16). Nasal inoculation was performed by spraying cell culture fluid into the recipients noses.

Result: Twenty (80%) out of 25 participants developed cold-like symptoms.

Notes: No controls were used. The participants were not blinded.

68. Transmission Route of Rhinovirus Type 39

Author(s): Bischoff, W.[68]   **Year:** 2010

Experiment 68.1

0	0 of 0 (0%)	0 of 10 (0%)
Sick donor(s)	Control recipient(s) became sick	Healthy recipient(s) became sick

Method: Ten healthy volunteers were experimentally infected with rhinovirus (HRV39). An aerosol generator was used to expose the participants to the cell culture fluid over twenty minutes.

Result: None of the recipients became unwell.

Notes: No controls were used. The participants were not blinded.

69. Use of a Human Influenza Challenge Model to Assess Person-to-Person Transmission

Author(s): Killingley, B., Enstone, J., Greatorex, J., et al.[69]   **Year:** 2011

Experiment 69.1

0	0 of 0 (0%)	4 of 9 (44%)
Sick donor(s)	Control recipient(s) became sick	Healthy recipient(s) became sick

Method: Nine healthy people were inoculated intranasally with a cultured strain of the influenza H3N2 'virus'. **Result:** Four of the nine (44%) recipients developed an influenza-like-illness. **Notes:** No controls were used. No mention of blinding.

Experiment 69.2

4	0 of 0 (0%)	10 of 15 (67%)
Sick donor(s)	Control recipient(s) became sick	Healthy recipient(s) became sick

Method: Four sick people from experiment 69.1 and two people with 'asymptomatic infections' were divided into three groups of two. Each group of two donors were housed with a group of five volunteers. They played games, watched television, and ate meals together for a total exposure time of 30 hours.
Result: Ten out of 15 recipients (67%) developed mild colds. Four of the 15 (27%) recipients developed an influenza-like illness, and three (20%) were 'laboratory-confirmed cases'.
Notes: No controls were used. No mention of blinding.

70. Minimal transmission in an influenza A (H3N2)

Author(s): Nguyen-Van-Tam, J., Killingley, B., et al.[70]   **Year:** 2020

Experiment 70.1

42	0 of 0	1 of 75
	(0%)	(1%)
Sick donor(s)	Control recipient(s) became sick	Healthy recipient(s) became sick

Method: A total of 52 healthy participants were experimentally infected with 'influenza', 42 of whom became sick. These infected volunteers were then directly exposed to two groups of healthy participants under controlled, household-like conditions for four days. One group of 40 people (protected) wore face shields and hand sanitised every fifteen minutes. They were only allowed to touch their face with a wooden spatula. The other group of 35 people (unprotected) did not wear any protective equipment, nor did they sanitise their hands.
Result: None of the 40 people in the protected group became sick. Only one (1%) of the 35 people in the unprotected group became sick.
Notes: No controls were used.

References

Chapter 1 References

1. Oliver C. 2022. *World's Dirtiest Man Dies Aged 94.* Daily Mail
2. Holmes O. 2022. *World's Dirtiest Man Dies in Iran at 94 a Few Months After First Wash.* The Guardian
3. Tahir T. 2022. *World's Dirtiest Man Dies Aged 94 - Months After Taking His First Shower in 67 Years.* News.com.au
4. Walker J. 1932. *Ann Intern Med.* 5(12):1526
5. Kruse W. 1914. *Munch Med Wschr.* 61:1547
6. Dold VH. 1917. *Munch Med Wschr.* 5:143–44
7. Foster G. 1916. *JAMA.* 66(16):1180
8. Nicolle C, Lebailly C. 1918. *Compt Rend.* 167:607–10
9. Lister F, et al. 1919. *Pub Sth African Inst Med Res.* 12(9):9–23
10. Shibley G, Mills K, Dochez A. 1930. *JAMA.* 95(21):1553
11. Cowan T, Fallon S. 2021. *The Contagion Myth.* Skyhorse
12. Engelbrecht T, Koehnlein C, de Harven E, Bailey S, Scoglio S. 2021. *Virus Mania.* Books on Demand. 3rd ed.
13. Bailey S. 2022. *Settling the Virus Debate.* drsambailey.com
14. Bailey M. 2022. *A Farewell to Virology.* drsambailey.com
15. Townsend J. 1924. *U.S Public Health Service.* 48:1–68
16. Hoyle F, et al. 1979. *Diseases from Space.* Harper & Row
17. Hoyle F, Wickramasinghe C. 2000. *Curr Sci.* 78(9):1057–59
18. Hoyle F, Wickramasinghe C. 1987. *Nature.* 327(6124):664–664
19. van Loghem JJ. 1928. *J Hyg.* 28(1):33–54
20. Semple A. 1951. *Proc Roy Soc Med.* 44:794–96
21. Deyle ER, et al. 2016. *Proc Natl Acad Sci.* 113(46):13081–86
22. Smith AE, Kenyon DH. 1972. *Perspect Biol Med.* 15(4):529–42
23. Lee WJ. 2019. In *Vitamin C in Human Health and Disease*, pp. 89–100. Dordrecht: Springer Netherlands

24. Weinstein R, et al. 2006. *Clin Inf Dis.* 42(5):737–737

25. Cannell JJ, Zasloff M, et al. 2008. *Virol J.* 5(1):29

26. Gregg MB. 1980. *Ann N Y Acad Sci.* 353(1):45–53

27. Chase R. 2021. *Drowning in a Sea of Dogma: Do Viruses Exist*

28. Hamade-Saad N. 2022. *Viruses May Be Endogenously-Generated Adaptive Particles That Facilitate Healing.* Quantum University

29. Bailey S, Bailey M. 2024. *The Final Pandemic.* drsambailey.com

30. Alison. 2021. *Sam Bailey on Isolating Viruses.* Waikato Uni.

31. Jarry J. 2020. *Psychiatrist Who Calmly Denies Reality.* McGill Uni.

32. Berezow À. 2021. *How Quacks Become Millionaires: "5G-COVID" Doctor Will Sell Supplements.* Am Council Health Sci

33. Stanton H. 2023. The Most Important Pediatrician in the World: Dr. Lawrence Palevsky

34. Massey C. 2023. *FOIs Reveal Institutions Around the World Have No Record of SARS-COV-2 Isolation.* fluoridefreepeel.com

35. Coppolino, E. 2022. *The COVID-19 Chronology.* planetwaves.fm

36. Rappoport J. 2020. *Covid Revisited.* nomorefakenews.com

37. Henningsen P. 2023. *21st Century Wire.* 21stcenturywire.com

38. Stewart GT. 1968. *Lancet.* 291(7551):1077–81

39. Charnley J. 1968. *Lancet.* 292(7559):101–2

40. Dubos R. 1955. *Sci Am.* 192(5):31–35

41. Richmond P. 1954. *J Hist Med Allied Sci.* 9(3):290–303

42. Papadopulos E, Turner V, et al. 1996. *Continuum (N Y).* 4(3):1–24

43. Farley J. 1977. *The Spontaneous Generation Controversy from Descartes to Oparin.* Baltimore: The Johns Hopkins University Press

44. Strick J. 1988. *Bull Sci Technol Soc.* 8(3):302–5

45. Reich W. 1979. *The Bion Experiments.* New York: Farrar & Straus

46. Morris B. 1987. *Immunol Cell Biol.* 65(1):49–55

47. Zumla A. 2011. *Curr Opin Pulm Med.* 17(3):131–33

48. Gardner MN, Brandt AM. 2006. *Am J Public Health.* 96(2):222–32

49. Kazan-Allen L. 2003. *Int J Occup Environ Health.* 9(3):173–93

50. Vargesson N, Stephens T. 2021. *Expert Opin Drug Saf.* 20(12):1455–57

51. Shy C. 1990. *World Health Stat Q.* 43(3):168–76

52. Moncrieff J, Cooper RE, Stockmann T, Amendola S, Hengartner MP, Horowitz MA. 2022. *Mol Psychiatry.* 28:3243–56

53. McNamara D. 2015. *Nutrients.* 7(10):8716–22

54. Malhotra A, et al. 2017. *Br J Sports Med.* 51(15):1111–12

55. McCallum L, et al. 2015. *Pflugers Arch*. 467(3):595–603

56. Terrier L-M, et al. 2019. *World Neurosurg*. 132:211–18

57. Zuckerman M. 2016. *Open Archaeology*. 2:42–55

58. Fraser S. 2020. *Can Fam Physician*. 66(6):389

59. Marshall A. 1933. *Sci Prog*. 40(157):71–77

60. Ling GN. 1969. *Int Rev Cytol*. 26(1):1–61

61. Baker JR. 1954. *J R Microsc Soc*. 74(3–4):217–21

62. Ling GN. 1997. *Physiol Chem Phys Med NMR*. 29(2):123–98

63. Hillman H, Peter S. 1980. *School Sci Rev*. 62(219):241–52

64. Hillman H. 2011. *Physiol Chem Phys Med NMR*. 41:61–63

65. Hillman H, Sartory P. 1977. *Perception*. 6(6):667–73

66. Rivers TM. 1937. *J Bacteriol*. 33(1):1–12

67. Kox M, van Eijk LT, Zwaag J, van den Wildenberg J, Sweep FCGJ, et al. 2014. *Proc Natl Acad Sci*. 111(20):7379–84

68. Lipton B. 2016. *The Biology of Belief: Unleashing the Power of Consciousness, Matter & Miracles*. Hay House. 10th Edition ed.

69. Dispenza J. 2014. *You Are the Placebo*. Hay House

70. Hadhazy A. 2016. *How it's Possible for an Ordinary Person to Lift a Car*. BBC

71. Ranganathan VK, Siemionow V, Liu JZ, Sahgal V, Yue GH. 2004. *Neuropsychologia*. 42(7):944–56

72. Slimani M, Tod D, Chaabene H, Miarka B, Chamari K. 2016. *J Sports Sci Med*. 15(3):434–50

73. Turek A. 2018. *Freedivers Routinely Achieve Impossible Feats, Achieved with a Special Reflex that Humans Share with Seals. What Exactly Does this Reflex do?* BBC

74. Lipscombe-Southwell A. 2023. *What's the Longest a Human can Hold their Breath Underwater?* BBC Science Focus

75. Collinge W, Yarnold P, Raskin E. 1998. *Subtle Energies & Energy Medicine*. 9(3):171–90

76. Sarnat R. 2018. *J Yoga Physiother*. 5(2):18–20

77. Ventegodt S, et al. 2004. *Sci World J*. 4:362–77

78. Gustafson C. 2017. *Integr Med (Encinitas)*. 16(6):44–50

79. Schmidt P. 1920. *Deutsch Med Wschr*. 46(43):1181–82

80. Jackson G, Dowling H, Spiesman I, Boand A. 1958. *AMA Arch Intern Med*. 101(2):267

81. Barrett B, Brown R, Rakel D, Rabago D, Marchand L, et al. 2011. *Ann Fam Med*. 9(4):312–22

Chapter 2 References

1. Moser M, Bender T, Margolis H, Gary N, Kendal A, Ritter D. 1979. *Am J Epidemiol.* 110(1):1–6

2. Zhang N, Li Y. 2018. *Int J Environ Res Public Health.* 15(8):1699

3. Leitmeyer K, Adlhoch C. 2016. *Epidemiology.* 27(5):743–51

4. Cannell JJ, Zasloff M, Garland CF, Scragg R. 2008. *Virol J.* 5(1):29

5. Macpherson J. 1876. *Edinb Med J.* 22(2):149–60

6. Carpenter KJ. 2012. *Ann Nutr Metab.* 61(3):259–64

7. Westphalen N. 2003. *JMVH.* 12(1):40–47

8. Lind J. 1757. *A Treatise on the Scurvy.* London: A. Millar in the Strand

9. Bhatt A. 2010. *Perspect Clin Res.* 1(1):6–10

10. Martini E. 2004. *Lancet.* 364(9452):2180

11. Milne I. 2012. *J R Soc Med.* 105(12):503–8

12. Baron JH. 2009. *Nutr Rev.* 67(6):315–32

13. Allan P. 2021. *U.S Naval Institute.* 35(1):1

14. Nault DM. 2020. In *Africa and the Shaping of International Human Rights*, pp. 38–63. Oxford University Press

15. Samudzi Z. 2021. *Capturing German South West Africa: Racial Production, Land Claims, and Belonging in the Afterlife of the Herero and Nama Genocide.* San Fransisco: University of California

16. Maedza P. 2018. Chains of Memory in the Postcolony: Performing and Remembering the Namibian Genocide. Cape Town

17. Schmitz S, Lowenstein EJ. 2019. *Int J Womens Dermatol.* 5(2):137–39

18. Voegtlin C. 1914. *JAMA.* LXIII(13):1094

19. Goldberger J. 1914. *Public Health Rep.* 29(26):119–22

20. Hegyi J, Schwartz RA, Hegyi V. 2004. *Int J Dermatol.* 43(1):1–5

21. Bay A. 2008. *Japan Review.* 20:111–56

22. Schmitz S, Lowenstein EJ. 2019. *Int J Womens Dermatol.* 5(2):137–39

23. Zimring C, Rathje W. 2012. *Encyclopedia of Consumption and Waste: The Social Science of Garbage, Volume 1.* Thousand Oaks: SAGE

24. Kraut A. 2004. *Goldberger's War: The Life and Work of a Public Health Crusader.* New York: Hill and Wang

25. Niles G. 1912. *J Am Med Assoc.* LVIII(18):1341

26. Wheeler GA. 1931. *Public Health Rep.* 46(38):2223

27. Akst D. 2000. *American Heritage Magazine.* 51(8):1–6

28. Unknown. 1912. *The Lancet.* 179(4630):1421

29. Etheridge E. 1972. *The Butterfly Caste: A Social History of Pellagra in the South*. Westport: Greenwood Publishing Company

30. Elmore JG. 1994. *Ann Intern Med.* 121(5):372

31. Robinson R. 1914. *Ky Med J.* 12(18):578

32. Tenney LP. 1915. *Tex Med J.* 30(10):449–54

33. Alschibaja K. 1929. *Vestnik Tropicheskoi Meditsiny*. 2(8):616–17

34. Leslie C. 2002. *J Med Humanit.* 23(3/4):187–202

35. Dewan J. 1941. *Am J Psychiatry*. 97(5):1188–93

36. Mooney SJ, Knox J, Morabia A. 2014. *Am J Epidemiol*. 180(3):235–44

37. Goldberger J. 1916. *Public Health Reports (1896-1970)*. 31(46):3159

38. Charartan F. 2004. *BMJ*. 329(7467):690

39. Goldberger J. 1927. *Public Health Rep*. 42(35):2193

40. Semba RD. 2012. *Int J Vitam Nutr Res*. 82(5):310–15

41. Bay A. 2012. *Beriberi in Modern Japan: The Making of a National Disease*. New York: University Rochester Press

42. Peder R, van der Watt L-M, Howkins A. 2016. *Antarctica and the Humanities*. London: Springer

43. Carter KC. 1977. *Med Hist*. 21(2):119–36

44. Evans AS. 1993. In *Causation and Disease*, pp. 123–46. Boston, MA: Springer US

45. Weisskopf M. 1987. *Los Angeles Times*

46. Hachiya N. 2006. *JMAJ*. 49(3):112–18

47. Yorifuji T. 2020. *J Epidemiol*. 30(1):12–14

48. Sakamoto M, Tatsuta N, Izumo K, et al. 2018. *Toxics*. 6(3):45

49. Minamata Disease - Its History and Lessons. 2007. Minimata

50. Miyo I. 2018. Exhibition, Document, Bodies: The (Re)presentation of the Minamata Disease

51. McCurry J. 2006. *Lancet*. 367(9505):99–100

52. Johnston E. 2006. *Asia-Pacific J*. 4(5):1–6

53. Atti SK, Silver EM, Chokshi Y, Casteel S, Kiernan E, et al. 2020. *Curr Probl Pediatr Adolesc Health Care*. 50(2):100758

Chapter 3 References

1. Townsend J. 1924. *U.S Public Health Service*. 48:1–68
2. Darwin E. 1818. *Zoonomia or the Laws of Organic Life*. Philadelphia: Edward Earle. Fourth Edition ed.
3. Woodforde J. 1803. *Med Phys J*. 9(52):505–9
4. Hirsch A. 1883. *Handbook of Geographical and Historical Pathology*. London: New Sydenham Society
5. *The Transactions of the Provincial Medical and Surgical Association*. 1838. London: John Churchill
6. Nightingale F. 1866. *National Archives*
7. Unknown. 1947. *Nature*. 160(4072):668–668
8. Creighton C. 1891. *A History of Epidemics in Britain*. Cambridge: Cambridge University Press
9. *Cold*. 2023. Online Etymology Dictionary
10. Eccles R, Wilkinson JE. 2015. *Rhinology*. 53(2):99–106
11. Hai-long Z, Shimin C, Yalan L. 2015. *J Tradit Complement Med*. 5(3):135–37
12. Huang W. 2020. *Pediatr Res Child Health*. 3(2):1–4
13. Dashtdar M, Dashtdar MR, Dashtdar B, Kardi K, Shirazi M khabaz. 2016. *J Pharmacopuncture*. 19(4):293–302
14. Pinghu Z, Yu S, Yuqian Z, Yingxin Z, Ronghua W. 2020. *J Clin Med Prac*. 24(12):1–5
15. Davey ML, Reid D. 1972. *J Epidemiol Community Health (1978)*. 26(1):28–32
16. Sisley R. 1891. *Epidemic Influenza: Notes on its Origin and Method of Spread*. London: Longman, Green and Co.
17. Kumate J. 2009. *Arch Neurocien*. 14(3):143
18. Hall CB. 2007. *Clin Infect Dis*. 45(3):353–59
19. Yousaf Kazmi S. 2022. *Saudi J Biol Sci*. 29(11):103454
20. Mackenzie M. 1884. *Diseases of the Throat and Nose*. London: J&A Churchill
21. Lower R. 1963. *De Catarrhis 1672*. London: Dawsons of Pall Mall
22. Sadler W. 1911. *The Cause and Cure of Colds*. Chicago: A. C. McClurg & Co
23. Smith W, Andrewes CH, Laidlaw PP. 1933. *Lancet*. 222(5732):66–68
24. Price WH. 1956. *Proc Natl Acad Sci*. 42(12):892–96
25. Clemow F. 1894. *Lancet*. 143(3673):139–43

26. Clemow F. 1894. *Lancet.* 143(3676):329–31
27. Rosenau M, Keegan W, Richey D, McCoy G, Goldberger J, et al. 1919. *Hygienic Laboratory.* 123:54–90
28. Hope-Simpson RE, Golubev DB. 1987. *Epidemiol Infect.* 99(1):5–54
29. Cannell J, Vieth R, Umahu J, Holick M, Grant W, et al. 2006. *Epidemiol Infect.* 134(6):1129–40
30. Deyle ER, Maher MC, Hernandez RD, Basu S, Sugihara G. 2016. *Proc Natl Acad Sci.* 113(46):13081–86
31. Hoyle F, Wickramasinghe C. 2000. *Curr Sci.* 78(9):1057–59
32. Hoyle F, Wickramasinghe C. 1979. *Diseases from Space.* Harper and Row
33. Cowan T, Fallon S. 2021. *The Contagion Myth.* Skyhorse
34. Engelbrecht T, Koehnlein C, de Harven E, Bailey S, Scoglio S. 2021. *Virus Mania.* Books on Demand. 3rd ed.
35. Smith AE, Kenyon DH. 1972. *Perspect Biol Med.* 15(4):529–42
36. Lee WJ. 2019. In *Vitamin C in Human Health and Disease*, pp. 89–100. Dordrecht: Springer Netherlands
37. Andrewes CH. 1942. *Proc R Soc Med.* 36(1):1–10
38. Fox JP, Kilbourne ED. 1973. *J Infect Dis.* 128(3):361–86
39. Cannell JJ, Zasloff M, Garland CF, Scragg R, Giovannucci E. 2008. *Virol J.* 5(1):29
40. Kelly J. 2011. *Common cold: The Centuries-old Battle Against the Sniffles.* BBC
41. Icard P, Simula L, Rei J, Fournel L, De Pauw V, Alifano M. 2021. *Biochimie.* 191:164–71
42. Rusnock A. 2002. In *Vital Accounts*, pp. 109–36. Cambridge University Press
43. Campbell FR. 1885. *Buffalo Med Surg J.* 26(5):193–214
44. Ballard E. 1879. *Trans Epidemiol Soc Lond.* 4(Pt 1):30–38
45. Anders HS. 1899. *Trans Am Climatol Assoc.* 15:286–303
46. Cormack J. 1853. *Assoc Med J.* 1(34):745–49
47. Wunderlich C. 1843. *Arch Physiol Heilk.* 2(321):6–62
48. Ackerknecht EH. 2009. *Int J Epidemiol.* 38(1):7–21
49. Leonard A. 1990. *J R Coll Physicians Lond.* 24(2):141–43
50. DeLacy M. 1993. *Bull Hist Med.* 67(1):74–118
51. Sydenham T. 1809. *The Works of Thomas Sydenham.* Philadelphia: Benjamin and Thomas Kite

52. Arbuthnot J. 1733. *An Essay Concerning the Effects of Air on Human Bodies*. London: Jacob Tonson

53. Diller T. 1909. *Aesculapian*. 1(2):65–84

54. van Loghem JJ. 1928. *J Hyg*. 28(1):33–54

55. Poling MI, Dufresne CR, Chamberlain RL. 2017. *Br J Gen Pract*. 67(654):32–33

56. Cuming R. 1803. *Med Phys J*. 10(56):312–15

57. Clarke J. 1808. *Edinb Med Surg J*. 4(16):422–40

58. Beddoes T. 1803. *Med Phys J*. 10(58):517–29

59. Beddoes T. 1803. *Med Phys J*. 10(57):385–410

60. Beddoes T. 1803. *Med Phys J*. 10(54):97–127

61. Beddoes T. 1803. *Med Phys J*. 10(56):303–12

62. Kinglake R. 1803. *Med Phys J*. 9(52):517–22

63. Rush B. 1805. *An Inquiry Into the Various Sources of the Usual Forms of Summer and Autumnal Disease in the United States, and the Means of Preventing Them: To Which Are Added, Facts, Intended to Prove the Yellow Fever Not to Be Contagious*. Philadelphia: J. Conrad & Co

64. Barnes D. 2021. *Harv Libr Bull*

65. Larkin C. 1825. *Lond Med Phys J*. 53(314):263–84

66. Jones A. 1827. *Philadelphia J Med Physical Sci*. 4(7):1

67. Ross G. 1845. *Lancet*. 45(1115):34–35

68. Prout W. 1836. *Chemistry, Meteorology and the Function of Digestion Considered with Reference to Natural Theology*. Philadelphia: Carey, Lead and Blanchard

69. Prout W. 1836. *The Bridgewater Treatises on the Power of Wisdom, and the Goodness of God, as Manifested in the Creation*. Philadelphia: Carey, Lea and Blanchard

70. Tytler R. 1834. *London Med Surg J*. 5(105):553–59

71. Bremer F. 1848. In *De permanente Comiteers Arbeider i Aarene 1846 og 1847*, pp. 213–21. Copenhagen: Reitzel

72. Skydsgaard MA. 2010. *Med Hist*. 54(2):215–36

73. Mussell J. 2007. *Endeavour*. 31(1):12–17

74. Simonds AK. 2018. *ERJ Open Res*. 4(1):00020–02018

75. Keegan J. 1918. *JAMA*. 71(13):1051

76. Taubenberger J, Morens D. 2009. *Rev Off Int Epizoot*. 28(1):187–202

77. John A. 1848. *Change of Air: Fallacies Regarding it*. London: John Ollivier

78. Atkinson JC. 1850. *Lancet*. 55(1382):240

79. Fibiger C. 1870. *Om Klimaets Virkninger paa Nosogenesen.* Copenhagen: Iversens Boghandel

80. Anders HS. 1899. *Trans Am Climatol Assoc.* 15:286–303

81. Davis N. 1890. *JAMA.* 14(23):817

82. Poore G. 1902. *The Earth in Relation to the Preservation and Destruction of Contagia.* London: Longmans, Green & Co

83. Sigelman CK. 2012. *Health Educ Behav.* 39(1):67–76

84. Nizame FA, Nasreen S, Unicomb L, Southern D, Gurley ES, et al. 2011. *BMC Public Health.* 11(1):901

85. Iyun BF, Tomson G. 1996. *Soc Sci Med.* 42(3):437–45

86. Helman CG. 1978. *Cult Med Psychiatry.* 2(2):107–37

87. Smith A. 1839. *An Account of the Yellow Fever which Appeared in the City of Galveston, Republic of Texas in the Autumn of 1839.* Galveston: Hamilton Stuart

88. Goldberg DS. 2012. *Can Bull Med Hist.* 29(2):351–71

89. Horlbeck HB. 1890. *Public Health Pap Rep.* 16:110–25

90. Choppin S. 1878. *Public Health Pap Rep.* 4:190–206

91. LeHardy JC. 1888. *Atlanta Med Surg J.* 5(10):605–16

92. Simon L V., Hashmi MF, Torp KD. 2023. *Yellow Fever*

93. Reese M. 1858. *Am Med Gaz J Health.* 10:618–19

94. Wiggins M. 2016. *Southwestern Hist Q.* 119(3):234–52

95. Smith N. 1831. *Medical and Surgical Memoirs.* Baltimore: William A. Francis

96. La Roche R. 1855. *Yellow Fever Considered in its Historical, Pathological, Etiological and Therapeutical Relations.* Philadelphia: Blanchard and Lea

97. Reese M. 1858. *Am Med Gaz J Health.* 10:544–45

98. Laicus. 1861. *BMJ.* 1(11):292

99. Richmond P. 1954. *J Hist Med Allied Sci.* 9(4):428–54

Chapter 4 References

1. Richmond P. 1954. *J Hist Med Allied Sci*. 9(3):290–303
2. Bennet J. 1868. *On The Atmospheric Germ Theory and the Origin of Infusoria*. Edinburgh: Adam & Charles Black
3. Béchamp A. 1855. *Compt Rend*. 40:436–38
4. Béchamp A. 1858. *Compt Rend*. 46:44–47
5. Béchamp A. 1883. *Les Microzymas*. Paris: J. B Bailerre
6. Béchamp A. 1912. *The Blood and its Third Anatomical Element*. London: John Ouseley Limited
7. Béchamp A. 1858. *Ann Chim*. 54:28–42
8. Pasteur L. 1861. *Mémoire sur les corpuscules organisés qui existent dans l'atmosphére. Examen de la doctrine des générations spontanées*. Paris: Mallet-Bachelier
9. Pasteur L. 1857. *Compt Rend*. 45:1032–36
10. Pasteur L. 1858. *Ann Chim*. 58:323–426
11. Pasteur L. 1857. *Compt Rend*. 45:1032–36
12. Hume E. 1923. *Béchamp or Pasteur? A Lost Chapter in the History of Biology*. London: C. W Daniel Company
13. Antoine Béchamp. 1870. *Les microzymas, la pathologie et la thérapeutique*. Paris: Boehm et Fils
14. Manchester KL. 2001. *Endeavour*. 25(2):68–73
15. Smith A. 1861. *Br Foreign Med Surg Rev*. 28(56):429–41
16. Joly N, Musset C. 1863. *Compt Rend*. 57:845–46
17. Pouchet F, Joly N, Musset C. 1863. *Compt Rend*. 57:558–61
18. Wanklyn JA. 1870. *Nature*. 2(38):234–35
19. Crellin JK. 1966. *Ann Sci*. 22(1):49–60
20. Pasteur L. 1878. *Théorie des germes et ses applications à la médecine et à la chirurgie*. G. Masson
21. Tulchinsky TH, Varavikova EA. 2014. In *The New Public Health*, pp. 1–42. Elsevier
22. Geison G. 2014. *The Private Science of Louis Pasteur*. New Jersey: Princeton University Press
23. Wright W. 1930. *De Contagione Et Contagiosis Morbis Et Eorum Curatione Libri III*. New York: Putnam
24. Torrey HB. 1938. *Osiris*. 5:246–75
25. Black G. 1884. *The Formation of Poisons by Micro-organisms: A Biological Study of the Germ*. Philadelphia: P. Blakiston Son & Co

26. Behrens C. 1947. *Hist Sci.* 57:172–77
27. Plenciz M. 2011. *Opera Medico-physica: De Contagio.* Nabu Press
28. Astier C. 1813. *Ann. Chem.* 87:271–85
29. Hameau J. 1895. *Etude sur les virus.* Paris: G. Masson
30. Cadeddu A. 1985. *Hist Philos Life Sci.* 7(1):87–104
31. Cadeddu A. 2000. *Hist Philos Life Sci.* 22(1):3–28
32. Cadeddu A. 1987. *Hist Philos Life Sci.* 9(2):255–76
33. Cavaillon J-M, Legout S. 2022. *Biomolecules.* 12(4):596
34. Debré P, Forster E. 1998. *Louis Pasteur.* Johns Hopkins University Press
35. Sturdy S. 1996. *Med Hist.* 40(3):380–82
36. Altman L. 1995. *The Doctor's World; Revisionist History Sees Pasteur As Liar Who Stole Rival's Ideas.* New York Times
37. Fee E. 1995. *NEJM.* 333:884–85
38. Anderson C. 1993. *Science (1979).* 259(5098):1117
39. Clause KC, Liu LJ, Tobita K. 2010. *Cell Commun Adhes.* 17(2):48–54
40. Enderlein E. 1925. *Bacteria Cyclogeny.* Prescott: Enderlein Enterprises Inc
41. Bird C. 1991. *The Persecution and Trial of Gaston Naessans.* Tiburon: H.J Kramer Inc
42. Reich W. 1979. *The Bion Experiments.* New York: Farrar, Straus and Giroux
43. Reich W, Du Teil R, Hahn A. 1938. *Die Bione: zur Entstehung des Vegetativen Lebens.* Oslo: Sexpol-Verlag
44. Leibniz G. 1935. *La Monadologia.* Firenze: Sansoni
45. Pasini E. 2017. *G.W. Leibniz's Anti-Death Perspective: Spontaneity of Death and Absolute Immortality.* Taiwan: Ria University Press
46. Leibnitz F, Hedge F. 1867. *J Speculative Monadology.* 1(3):129–37
47. Dallinger WH, Drysdale J. 1873. *Monthly Microscopical J.* 10(2):53–58
48. Zumla A. 2011. *Curr Opin Pulm Med.* 17(3):131–33
49. Evans AC. 1929. *J Bacteriol.* 17(2):63–77
50. Houston A. 1900. *Nature.* 62(1611):465–66
51. Bernard C. 1878. *Lefons sur tes Phenomenes de la Vie Communs aux Animaux et aux Vegetaux,* Vol. 1. Paris: J. B Bailliere
52. McLaughlin RW, Vali H, Lau PCK, Palfree RGE, De Ciccio A, et al. 2002. *J Clin Microbiol.* 40(12):4771–75
53. Tedeschi GG, Amici D. 1972. *Ann Sclavo.* 14(4):430–42

54. Tedeschi G, Amici D, Paparelli M. 1969. *Nature.* 222(5200):1285–86

55. Pease PE, Bartlett R, Farr M. 1981. *Experientia.* 37(5):513–15

56. Almquist E. 1917. *Zeitschrift für Hygiene und Infektionskrankheiten.* 83:1–18

57. Mellon RR. 1925. *J Bacteriol.* 10(5):481–511

58. Villequez E. 1955. *Librarie Maloine*

59. Villequez E. 1965. *Gaz Méd France.* 12:535–41

60. Villequez E. 1966. In *Biochemistry of Blood Cells and their Preservation.* 23:752–55. New York: Basel

61. Wilson WJ. 1906. *J Pathol Bacteriol.* 11(4):394–404

62. Walker EWA, Murray W. 1904. *BMJ.* 2(2270):16–18

63. Hort EC. 1916. *Journal of the Royal Microscopical Society.* 36(6):528–33

64. Mellon RR. 1922. *Exp Biol Med.* 20(3):191–191

65. Ransome A. 1908. *Lancet.* 171(4402):90–94

66. Tedeschi G, Amici D, Paparelli M. 1970. *Haematologia (Budap).* 4(1):27–47

67. Lohnis F, Smith R. 1916. *J Agric Res.* 18(6):675–702

68. Spencer R, Workman W. 1932. *Public Health Rep.* 47(7):377–425

69. Lohnis F, Smith N. 1923. *J Agric Res.* 23(6):

70. Lundie Alex, Thomas DJ, Fleming S. 1915. *Lancet.* 186(4804):693–94

71. Ayoade MS. 2017. *JOJ Nursing & Health Care.* 4(2):555631

72. Fazel S, Baillargeon J. 2011. *Lancet.* 377(9769):956–65

73. Antelman SM, Chiodo LA. 1984. In *Drugs, Neurotransmitters, and Behavior*, pp. 279–341. Boston, MA: Springer US

74. Youssef D. 2012. *The Sanitized City and Other Urban Myths: Fantasies of Risk and Illness in the Twentieth Century Metropolis.* University of California. 1–336 pp.

Chapter 5 References

1. Heaman EA. 1995. *Can Bull Med Hist.* 12(1):3–25
2. Leviton R. 2000. *Physician: Medicine and the Unsuspected Battle for Human Freedom.* Hampton Roads Publishing
3. Cordingley E. 1924. *Principles and Practice of Naturopathy.* Health Research
4. Stewart GT. 1968. *Lancet.* 291(7551):1077–81
5. Dickinson W. 1902. *Lancet,* pp. 1297–1301
6. Collins WJ. 1902. *J Sanitary Inst.* 23(3):335–56
7. Hodge J. 1905. *Eclectic Med J.* 65:605–7
8. Richmond P. 1954. *J Hist Med Allied Sci.* 9(4):428–54
9. Hayes R. 1948. *Hahnemannian Gleanings,* pp. 129–35
10. Shafi H. 1955. *Hahnemannian Gleanings,* pp. 296–304
11. Richmond P. 1954. *J Hist Med Allied Sci.* 9(3):290–303
12. Laicus. 1861. *BMJ.* 1(11):292
13. Dubos R, Brock T. 1988. *Pasteur and Modern Science.* Heidelberg: Springer Berlin
14. Balloux F, van Dorp L. 2017. *BMC Biol.* 15(1):91
15. Marshall JS, Warrington R, Watson W, Kim HL. 2018. *Allergy, Asthma & Clin Immunol.* 14(S2):49
16. Zachary JF. 2017. In *Pathologic Basis of Veterinary Disease,* pp. 132-241.e1. Elsevier
17. Igea J. 2015. *Curr Immunol Rev.* 11(1):55–65
18. El-Gilany A-H. 2021. *Int J Health Allied Sci.* 10(1):11
19. Ribeiro da Cunha, Fonseca, Calado. 2019. *Antibiotics.* 8(2):45
20. O'Hare R. 2020. *'Vaccines have saved more lives than any other medicines'- Robin Shattock.* Imperial College London
21. Andrei G. 2021. *Front Virol.* 1(666548):1–8
22. 2011. *Nat Rev Microbiol.* 9(9):628–628
23. Casanova J-L. 2023. *Proc Natal Acad Sci.* 120(26):
24. Béchamp A. 1912. *The Blood and its Third Anatomical Element.* London: John Ouseley Limited
25. Béchamp A. 1883. *Les Microzymas.* Paris: J. B Bailerre
26. Morris B. 1987. *Immunol Cell Biol.* 65(1):49–55
27. Bernard C. 1878. *Lefons sur tes Phenomenes de la Vie Communs aux Animaux et aux Vegetaux,* Vol. 1. Paris: J. B Bailliere

28. Cannon W. 1932. *The Wisdom of the Body*. New York: Norton & Company

29. Cannon W. 1926. In *A Charles Richet: ses amis, ses collègues, ses élèves*, ed A Petit. Paris: Les Éditions Médicales

30. Shelton H. 2010. *Human Life Its Philosophy and Laws: An Exposition of the Principles and Practices of Orthopathy*. Kessinger Publishing

31. Sydenham T. 1809. *The Works of Thomas Sydenham*. Philadelphia: Benjamin and Thomas Kite

32. Braithwaite W. 1860. *Principles of Homeopathy with a Few Hints on the Nature and Cure of Disease*. London: Simpkin Marshall & Co. 17–20 pp.

33. Antoine Béchamp. 1870. *Les microzymas, la pathologie et la thérapeutique*. Paris: Boehm et Fils

34. Campbell F. 1885. *Buffalo Med Surg J*. 24(11):483–99

35. Bashore H. 1904. *Sanitarian*. 50(410):42

36. Liebig J. 1842. *Chemistry in its Application to Agriculture and Physiology*. London: Taylor and Walton

37. Hamlin C. 1990. *A Science of Impurity: Water Analysis in Nineteenth Century Britain*. Berkley: University of California Press. 130–133 pp.

38. Frenchstone R. 1886. *Zymotic Diseases: Considered with Reference to their Cause, Extent and Prevention*. Indianapolis: WM. B. Burford, Printer and Binder

39. Carpenter W. 1884. In *The Nineteenth Century: A Monthly Review*. Philadelphia: Leonard Scott Publishing Company

40. Ransome A. 1908. *Lancet*. 171(4402):90–94

41. Ayres P. 1848. *Lancet*. 2:445–47

42. King LS. 1983. *JAMA*. 249(6):794

43. Eyler J. 1973. *J Hist Med Allied Sci*. XXVIII(2):79–100

44. Bastian HC. 1875. *BMJ*. 1(745):469–76

45. Richardson B. 1858. *The Cause of the Coagulation of the Blood, being the Astley Cooper Prize Essay for 1856*. London: J Churchill

46. Tait L. 1882. *BMJ*. 2(1139):830–32

47. Tait L. 1890. *BMJ*. 2(1552):728–32

48. White W. 1891. *Ann Surg*. 13(1):1–30

49. Das K. 1895. *Indian Med Gaz*. 30(4):162–65

50. Wilson G. 1899. *BMJ*. 2(2014):347–48

51. Tait L. 1887. *BMJ*. 2(1386):166–70

52. Mammas I, Drysdale S, Theodoridou M, Greenough A, Spandidos D. 2020. *Exp Ther Med*. 20(6):1–1

53. Sokullu E, Soleymani Abyaneh H, Gauthier MA. 2019. *Pharmaceutics*. 11(5):211

54. van der Want JPH, Dijkstra J. 2006. *Arch Virol*. 151(8):1467–98

55. Ravenel M. 1935. *Sedgwick's Principles of Sanitary Science and Public Health*. New York: Samuel C. Prescott and Murray P. Horwood

56. Mullet C. 1952. *Osiris*. 10:224–51

57. Ackerknecht EH. 2009. *Int J Epidemiol*. 38(1):7–21

58. Tulchinsky TH, Varavikova EA. 2014. In *The New Public Health*, pp. 1–42. Elsevier

59. Kingzett C. 1877. *J Soc Arts*. 26:311

60. Barnard FA. 1873. *Public Health Pap Rep*. 1:70–87

61. Hurd EP. 1874. *Boston Med Surg J*. 91(5):97–110

62. Last J. 2001. *Encyclopedia of Public Health*. New York: Macmillan. 765 pp.

63. Andam CP, Worby CJ, Chang Q, Campana MG. 2016. *Trends Microbiol*. 24(12):978–90

64. Brown TM, Fee E. 2006. *Am J Public Health*. 96(12):2104–5

65. Eisenberg L. 1986. *Med War*. 2(4):243–50

66. Lange KW. 2021. *Global Health J*. 5(3):149–54

67. Walter E, Scott M. 2017. *J Intensive Care Soc*. 18(3):234–35

68. Hume E. 1923. *Béchamp or Pasteur? A Lost Chapter in the History of Biology*. London: C. W Daniel Company

69. Powell T. 1897. *Los Angeles Herald*. 25(52):36

70. Bennet J. 1868. *On The Atmospheric Germ Theory and the Origin of Infusoria*. Edinburgh: Adam & Charles Black

71. Dean T. 1913. *The Crime of Vaccination: Or Bacteria, X.Y.Z.* San Fransisco: Kessinger Publishing

72. Smith A. 1839. *An Account of the Yellow Fever which Appeared in the City of Galveston, Republic of Texas in the Autumn of 1839*. Galveston: Hamilton Stuart

73. Strueh C. 1904. *Naturopath Herald Health*. 5(4):81–83

74. Lust B. 1907. *Naturopath Herald Health*. 8(5):129–34

75. Fraser J. 1916. *Canada Lancet*. 49(10):447–48

76. Rodermund M. 1901. *Fads in the Practice of Medicine and the Cause and Prevention of Disease*. Chicago: Twentieth Century Publishing Co.

77. Hodge J. 1902. *The Vaccination Superstition*. New York: Forgotten Books

78. Unknown. 1901. *The New York Times*, p. 8

79. Golden J. 2021. *Aaron Rodgers isn't the First Big-name Wisconsin Anti-vaccine Voice*. The Washington Post

80. Victor von B. 1880. *Berl Klin Wschr.* 17(43):609–11

81. Lowe J. 1883. *BMJ*. 2(1176):53–57

82. Keith T. 1885. *BMJ*. 1(1257):214–15

83. Bantock G. 1881. *BMJ*. 1(1045):70

84. Tait L. 1868. *Med Times Gaz*. 2:465

85. Bantock GeoG. 1899. *BMJ*. 1(1997):846–48

86. Ormiston R. 1889. *Am J Dent Sci*. 23(2):49–64

87. Cabot H. 1921. *Can Med Assoc J*. 11(9):610–14

Chapter 6 References

1. Bailey CH. 1938. *J Chem Educ.* 15(8):399

2. Fearon W. 1928. *Irish Q Rev.* 17(65):72–81

3. Redi F. 1745. *Opere di Francesco Redi.* Lyon Public Library

4. Hill LR. 1981. *Aslib Proc.* 33(4):137–40

5. Horowitz N. 1956. *Caltech Magazine.* 20(2):21–25

6. Reed G. 1916. *Sci Am*, Nov. 18

7. Folkes M, Needham JT. 1749. *Observations upon the generation, composition, and decomposition of animal and vegetable substances.* London

8. Spallanzani L. 1914. *Saggio di osservazioni microscopiche concernenti il sistema della generazione dei signori di Needham e Buffon.* Società Tipografica Editrice Barese

9. Roll-Hansen N. 2018. *Hist Philos Life Sci.* 40(4):68

10. Pouchet F. 1858. *Compt Rend.* 47:979–82

11. Pouchet F. 1859. *Hétérogénie Ou Traité De La Génération Spontanée Basé Sur De Nouvelles Expériences.* Paris: J. B. Bailliere Et Fils

12. Antoine Béchamp. 1870. *Les microzymas, la pathologie et la thérapeutique.* Paris: Boehm et Fils

13. Farley J. 1977. *The Spontaneous Generation Controversy from Descartes to Oparin.* Baltimore: The Johns Hopkins University Press

14. Strick J. 1988. *Bull Sci Technol Soc.* 8(3):302–5

15. Hume E. 1923. *Béchamp or Pasteur? A Lost Chapter in the History of Biology.* London: C. W Daniel Company

16. Pasteur L. 1858. *Ann Chim.* 58:323–426

17. Spalding D. 1876. *Nature.* 14(342):44–47

18. Joly N, Musset C. 1863. *Compt Rend.* 57:845–46

19. Pouchet F, Joly N, Musset C. 1863. *Compt Rend.* 57:558–61

20. Meunier V. 1865. *Compt Rend.* 61:1060–63

21. Meunier V. 1856. *Compt Rend.* 61:991–92

22. Meunier V. 1865. *Compt Rend.* 61:449–51

23. Meunier V. 1865. *Compt Rend.* 61:377–78

24. Bennet J. 1868. *On The Atmospheric Germ Theory and the Origin of Infusoria.* Edinburgh: Adam & Charles Black

25. Parfitt E. 1869. *Monthly Microscopical J.* 2(5):253–68

26. Richmond P. 1954. *J Hist Med Allied Sci.* 9(3):290–303

27. Huizinga D. 1873. *Pflüger, Archiv für die Gesammte Physiologie des Menschen und der Thiere.* 7(1):549–74
28. Pammel L. 1893. *Proc Iowa Acad Sci.* 1(4):66–91
29. Wigand A. 1884. *Entstehung und Fermentwirkung der Bakterien; Vorläufige Mittheilung.* Marburg: N. G. Elwert
30. Bastian H. 1876. *Compt Rend.* 83:362–64
31. Bastian H. 1876. *Compt Rend.* 83:159–60
32. Bastian H. 1877. *Proc R Soc London.* 25(171–178):149–56
33. Bastian H. 1872. *The Beginnings of Life: Being Some Account of the Nature, Modes of Origin and Transformation of Lower Organisms.* London: Macmillan
34. Bastian H. 1871. *The modes of origin of lowest organisms.* London: Macmillan
35. Bastian H. 1870. *Nature.* 2(35):170–77
36. Bastian HC. 1876. *BMJ.* 1(788):157–59
37. Tan S, Rogers L. 2007. *Singapore Med J.* 48(1):4–5
38. Farley J, Geison GL. 1974. *Bull Hist Med.* 48(2):161–98
39. Roll-Hansen N. 1979. *J Hist Med Allied Sci.* XXXIV(3):273–92
40. Pasteur L. 1876. *Etudes sur la bière, ses maladies avec une théorie nouvelle de la fermentation.* Paris: Gauthier-Villars
41. Duclaux E. 1896. *Pasteur, histoire d'un esprit*, Vol. 1. Sceaux: impr. de Charaire et Cie
42. Dagognet F. 1967. *Méthodes et doctrine dans l'oeuvre de Pasteur.* Paris: Presses universitaires de France
43. Dubos R. 1976. *Louis Pasteur, Free Lance of Science.* New Jersey: Scribner, Armstrong, & Co
44. Pasteur L. 1861. *Mémoire sur les corpuscules organisés qui existent dans l'atmosphére. Examen de la doctrine des générations spontanées.* Paris: Mallet-Bachelier
45. Pasteur L. 1878. *Théorie des germes et ses applications à la médecine et à la chirurgie.* G. Masson
46. Parkes E. 1883. *A Manual of Practical Hygiene.* New York: William Wood & Company. Sixth Edition ed.
47. *Eight Annual Report Sanitary Commissioner with the Government of India.* 1872. Calcutta: Superintendent Government Printing
48. Pouchet F. 1860. *Compt Rend.* 50:748–50
49. Bell J, Leishman W. 1862. *Glasgow Med J.* 9:202–22

50. Debré P. 20000. *Louis Pasteur.* Baltimore: Johns Hopkins University Press

51. Roll-Hansen N. 1983. *Soc Stud Sci.* 13(4):481–519

52. Wanklyn JA. 1870. *Nature.* 2(38):234–35

53. Child G. 1865. *Proc R Soc London.* 14:178–86

54. Doetsch R. 1962. *J Hist Med Allied Sci.* 17(3):325–32

55. Unknown. 1876. *Boston Med Surg J.* 94(9):249–51

56. Bastian HC. 1912. *BMJ.* 2(2709):1542–47

57. Hewlett R. 1914. *Nature.* 92(2308):579–83

58. Frankland E. 1871. *Nature.* 3(64):225–225

59. Sanderson J. 1873. *Nature.* 7(167):180–81

60. Beale L. 1872. *Disease Germs: Their Nature and Origin.* Philadelphia: Lindsay & Blakiston. Second ed.

61. Crellin JK. 1966. *Ann Sci.* 22(1):49–60

62. Weed LA. 1942. *Ann Med Hist.* 4(1):55–62

63. Pickett MJ, Nelson EL. 1951. *J Bacteriol.* 61(2):229–37

64. Nelson EL, Pickett MJ. 1951. *J Infect Dis.* 89(3):226–32

65. Pasteur L. 1876. *Compt Rend.* 83:377–78

66. Strick J. 1999. *J Hist Biol.* 32(1):51–92

67. Unknown. 1915. *BMJ.* 27(2):795–96

68. Bastian H. 1913. *The Origin of Life: Experiments with Superheated Saline Solutions in Hermetically Sealed Vessels.* London: Watts & Co.

69. Burdon-Sanderson J. 1871. *J Cell Sci.* 11(44):323–52

70. Sanderson JB. 1877. *BMJ.* 2(886):879–81

71. Sanderson JB. 1878. *BMJ.* 1(893):179–83

72. Burdon-Sanderson J. 1873. *Nature.* 8(190):141–43

73. Roberts W. 1873. *Nature.* 7(173):302–302

74. Bastian HC. 1875. *BMJ.* 1(745):469–76

75. Burdon-Sanderson J. 1875. *Lancet.* 105(2695):592–93

76. Campbell F. 1885. *Buffalo Med Surg J.* 24(11):483–99

77. Reich W. 1979. *The Bion Experiments.* New York: Farrar, Straus and Giroux

78. Reich W, Du Teil R, Hahn A. 1938. *Die Bione: zur Entstehung des Vegetativen Lebens.* Oslo: Sexpol-Verlag

79. Strick J. 2015. *Wilhelm Reich, Biologist.* Cambridge: Harvard University Press

80. Nelson EL. 1958. *J Experimental Med.* 107(5):769–82

81. Burke J. 1906. *Nature.* 74(1905):1–3

82. Bonifas V. 1963. *Pathologia et Microbiologia* . 26(5):696–710

83. Zwillenberg LO, Bonifas VH. 1964. *Pathobiology*. 27(1):95–102

84. Činátl J. 1967. *Exp Cell Res*. 47(1–2):123–31

85. Činátl J. 1969. *J Theor Biol*. 23(1):1–10

86. Crile G, Telkes M, Rowland AF. 1932. *Protoplasma*. 15(1):337–60

87. Bungenberg de Jong M, Kruyt H. 1949. *Elsevier*, pp. 232–58

88. Nelson E. 1958. *J Experimental Med*. 107(5):755–68

89. Smith AE, Kenyon DH. 1972. *Perspect Biol Med*. 15(4):529–42

90. Laidlaw P. 1925. *Brit J Exp Path*. 6(1):36–39

91. Brown T, Swift H, Watson R. 1940. *J Bact*. 40:857

92. Keosian J. 1960. *Science (1979)*. 131(3399):479–82

93. Smith A, Kenyon D. 1970. *University of California*

94. Richardson B. 1877. *Nature*. 16(414):480–86

95. Engelkirk P, Engelkirk-Duben J, Fader R. 2020. *Burton's Microbiology for the Health Sciences, Enhanced Edition*. Burlington: Jones & Bartlett Learning

96. Secord JA. 2018. In *Reproduction*, pp. 672–672. Cambridge University Press

97. Dubos R. 1950. *Louis Pasteur*. New York: Little Brown & Co

98. Nelson CH. 1954. *Am J Phys*. 22(4):244–244

99. Conant J. 1953. *Pasteur's and Tyndall's study of spontaneous generation*. Cambridge: Harvard University Press

100. López Cerezo JA. 2015. *J Gen Phil Sci*. 46(2):301–18

101. Rashevsky N. 1943. *Bull Math Biophys*. 5(4):165–69

Chapter 7 References

1. Richmond P. 1954. *J Hist Med Allied Sci.* 9(4):428–54
2. Richmond P. 1954. *J Hist Med Allied Sci.* 9(3):290–303
3. Koch R. 1882. *Berliner Klin Wschr.* 251(3):287–96
4. King L. 1952. *J Hist Med Allied Sci.* VII(4):350–61
5. Berman JJ. 2019. In *Taxonomic Guide to Infectious Diseases*, pp. 321–65. Elsevier
6. Tan S, Berman E. 2008. *Singapore Med J.* 49(11):854
7. Osterhaus ADME, Fouchier RAM, Kuiken T. 2004. *Philos Trans R Soc Lond B Biol Sci.* 359(1447):1081–82
8. Fouchier RAM, Kuiken T, Schutten M, van Amerongen G, van Doornum GJJ, et al. 2003. *Nature.* 423(6937):240–240
9. Segre JA. 2013. *J Invest Dermatol.* 133(9):2141–42
10. Grimes D. 2006. *Microbe.* 1(5):223–28
11. Gradmann C. 2014. *Microbes Infect.* 16(11):885–92
12. Gradmann C. 2008. *Medizinhist J.* 43(2):121–48
13. Henle J. 1840. *Von den Miasmen und Contagien und von den miasmatisch kontagiosen 1840. Leipzig, 1910.* Barth: Krankheiten
14. Evans AS. 1993. In *Causation and Disease*, pp. 123–46. Boston, MA: Springer US
15. Klebs E. 1878. *Uber die Umgestaltung der medicinischen Anschauungen in den letzten drei Jahrzehnten.* Leipzig: F.C.W.Vogel
16. Klebs E. 1883. *Verh. Kongr. Innere Med.* 2:139–54
17. Loffler F. 1884. *Mitt. Kaiserl. Gesundheitsamt.* 2:421–99
18. Duhé RJ. 2008. In *Encyclopedia of Cancer*, pp. 1611–13. Berlin, Heidelberg: Springer Berlin Heidelberg
19. Koch R. 1884. *BMJ.* 2(1236):453–59
20. Hill A. 1915. *Lancet.* 186(4814):1271
21. Black G. 1884. *The Formation of Poisons by Micro-organisms: A Biological Study of the Germ.* Philadelphia: P. Blakiston Son & Co
22. Tabrah FL. 2011. *Hawaii Med J.* 70(7):144–48
23. Wall J. 1891. *Atlanta Med Surg J.* 8(2):74–86
24. Leverson M. 1898. *Homeopathic Physician.* 18(6):263–69
25. Horsley V, Hadwen W. 1892. A Correspondence in the Daily Mail Between Sir Victor Horsley and Dr. Walter R. Hadwen. Charing Cross
26. Beale L. 1872. *Disease Germs: Their Nature and Origin.* Philadelphia: Lindsay & Blakiston. Second ed.

27. Von Pettenkofer M. 1892. *Lancet.* 140(3612):1182–85

28. Dubovsky H. 1982. *S Afr Med J.* Spec No:3–5

29. Ackerknecht EH. 2009. *Int J Epidemiol.* 38(1):7–21

30. Mockett J, Meymott H. 1884. *BMJ.* 2(1240):675–77

31. Koch R. 1891. *Vortrag in der 1.* 1(35):650–60

32. Drexler M. 2010. *What You Need to Know About Infectious Disease.* Washington DC: National Academies Press

33. Shanmuganathan R, et al. 2015. *Glob J Health Sci.* 7(4):110–20

34. Kaufmann S. 2002. *Ann Rheum Dis.* 61(S2):54–58

35. Zumla A, Maeurer M. 2015. *Clin Infect Dis.* 61(9):1432–38

36. World Health Organisation. 2022. Tuberculosis

37. Cegielski J, McMurray D. 2004. *Int J Tuberc Lung Dis.* 8(3):286–98

38. Mariana M, et al. 2020. *Majalah Kedokteran Sriwijaya.* 52(1):275–82

39. Moutinho S. 2022. *Sci Am.* 605(7910):16–20

40. Li A, Yuan S, Li Q, Li J, Yin X, Liu N. 2023. *Front Med.* 10:1–14

41. Short FL, MacInnes JI. 2022. In *Pathogenesis of Bacterial Infections in Animals*, pp. 57–78. Wiley

42. Unknown. 2006. *Nat Rev Microbiol.* 4(6):414–414

43. Knipe D, Howley P. 2007. *Fields' Virology.* Philadelphia: Lippincott Williams & Wilkins

44. Fildes P, McIntosh J. 1920. *Br J Exp Pathol.* 1(3):159–74

45. Rivers TM. 1937. *J Bacteriol.* 33(1):1–12

46. Shors T. 2009. *Understanding Viruses.* Sudbury: Jones & Bartlett

47. Rivers T, Benison S. 1967. *Tom Rivers: Reflections on a Life in Medicine and Science.* Cambridge: M.I.T Press

48. Van Helvoort T. 1996. *ASM News.* 62(3):142–45

49. Guttman B. 2013. In *Brenner's Encyclopedia of Genetics*, pp. 291–94. Elsevier

50. Méthot P-O. 2016. *Studies in History and Philosophy of Science Part C: Studies in History and Philosophy of Biological and Biomedical Sciences.* 59:145–53

Chapter 8 References

1. Begley CG, Ellis LM. 2012. *Nature*. 483(7391):531–33

2. Ioannidis J. 2005. *PLoS Med*. 2(8):e124

3. Smith R. 2013. *BMJ*, p. 1

4. Flood L, Mintzes B, Chiu K, Dai Z, Karanges EA, Holman B. 2022. *J Gen Intern Med*. 37(12):3196–98

5. Chopra SS. 2003. *JAMA*. 290(1):113

6. Demasi M. 2022. *BMJ*, p. 1538

7. Dyer O. 2022. *BMJ*, p. 2549

8. Poutoglidou F, Stavrakas M, Tsetsos N, Poutoglidis A, Tsentemeidou A, et al. 2022. *Voices in Bioethics*. 8:1–6

9. Gupta A. 2013. *Perspect Clin Res*. 4(2):144

10. George SL, Buyse M. 2015. *Clin Investig (Lond)*. 5(2):161–73

11. Sarwar U, Nicolaou M. 2012. *J Res Med Sci*. 17(11):1077–81

12. Oransky I, Marccus A. 2023. *The Guardian*

13. Smith R. 2021. *BMJ Blogs*

14. Angell M. 2009. *Drug Companies & Doctors: A Story of Corruption*. The New York Review of Books magazine

15. Horton R. 2015. *Lancet*. 385(9976):1380

16. Fleck L. 1979. *Genesis and Development of a Scientific Fact*. Chicago: University of Chicago Press. 100 pp.

17. Armstrong J, Green K. 2022. *The Scientific Method*. Cambridge: Cambridge University Press

18. Chang M. 2014. *Principles of Scientific Methods*. London: CRC Press

Chapter 9 References

1. Kurtz TW, Al-Bander HA, Morris RC. 1987. *NEJM*. 317(17):1043–48
2. Shore AC, Markandu ND, MacGregor GA. 1988. *J Hypertens*. 6(8):613–17
3. Whitescarver SA, Ott CE, Jackson BA, Guthrie GP, Kotchen TA. 1984. *Science (1979)*. 223(4643):1430–32
4. Kurtz TW, Morris RC. 1983. *Science (1979)*. 222(4628):1139–41
5. Sniecinski RM, Wright S, Levy JH. 2007. In *Cardiothoracic Critical Care*, pp. 33–52. Elsevier
6. Overlack A, Maus B, Ruppert M, Lennarz M, Kolloch R, Stumpe KO. 2008. *Deutsche Med Wschr*. 120(18):631–35
7. McCallum L, Lip S, Padmanabhan S. 2015. *Pflugers Arch*. 467(3):595–603
8. *Sodium*. 2023. Royal Society of Chemistry
9. Winter M. 2023. *Sodium - 11Na*. Department of Chemistry, The University of Sheffield
10. Jeevanandam J, Pal K, Danquah MK. 2019. *Biochimie*. 157:38–47
11. Louten J. 2016. In *Essential Human Virology*, pp. 19–29. Elsevier
12. Kutter JS, Spronken MI, Fraaij PL, Fouchier RA, Herfst S. 2018. *Curr Opin Virol*. 28:142–51
13. Killingley B, Nguyen-Van-Tam J. 2013. *Influenza Other Respir Viruses*. 7:42–51
14. Radigan K, Budinger S, Misharin A, Chi M. 2015. *Infect Drug Resist*, p. 311
15. Bailey M. 2022. *A Farewell to Virology (Expert Edition)*. www.drsambailey.com
16. Taylor MW. 2014. In *Viruses and Man: A History of Interactions*, pp. 23–40. Cham: Springer International Publishing
17. Hassan Z, Kumar ND, Reggiori F, Khan G. 2021. *Cells*. 10(10):2535
18. Pellett PE, Mitra S, Holland TC. 2014. *Handb Clinc Neurol*. 123:45–66
19. Thaker SK, Ch'ng J, Christofk HR. 2019. *BMC Biol*. 17(1):59
20. Cassedy A, Parle-McDermott A, O'Kennedy R. 2021. *Front Mol Biosci*. 8(637559):1–21
21. Racaniello V. 2021. *Understanding virus isolates, variants, and strains*. Virology Blog

22. Wang T-E, Chao T-L, Tsai H-T, Lin P-H, Tsai Y-L, Chang S-Y. 2020. *PLoS Comput Biol.* 16(5):e1007883

23. Petersen LR, Ksiazek TG. 2017. In *Infectious Diseases*, pp. 1493-1508.e2. Elsevier

24. Tyrrell DAJ, Bynoe ML. 1965. *BMJ.* 1(5448):1467–70

25. Tyrrell DAJ. 1966. *Proc R Soc Med.* 59(7):637–38

26. Kendall EJC, Bynoe ML, Tyrrell DAJ. 1962. *BMJ.* 2(5297):82–86

27. Tyrrell D. 1979. *Postgrad Med J.* 55(640):117–21

28. Tyrrell D, Parsons R. 1960. *Lancet.* 275(7118):239–42

29. Rustigian R, Johnston P, Reihart H. 1955. *Exp Biol Med.* 88(1):8–16

30. Enders JF, Peebles TC. 1954. *Exp Biol Med.* 86(2):277–86

31. Kovacik A, Tvrda E, Fulopova D, Cupka P, Kovacikova E, et al. 2017. *Advanced Research in Life Sciences.* 1(1):111–16

32. Gadea I, Zapardiel J, Ruiz P, Gegúndez MI, Esteban J, Soriano F. 1993. *J Clin Microbiol.* 31(9):2517–18

33. Baer A, Kehn-Hall K. 2014. *J Vis Exp.* 93(52065):1–10

34. Christie GE. 1999. In *Encyclopedia of Virology*, pp. 1413–18. Elsevier

35. Ryu W-S. 2017. In *Molecular Virology of Human Pathogenic Viruses*, pp. 47–62. Elsevier

36. Santos SB, Carvalho CM, Sillankorva S, Nicolau A, Ferreira EC, Azeredo J. 2009. *BMC Microbiol.* 9(1):148

37. Hassan SN, Ahmad F. 2020. *Gulhane Med J.* 62(4):224–30

38. Morgan C, Hsu KC, Rifkind RA, Knox AW, Rose HM. 1961. *J Exp Med.* 114(5):833–36

39. Haynes M, Rohwer F. 2011. In *Metagenomics of the Human Body*, pp. 63–77. New York, NY: Springer New York

40. Mokili JL, Rohwer F, Dutilh BE. 2012. *Curr Opin Virol.* 2(1):63–77

41. Liang G, Bushman FD. 2021. *Nat Rev Microbiol.* 19(8):514–27

42. Porto BN. 2022. *Front Immunol.* 13(885341):1–6

43. Wylie KM. 2017. *Clin Chest Med.* 38(1):11–19

44. Khamson S, Kaewnaphan B, Horthongkham N, Kantakamalakul W, Chaimayo C. 2022. *Mal J Med Health Sci.* 18(3):59–65

45. Chong YM, Tan XH, Hooi PS, Lee LM, Sam I, Chan YF. 2019. *J Med Virol.* 91(8):1562–65

46. Toda S, Okamoto R, Nishida T, Nako T. 2006. *Jpn J Infect Dis.* 59(2):142–43

47. Prescott J, Feldmann H, Safronetz D. 2017. *Antiviral Res.* 137:1–5

48. Du Y, Wang C, Zhang Y. 2022. *Viruses.* 14(12):2645

49. Kumar N, Sharma S, Barua S, Tripathi BN, Rouse BT. 2018. *Clin Microbiol Rev.* 31(4):111–17

50. Leland DS, Ginocchio CC. 2007. *Clin Microbiol Rev.* 20(1):49–78

51. Govorkova EA, Kaverin N V., Gubareva L V., Meignier B, Webster RG. 1995. *J Infect Dis.* 172(1):250–53

52. Hematian A, Sadeghifard N, Mohebi R, Taherikalani M, Nasrolahi A, et al. 2016. *Osong Public Health Res Perspect.* 7(2):77–82

53. Timbury M. 1995. *Rev Med Virol.* 5:187–91

54. Smith W, Andrewes CH, Laidlaw PP. 1933. *Lancet.* 222(5732):66–68

55. Hall E. 2021. *Influenza.* Centers for Disease Control and Prevention

56. Andrewes C, Smith W, Laidlaw P. 1935. *Br J Exp Pathol.* 16(6):566–82

57. Magill TP. 1940. *Exp Biol Med.* 45(1):162–64

58. Francis T. 1940. *Science (1979).* 92(2392):405–8

59. Dochez AR, Shibley GS, Mills KC. 1930. *J Exp Med.* 52(5):701–16

60. Dochez AR, Mills KC, Kneeland Y. 1931. *Exp Biol Med.* 28(5):513–16

61. Dochez AR, Mills KC, Kneeland Y. 1931. *Exp Biol Med.* 29(1):64–66

62. Guy JS. 2015. In *Coronaviruses: Methods and Protocols, Methods in Molecular Biology*, pp. 63–71. New York: Humana

63. Rasmussen AF, Stokes JC. 1951. *J Immunol.* 66(2):237–47

64. Dolskiy AA, Grishchenko I V., Yudkin D V. 2020. *Int J Mol Sci.* 21(21):7978

65. Davison N. 2017. *Why Can't We Cure the Common Cold?* The Guardian

66. Price WH. 1956. *Proc Natl Acad Sci.* 42(12):892–96

67. McIntyre CL, Knowles NJ, Simmonds P. 2013. *J Gen Virol.* 94(8):1791–1806

68. Choi T, Devries M, Bacharier LB, Busse W, Camargo CA, et al. 2021. *Am J Respir Crit Care Med.* 203(7):822–30

69. Rivers TM. 1937. *J Bacteriol.* 33(1):1–12

70. Almeida JD, Tyrrell DAJ. 1967. *J Gen Virol.* 1(2):175–78

71. King L. 1952. *J Hist Med Allied Sci.* VII(4):350–61

72. Williams R. 1957. *Int Rev Cytol.* 6:129–91

73. Hillier J. 1950. *Annu Rev Microbiol.* 4(1):1–20

74. Angulo J. 1950. *To be published*

75. Dittmayer C, Laue M. 2022. *Eur Resp J.* 60(3):2200266

76. Miller SE, Goldsmith CS. 2020. *J Am Soc Nephrol.* 31(9):2223–24

77. Dolhnikoff M, Ferreira Ferranti J, de Almeida Monteiro RA, Duarte-Neto AN, Soares Gomes-Gouvêa M, et al. 2020. *Lancet Child Adolesc Health*. 4(10):790–94

78. Neil D, Moran L, Horsfield C, Curtis E, Swann O, et al. 2020. *J Pathol*. 252(4):346–57

79. Bradley BT, Maioli H, Johnston R, Chaudhry I, Fink SL, et al. 2020. *Lancet*. 396(10247):320–32

80. Tavazzi G, Pellegrini C, Maurelli M, Belliato M, Sciutti F, et al. 2020. *Eur J Heart Fail*. 22(5):911–15

81. Caly L, Druce J, Roberts J, Bond K, Tran T, et al. 2020. *Med J Aust*. 212(10):459–62

82. Miller SE, Brealey JK. 2020. *Kidney Int*. 98(1):231–32

83. Goldsmith CS, Miller SE, Martines RB, Bullock HA, Zaki SR. 2020. *Lancet*. 395(10238):e99

84. Bawden F. 1951. *Sci Prog*. 39(153):1–12

85. Sharp DG, Taylor AR, McLean IW, Beard D, Beard JW, et al. 1943. *Science (1979)*. 98(2544):307–8

86. Taylor AR, Sharp DG, Beard D, Beard JW, Dingle JH, Feller AE. 1943. *J Immunol*. 47(3):261–82

87. Sharp DG, Taylor AR, McLean IW, Beard D, Beard JW, et al. 1944. *J Immunol*. 48(2):129–53

88. Heinmets F. 1948. *J Bacteriol*. 55(6):823–31

89. Angulo JJ. 1951. *Archiv for die gesamte Virusforschung*. 4(3):199–206

90. Nakata S, Petrie BL, Calomeni EP, Estes MK. 1987. *J Clin Microbiol*. 25(10):1902–6

91. McFarlane AS. 1949. *BMJ*. 2(4639):1247–50

92. Korsman SNJ, van Zyl GU, Nutt L, Andersson MI, Preiser W. 2012. In *Virology*, pp. 26–27. Elsevier

93. Hopfer H, Herzig MC, Gosert R, Menter T, Hench J, et al. 2021. *Histopathology*. 78(3):358–70

94. Perry A, Brat DJ. 2018. In *Practical Surgical Neuropathology: A Diagnostic Approach*, pp. 1–17. Elsevier

95. Turgeon M. 2022. In *Clinical Laboratory Science: Concepts, Procedures, and Clinical Applications*. St. Louis: Elsevier

96. Iwata H, Hayashi Y, Hasegawa A, Terayama K, Okuno Y. 2022. *Int J Pharm X*. 4:100135

97. Ayub B, Wani H, Shoukat S, Para P, Ganguly S, Ali M. 2017. *J Envir Life Sci*. 2(3):91–94

98. Rhian M, Lensen S, Williams R. 1949. *J Immunol*. 62(4):487–504

99. Francis T. 1948. *JAMA*. 136(17):1088

100. Angulo JJ, Watson JHL, Olarte J. 1950. *J Bacteriol*. 60(2):129–38

101. Payne S. 2017. In *Viruses*, pp. 37–52. Elsevier

102. Roingeard P, Raynal P-I, Eymieux S, Blanchard E. 2019. *Rev Med Virol*. 29(1):e2019

103. Golding CG, Lamboo LL, Beniac DR, Booth TF. 2016. *Sci Rep*. 6(1):26516

104. Beniac D, Siemens C, Wright C, Booth T. 2014. *Viruses*. 6(9):3458–71

105. Pan Y, Zhang D, Yang P, Poon LLM, Wang Q. 2020. *Lancet Infect Dis*. 20(4):411–12

106. Whitford W, Guterstam P. 2019. *Future Med Chem*. 11(10):1225–36

107. Li M, Liao L, Tian W. 2020. *Front Cell Dev Biol*. 8(573511):1–12

108. Badierah RA, Uversky VN, Redwan EM. 2021. *J Biomol Struct Dyn*. 39(8):3034–60

109. Val S, Jeong S, Poley M, Krueger A, Nino G, et al. 2017. *Pediatr Res*. 81(6):911–18

110. Brennan K, Martin K, FitzGerald SP, O'Sullivan J, Wu Y, et al. 2020. *Sci Rep*. 10(1):1039

111. Kesimer M, Scull M, Brighton B, DeMaria G, Burns K, et al. 2009. *FASEB J*. 23(6):1858–68

112. McNamara RP, Dittmer DP. 2020. *J Neuroimmune Pharmacol*. 15(3):459–72

113. Welch JL, Stapleton JT, Okeoma CM. 2019. *J Gen Virol*. 100(3):350–66

114. Zabrodskaya Y, Plotnikova M, Gavrilova N, Lozhkov A, Klotchenko S, et al. 2022. *Viruses*. 14(12):2690

115. Deschamps T, Kalamvoki M. 2018. *J Virol*. 92(18):1102–18

116. Wang J, Wu F, Liu C, Dai W, Teng Y, et al. 2019. *Virol Sin*. 34(1):59–65

117. Nolte-'t Hoen E, Cremer T, Gallo RC, Margolis LB. 2016. *Proc Natl Acad Sci*. 113(33):9155–61

118. Giannessi F, Aiello A, Franchi F, Percario ZA, Affabris E. 2020. *Viruses*. 12(5):571

119. Martins S de T, Alves LR. 2020. *Front Cell Inf Micro*. 10(593170):1–14

120. Pan B-T, Johnstone RM. 1983. *Cell*. 33(3):967–78

121. Harding C, Heuser J, Stahl P. 1983. *J Cell Biol*. 97(2):329–39

122. Bouvier NM, Palese P. 2008. *Vaccine*. 26:D49–53

123. Kumar B, Asha K, Khanna M, Ronsard L, Meseko CA, Sanicas M. 2018. *Arch Virol*. 163(4):831–44

124. Goldsmith CS, Miller SE. 2009. *Clin Microbiol Rev*. 22(4):552–63

125. Borger P, Malhorta B, Yeadon M. 2020. *Corman Drosten Review Report*. Corman Drosten Review

126. Borger P, Malhorta R, Yeadon M, Clare C, McKernan K, et al. 2021. *Zenodo*

127. Corman VM, Landt O, Kaiser M, Molenkamp R, Meijer A, et al. 2020. *Eurosurveillance*. 25(3):2000045

128. Weller T, Robbins F, Enders J. 1949. *Exp Biol Med*. 72(1):153–55

129. Enders JF, Weller TH, Robbins FC. 1949. *Science (1979)*. 109(2822):85–87

130. Norrby E, Prusiner SB. 2007. *Ann Neurol*. 61(5):385–95

Chapter 10 References

1. Stallybrass C. 1938. *J R Inst Public Health*. 1(13):769–80
2. Erkoreka A, Hernando-Pérez J, Ayllon J. 2022. *Infect Dis Rep*. 14(3):453–69
3. Berche P. 2022. *Presse Med*. 51(3):104111
4. Le Goff J. 2011. *Genus*. 67(2):77–99
5. Parsons H. 1891. *BMJ*. 2(1597):303–8
6. Pineo R. 2021. *J Dev Soc*. 37(4):398–448
7. Crosby A. 2003. *America's Forgotten Pandemic: The Influenza of 1918*. Cambridge: Cambridge University Press
8. Dunn FL. 1958. *JAMA*. 166(10):1140
9. Yang Y, Peng F, Wang R, Guan K, Jiang T, et al. 2020. *J Autoimmun*. 109:102434
10. Latiff LA, Parhizkar S, Zainuddin H, Chun GM, Rahiman MAA, et al. 2012. *Glob J Health Sci*. 4(2):
11. Unknown. 2020. Coronavirus: The First Three Months as it Happened
12. Hoyle F, Wickramasinghe C. 2000. *Curr Sci*. 78(9):1057–59
13. Kimmerly V, Mehfoud N, Shipe M. 2014. *Mapping the 1889-1894 Russian Flu*. National Institute of Health
14. Mummert A, Weiss H, Long L-P, Amigó JM, Wan X-F. 2013. *PLoS One*. 8(4):e60343
15. Herring D, Carraher S. 2011. Miasma to Microscopes: The Russian Influenza in Hamilton. Ontario
16. Tulchinsky TH, Varavikova EA. 2014. In *The New Public Health*, pp. 1–42. Elsevier
17. Assmann R. 1890. *Am Meteorol J*. 7(1):37
18. Thomson RS. 1890. *Glasgow Med J*. 33(3):187–91
19. Valleron A-J, Cori A, Valtat S, Meurisse S, Carrat F, Boëlle P-Y. 2010. *Proc Natl Acad Sci*. 107(19):8778–81
20. Mennaberg J, Leichenstern O. 1905. *Malaria, Influenza And Dengue*. W.B. Saunders and Co
21. Althaus J. 1892. *Influenza: Its Pathology, Symptoms, Complications and Sequels*, Vol. 266. London: Longman & Co
22. Brüssow H, Brüssow L. 2021. *Microb Biotechnol*. 14(5):1860–70
23. Egerton F. 1890. *Lancet*. 135(3464):167
24. Manby A, Rowell H. 1890. *Lancet*. 135(3462):51

25. Bertillon J. 1891. *Trans Epidemiol Soc Lond.* 9:103

26. Fitzgerald C. 1893. *Lancet.* 142(3655):718

27. Ulrich C. 1890. *JAMA.* XV(14):495

28. Egerton Fitzgerald C. 1890. *Lancet.* 136(3504):871–72

29. Hagan H. 1890. *Southern Med Rec.* 20(3):126–30

30. Brakenridge D. 1890. *Trans Med Chir Soc Edinb.* 9:117–43

31. Clemow F. 1889. *BMJ.* 2(1510):1305

32. Pryor HB. 1964. *Clin Pediatr (Phila).* 3(1):19–24

33. Brakenridge D. 1890. *Edinb Med J.* 35(11):996–1011

34. Ewing ET. 2019. *Influenza Other Respir Viruses.* 13(3):279–87

35. 1893. *Br Med J.* 2(1720):1346

36. Parsons H. 1891. *Report on the Influenza Epidemic of 1889-90.* H.M Stationary Office. 96 pp.

37. Honigsbaum M. 2011. *Vaccine.* 29:B11–15

38. Clemow F. 1894. *Lancet.* 143(3676):329–31

39. Clemow F. 1894. *Lancet.* 143(3673):139–43

40. Moir DM. 1890. *Ind Med Gaz.* 25(12):353–58

41. Siegfried C. 1891. *Medical Record.* 39(19):531

42. Hilderbrandsson H. 1891. *Am Meteorol J.* 8(1):13

43. Anders HS. 1899. *Trans Am Climatol Assoc.* 15:286–303

44. Curtin RG, Watson EW. 1892. *Annu Meet Amer Climatol Assoc.* 8:88–97

45. Sisley R. 1891. *Epidemic Influenza: Notes on its Origin and Method of Spread.* London: Longman, Green and Co.

46. Richmond W. 1890. *Lancet.* 135(3464):127–28

47. Parsons H. 1890. *BMJ.* 1(1515):102–3

48. Mulhall JC. 1892. *Annu Meet Amer Climatol Assoc.* 8:197–201

49. Pfeiffer R. 1892. *Deutsche Med Wschr.* 18:28

50. Pfeiffer R. 1892. *BMJ.* 1(1620):128–128

51. Canon P. 1892. *BMJ.* 1(1620):129–129

52. Kitasato S. 1892. *BMJ.* 1(1620):128–128

53. Borchardt M. 1894. *Berl. klin. Wochenschr.* 2:

54. Kruse W. 1894. *Deutsche Med Wschr.* 20(24):513–15

55. Weichselbaum A. 1892. *Wiener Klin Wschr.* 32(33):

56. Shelbourne I. 2021. *The Influenza Problem: Paradigms, a Pandemic, and the Search for Pfeiffer's Bacillus. Institute of Historical Research.* University of London

57. Van Epps HL. 2006. *Journal of Experimental Medicine*. 203(4):803–803

58. Walker J. 1928. *J Infect Dis*. 43(4):300–305

59. Rosenau M, Keegan W, Goldberger G. 1918. *Hygienic Laboratory*. 123:5–30

60. McCoy G, Richey D. 1918. *Hygienic Laboratory*. 123:42–51

61. Rosenau M, Keegan W, Richey D, McCoy G, Goldberger J, et al. 1919. *Hygienic Laboratory*. 123:54–90

62. Cecil R, Steffen G. 1921. *J Infect Dis*. 28(3):201–25

63. Lister F, Taylor E. 1919. *Public South African Inst Med Res*. 12(9):9–23

64. Cautley E. 1894. Report of M.O.H. to Local Government Board

65. White R. 1906. *Catarrhal Fevers, Commonly Called Colds: Their Causes, Consequences, Control and Cure*. Edinburgh

66. White R. 1906. *BMJ*. 2(2375):54

Chapter 11 Refereces

1. Townsend J. 1924. *U.S Public Health Service.* 48:1–68
2. Pfeiffer R. 1892. *BMJ.* 1(1620):128–128
3. Tinnerholm Ljungberg H. 2021. *Eur J Hist Med Health.* 78(2):267–86
4. Hedgecoe A. 2009. *Med Hist.* 53(3):331–50
5. Harris JC. 2006. *Arch Gen Psychiatry.* 63(5):482
6. Kelly C. 2010. *Can Bull Med Hist.* 27(2):321–42
7. Coudray F. 1926. *Arch. Med. et Pharm. Milit.* 85(4):387–403
8. Winterbottom T. 1828. *Edinb Med Surg J.* 30(97):321–44
9. Bulmus B. 2012. In *Plague, Quarantines and Geopolitics in the Ottoman Empire*, pp. 130–51. Edinburgh University Press
10. Weisse AB. 2012. *Tex Heart Inst J.* 39(1):51–54
11. Ackerknecht EH. 2009. *Int J Epidemiol.* 38(1):7–21
12. Davis D. 1906. *J Infect Dis.* 3(1):1–36
13. Kruse W. 1914. *Munch Med Wschr.* 61:1547
14. Morton HE. 1938. *Am J Clin Pathol.* 8(ts2_6):185–205
15. Robinson WL. 1928. *Ann Surg.* 88(3):333–34
16. Mudd S. 1923. *J Bacteriol.* 8(5):459–81
17. Foster G. 1916. *JAMA.* 66(16):1180
18. Dold VH. 1917. *Munch Med Wschr.* 5:143–44
19. Walker JE. 1928. *J Infect Dis.* 43(4):300–305
20. Park WH, Cooper G. 1921. *J Immunol.* 6(1):81–85
21. Grafe A. 1991. *A History of Experimental Virology.* Heidelberg: Springer Berlin
22. Aronson J. 2021. *When I Use a Word...Viruses.* British Medical Journal
23. Simon C. 1926. *Sci Mon.* 23(5):407–13
24. van der Want JPH, Dijkstra J. 2006. *Arch Virol.* 151(8):1467–98
25. Mammas I, Drysdale S, Theodoridou M, Greenough A, Spandidos D. 2020. *Exp Ther Med.* 20(6):1–1
26. Schmidt P. 1920. *Deutsch Med Wschr.* 46(43):1181–82
27. Dochez AR, Shibley GS, Mills KC. 1930. *J Exp Med.* 52(5):701–16
28. Kerr W. 1950. *Ann Intern Med.* 33(2):333
29. Walker J. 1932. *Ann Intern Med.* 5(12):1526
30. Yuta A, Doyle WJ, Gaumond E, Ali M, Tamarkin L, et al. 1998. *Am J Physiol Lung Cell Mol Physiol.* 274(6):L1017–23
31. Doyle WJ, Skoner DP, Gentile D. 2005. *Curr Allergy Asthma Rep.* 5(3):173–81

32. Gwaltney JM. 2002. *Am J Med.* 112(6):13–18

33. Andrewes C. 1953. *Br Med Bull.* 9(3):206–7

34. Andrewes CH. 1949. *Lancet.* 253(6541):71–75

35. Andrewes CH. 1950. *NEJM.* 242(7):235–40

36. Troescher-Elam E, Ancona GR, Kerr WJ. 1945. *Am J Physiol.* 144(5):711–16

37. Parvez L, Hilberg O, Vaidya M, Noronha A. 2000. *Rhinol Suppl.* 16:45–50

38. Doyle WJ, Boehm S, Skoner DP. 1990. *J Allergy Clin Immunol.* 86(6):924–35

39. Grandjean LC. 1949. *Acta Pharmacol Toxicol (Copenh).* 5(1):45–52

40. Naclerio RM, Proud D, Lichtenstein LM, Kagey-Sobotka A, Hendley JO, et al. 1988. *J Infect Dis.* 157(1):133–42

41. Simonsson BG, Skoogh B-E, Bergh NP, Andersson R, Svedmyr N. 1973. *Respiration.* 30(4):378–88

42. Fuller RW, Jackson DM. 1990. *Thorax.* 45(6):425–30

43. Nagaki M, Shimura S, Irokawa T, Sasaki T, Oshiro T, et al. 1996. *Am J Physiol Lung Cell Mol Physiol.* 270(6):L907–13

44. Proud D, Reynolds CJ, Lacapra S, Kagey-Sobotka A, Lichtenstein LM, Naclerio RM. 1988. *Am Rev Resp Dis.* 137(3):613–16

45. Shibayama Y, Skoner D, Suehiro S, Konishi J-E, Fireman P, Kaplan AP. 1996. *Immunopharmacology.* 33(1–3):311–13

46. Hobbs B. 2017. *ABC News*

47. Yodaiken RE. 1981. *JAMA.* 246(15):1677

48. Rogers DF. 1996. *Clin Exp Allergy.* 26(4):365–67

49. Cheng J, Zens MS, Duell E, Perry AE, Chapman MS, Karagas MR. 2015. *Cancer Epidemiol Biomarkers Prev.* 24(4):749–54

50. Eccles R. 2021. *Clin Otolaryngol.* 46(1):4–8

51. Jawetz E, Talbot JC. 1950. *Calif Med.* 73(5):379–83

52. Pappas DE. 2018. In *Principles and Practice of Pediatric Infectious Diseases*, pp. 199-202.e1. Elsevier

Chapter 12 Refereces

1. Weinstein L. 1976. *NEJM*. 294(19):1058–60
2. Martini M, Gazzaniga V, et al. 2019. *J Prev Med Hyg*. 60(1):E64–67
3. Erkoreka A. 2009. *J Mol Genetic Med*. 03(02):
4. Hobday RA, Cason JW. 2009. *Am J Public Health*. 99(S2):S236–42
5. Unknown. 2019. *1918 Pandemic (H1N1 Virus)*. Centers for Disease Control and Prevention
6. Jordan E. 1927. *Epidemic Influenza: A Survey* . Chicago: American Medical Association
7. Humphries MO. 2014. *War Hist*. 21(1):55–81
8. Oxford JS. 2001. *Philos Trans R Soc Lond B Biol Sci*. 356(1416):1857–59
9. Hoyle F, Wickramasinghe C. 2000. *Curr Sci*. 78(9):1057–59
10. Riggs T. 1919. *Influenza in Alaska and Puerto Rico: Hearings Before the Subcommittee of House Committee on Appropriations, 65th Congress*. Washington DC: Government Printing Services
11. Tuttle T. 1918. *Twelfth Biennial Report of the State Board of Health*. Washington: Frank M. Lamborn
12. Carney J. 2020. *The Spanish Flu in Alaska: Why Some Villages Were Devastated and Others Unscathed*. Anchorage: Anchorage Press
13. Amundsen R, Ellsworth L. 1927. *First Crossing of the Polar Sea*. George H. Doran Company
14. Unknown. 2021. *The Flu Pandemic Hit Nenana 100 Years Ago*. National Park Service
15. Troll T. 2019. *Bristol Bay Remembers: The Great Flu of 1919*. Bristol Bay Native Corporation and Bristol Bay Land Heritage Trust
16. Liang ST, Liang LT, et al. 2021. *Postgrad Med J*. 97(1147):273–74
17. Isador A. 1920. *Med Rec*. 98(24):969
18. Taubenberger JK. 2006. *Proc Am Philos Soc*. 150(1):86–112
19. Knobler S, Mack A, Mahmoud A. 2005. The Threat of Pandemic Influenza: Are We Ready? Workshop Summary
20. Gagnon A, Miller MS, et al. 2013. *PLoS One*. 8(8):e69586
21. Fornasin A, Breschi M, Manfredni M. 2018. *Infez Med*. 26(1):97–106
22. Shanks GD, Brundage JF. 2012. *Emerg Infect Dis*. 18(2):201–7
23. Shanks GD, et al. 2011. *Influenza Respir Viruses*. 5(3):213–19
24. Shanks GD, MacKenzie A, et al. 2010. *J Inf Dis*. 201(12):1880–89
25. Folley E. 1919. *Lancet*. 193(4990):656–57
26. Oliver W. 1919. *Sci Am*. 12-(9):212–13

27. Barry JM. 2009. *Nature.* 459(7245):324–25

28. Pryor HB. 1964. *Clin Pediatr (Phila).* 3(1):19–24

29. Robertson E. 1919. *Can Med Assoc J.* 9(2):155–59

30. Edington A. 1919. *Lancet.* 194(5017):730–31

31. Influenza Committee Advisory Board. 1918. *BMJ.* 2(3019):505–9

32. Howitt H. 1919. *Pub Health J.* 10(11):508–10

33. Barry J. 1999. *The Great Influenza.* London: Penguin Books

34. Le Count E. 1919. *JAMA.* 72:650–52

35. Keeping J. 2015. *The Oklahoman*

36. *Profiting from the Pandemic.* 2018. University of North Carolina

37. Honigsbaum M. 2019. *The Pandemic Century One Hundred Years of Panic, Hysteria and Hubris.* London: Hurst & Company

38. Cox J, Gill D, et al. 2019. *Lancet Infect Dis.* 19(4):360–61

39. Wever PC, et al. 2014. *Influenza Respir Viruses.* 8(5):538–46

40. Fleury B. 2020. *The 1918 Spanish Flu—Why We Were So Vulnerable.* Wondrium Daily

41. Barry J. 2005. *Lessons from the 1918 Flu.* Time Magazine

42. Cipriano PF. 2018. *Int Nurs Rev.* 65(3):305–6

43. Marsh P. 2021. *The Spanish Flu in Ireland.* Cham: Springer International Publishing

44. McCord CP. 1966. *J Occup Med.* 8(11):593–98

45. Wilson M, Wilson PJK. 2021. In *Close Encounters of the Microbial Kind*, pp. 175–84. Cham: Springer International Publishing

46. Catherine Belling. 2009. *Lit Med.* 28(1):55–81

47. Preston J. 2017. *"More deadly than bullets or bombs": In just three years the Spanish flu wiped out 100 million people.* Daily Mail

48. Cairns P. 1918. *South African Med J*

49. Ferrari L. 2020. *Pathologica.* 112(02):110–14

50. Mills CE, Robins JM, Lipsitch M. 2004. *Nature.* 432(7019):904–6

51. Brundage JF, Shanks GD. 2008. *Emerg Infect Dis.* 14(8):1193–99

52. Klugman KP, Astley CM, Lipsitch M. 2009. *Emerg Infect Dis.* 15(2):346–47

53. Kaplan M, Webster R. 1977. *Sci Am.* 237(6):88–107

54. Byerly CR. 2010. *Public Health Rep.* 125 Suppl 3(Suppl 3):82–91

55. Oxford J, Sefton A, Jackson R, Innes W, Daniels R, Johnson N. 2002. *Lancet Infect Dis.* 2(2):111–14

56. Knowles R. 1925. *Ind Med Gaz.* 60(7):329–32

57. Freemantle M. 2015. *The Chemists' War.* R Soc Chem

58. Reddy G, Lee SH. 2015. In *Wildlife Toxicity Assessments for Chemicals of Military Concern*, pp. 617–36. Elsevier

59. Vaish A, Consul S, Agrawal A, Chaudhary S, Gutch M, et al. 2013. *J Emerg Trauma Shock*. 6(4):271

60. Herringham W. 1920. *Lancet*. 195(5034):423–24

61. Unknown. 1919. *Lancet*, pp. 471–72

62. Glarum J, Birou D, Cetaruk E. 2010. In *Hospital Emergency Response Teams*, pp. 19–83. Elsevier

63. Wagner F. 1934. *Army Ordnance*. 15(85):19–22

64. Padley AP. 2016. *Anaesth Intensive Care*. 44(1_suppl):24–30

65. Herringham W. 1920. *Proc R Soc Med*. 13(War Sect):31–36

66. Cao C, Zhang L, Shen J. 2022. *Front Immunol*. 13(917395):1–12

67. Kumar A, Chaudhari S, et al. 2012. *Indian J Occup Environ Med*. 16(2):88

68. Oxford JS, Gill D. 2019. *Hum Vaccin Immunother*. 15(9):2009–12

69. Ross S, Henderson A. 1918. *JAMA*. 71(9):770

70. Starr I. 2006. *Ann Intern Med*. 145(2):138

71. Shanks GD. 2015. *Travel Med Infect Dis*. 13(3):217–22

72. McCowen G. 1924. *J State Med*. 32(6):277–93

73. Hammond J, Rolland W, Shore T. 1917. *Lancet*. 2:41–45

74. Covey G, Barron M. 1919. *Am J Med Sci*. 157(6):808

75. Reeves J. 2016. *Huntsville Hist Rev*. 41(1):1–12

76. Berghoff R. 1919. *Arch Intern Med*. 24(6):678

77. *Medical Management Guidelines for Phosgene*. 2014. Agency for Toxic Substances and Disease Registry

78. Sciuto AM, Kodavanti UP. 2020. In *Handbook of Toxicology of Chemical Warfare Agents*, pp. 515–44. Elsevier

79. *Signs & Symptoms of Exposure to Sulfur Mustard*. 2019. Centers for Disease Control and Prevention

80. Von Zimmerman MA, Arnold TC. 2023. *Phosgene Toxicity*

81. Maranda EL, Ayache A, Taneja R, Cortizo J, Nouri K. 2016. *JAMA Dermatol*. 152(8):933

82. Oxford JS, Lambkin R, Sefton A, Daniels R, Elliot A, et al. 2005. *Vaccine*. 23(7):940–45

83. Honigsbaum M. 2018. *Spanish Flu: The Killer that Still Stalks Us, 100 Years On*. The Guardian

84. Brundage JF. 2006. *Lancet Infect Dis*. 6(5):303–12

85. Shanks GD. 2019. *Intern Med J*. 49(7):919–23

86. Winternitz M, Wason I, McNamara F. 1920. *The Pathology of Influenza*. New Haven: Yale University Press

87. McCordock HA, Muckenfuss RS. 1933. *Am J Pathol*. 9(2):221-252.7

88. Winternitz MC, Smith GH, McNamara FP. 1920. *J Exp Med*. 32(2):211–17

89. Kashgarian M, Gordon M. 2007. *Yale Medicine Magazine*

90. Kilbourne ED. 1987. *Influenza*. Boston, MA: Springer US

91. Winternitz MC, et al. 1920. *J Exp Med*. 32(2):199–204

92. Bristow NK. 2010. *Pub Health Rep*. 125(S3):134–44

93. *History of United States' Involvement in Chemical Warfare*. 2023. DoD Environment, Safety & Occupational Health Network and Information Exchange

94. *First Usage of Poison Gas*. 2023. The National WWI Museum and Memorial

95. Shufflebotham F. 1919. *BMJ*. 1(3042):478–79

96. Carr D. 1991. *Hist J Mass*. 19(1):43–62

97. Kraut AM. 2010. *Pub Health Rep*. 125(S3):123–33

98. Kolata G. 1999. *The Story of the Great Influenza Pandemic of 1918 and the Search for the Virus That Caused It*. Atria

99. Goulart A da C. 2005. *Hist Cienc Saude Manguinhos*. 12(1):101–42

100. Viboud C, Simonsen L, Fuentes R, Flores J, Miller MA, Chowell G. 2016. *J Inf Dis*. 213(5):738–45

101. Starko KM. 2009. *Clinical Infectious Diseases*. 49(9):1405–10

102. Unknown. 1918. *Take Steps to Stop Influenza Spread*. New York Times. 13–14 pp.

103. Unknown. 1918. *Division of Sanitation Department of the Navy*, Vol. 3. Annual Report of the Secretary of the Navy 1919

104. Bakalar N. 2009. *In 1918 Pandemic, Another Possible Killer: Aspirin*. New York Times

105. Shimazu T. 2009. *BMJ*. 338(jun15 1):b2398–b2398

Chapter 13 References

1. Davis D. 1906. *J Inf Dis*. 3(1):1–36
2. Brackeen TC. 1919. *J Natl Med Assoc*. 11(4):146–48
3. Nuzum J, Pilot I, Bonar B, Stangl F. 1918. *JAMA*. 71(19):1562
4. Selter H. 1918. *Deutsche Med Wschr*. 44(34):932–33
5. Dujarric de la Rivière R. 1918. *Compt Rend*. 167:606–7
6. Nicolle C, Lebailly C. 1918. *Compt Rend*. 167:607–10
7. Rosenau M, Keegan W. 1918. *Hygienic Laboratory*. 123:5–30
8. McCoy G, Richey D. 1918. *Hygienic Laboratory*. 123:42–51
9. Rosenau M, Keegan W, et al. 1919. *Hygienic Laboratory*. 123:54–90
10. Riley R. 2020. *A Review of the Impacts of the 1918 Spanish Flu Pandemic*. University of Birmingham
11. Yamanouchi T, Sakakami K. 1919. *Lancet*. 193(4997):971
12. *Lactated Ringers solution*. 2020. MIMs
13. Michelli F, Satta G. 1919. *J R Acad Med Turin*, pp. 115–36
14. Schofield F, Cynn HC. 1919. *JAMA*. 72(14):981
15. Lister F. 1919. *Public South African Inst Med Res*. 12(9):9–23
16. Wahl HR, White GB, Lyall HW. 1919. *J Inf Dis*. 25(5):419–26
17. Bloomfield A. 1920. *John's Hopkins Hospital Bulletin*. 31(349):1
18. Gordon M. 1922. *J R Army Med Corps*. 39(1):400–401
19. Kraus S. 1922. *Gaz. Clinica de Janeiro*, p. 10
20. Large SH. 1924. *Ann Otology Rhinol Laryngol*. 33(4):1350–55
21. Schmidt P. 1920. *Deutsch Med Wschr*. 46(43):1181–82
22. Cecil R, Steffen G. 1921. *J Inf Dis*. 28(3):201–25
23. Williams A, Nevin M, et al. 1921. *J Immunol*. 6(1):5–24
24. Robertson R, Groves R. 1924. *J Inf Dis*. 34(4):400–406
25. Walker J. 1929. *J Inf Dis*. 1929:254–56
26. Costa-Mandry O, Morales-Otero P, Suarez J. 1932. *Puerto Rico J Public Health Trop Med*. 8:205–19
27. Smorodintseff AA, et al. 1937. *Am J Med Sci*. 194(2):159–70

Chapter 14 References

1. Tyrrell D. 1990. *J R Coll Physicians Lond*. 24(2):137–40
2. Andrewes CH. 1949. *Lancet*. 253(6541):71–75
3. Andrewes C. 1953. *Br Med Bull*. 9(3):206–7
4. Andrewes CH, Lovelock JE, Sommerville T. 1951. *Lancet*. 257(6645):25–27
5. Oransky I. 2005. *Lancet*. 365:2084
6. Epps G. 1982. *Stalking the Common Cold*, Vol. 6. New York Times. 75 pp.
7. Wilson M, Wilson PJK. 2021. In *Close Encounters of the Microbial Kind*, pp. 159–73. Cham: Springer International Publishing
8. Wang K, Xi W, Yang D, Zheng Y, Zhang Y, et al. 2017. *J Thorac Dis*. 9(11):4502–11
9. Barker J, Stevens D, Bloomfield SF. 2001. *J Appl Microbiol*. 91(1):7–21
10. Jawetz E, Talbot J. 1950. *Calif Med*. 73(5):379–83
11. Lovelock JE, Roden AT, Porterfield JS, Sommerville T, Andrewes CH. 1952. *Lancet*. 260(6736):657–60
12. Andrewes CH, Chaproniere DonnaM, Compels AnnetteEH, Pereira HG, Roden AT. 1953. *Lancet*. 262(6785):546–47
13. Tyrrell DAJ, Bynoe ML. 1961. *BMJ*. 1(5223):393–97
14. Tyrrell DAJ, Parsons R. 1960. *Lancet*. 275(7118):239–42
15. Dabin K. 2020. *Revealing the First Coronavirus*. Science Museum Group
16. Walker J. 1932. *Ann Intern Med*. 5(12):1526
17. Boring EG. 1954. *Am J Psychol*. 67(4):573
18. Jackson G, Dowling H, Anderson T, Riff L, Saporta J. 1960. *Ann Intern Med*. 53(4):719
19. Topping NH, Atlas LT. 1947. *Science (1979)*. 106(2765):636–37
20. Dochez AR, Shibley GS, Mills KC. 1930. *J Exp Med*. 52(5):701–16
21. Vaughan V, Vaughan H, Palmer G. 1922. *Epidemiology and Public Health: A Text and Reference Book for Physicians, Medical Students and Health Workers*, Vol. 1. Michian: C. V Mosby Company
22. Misra S. 2012. *Indian J Sex Transm Dis AIDS*. 33(2):131
23. Kaptchuk TJ. 2002. *Ann Intern Med*. 136(11):817
24. Kaptchuk TJ. 2011. *Philosophical Transactions of the Royal Society B: Biological Sciences*. 366(1572):1849–58
25. Benedetti F. 2012. *J Acupunct Meridian Stud*. 5(3):97–103

26. Andrewes CH. 1950. *NEJM*. 242(7):235–40

27. Kerr JR, Taylor-Robinson D. 2007. *Biographical Memoirs of Fellows of the Royal Society*. 53:349–63

28. Schmelzer D, Schlemmer P, Schobersberger W, Blank C. 2023. *World Leis J*. 65(3):408–26

29. Vingerhoets AJJM, van Huijgevoort M, van Heck GL. 2002. *Psychother Psychosom*. 71(6):311–17

30. Mwale S. 2017. *Healthy Volunteers in Commercial Clinical Drug Trials: When Human Beings Become Guinea Pigs*. Brighton: Springer

Chapter 15 References

1. Killingley B, et al. 2013. *Influenza Respir Viruses*. 7:42–51
2. Kutter JS, Spronken MI, et al. 2018. *Curr Opin Virol*. 28:142–51
3. Cowan T, Fallon S. 2021. *The Contagion Myth*. Skyhorse
4. Engelbrecht T, Koehnlein C, de Harven E, Bailey S, Scoglio S. 2021. *Virus Mania*. Books on Demand. 3rd ed.
5. Weinstein R, et al. 2006. *Clin Inf Dis*. 42(5):737–737
6. Nguyen-Van-Tam JS, et al. 2020. *PLoS Pathog*. 16(7):e1008704
7. *Key Facts About Influenza*. 2021. Centers for Disease Control
8. *Prevention Strategies for Seasonal Influenza in Healthcare Settings*. 2021. Centers for Disease Control
9. Brankston G, Gitterman L, Hirji Z, Lemieux C, Gardam M. 2007. *Lancet Infect Dis*. 7(4):257–65
10. Chen W, Zhang N, et al. 2020. *Build Environ*. 176:106859
11. Myatt TA, Johnston SL, et al. 2003. *BMC Public Health*. 3(1):5
12. Jennings LC, Dick EC, et al. 1988. *J Infect Dis*. 158(4):888–92
13. Dick EC, Jennings LC, Mink KA, Wartgow CD, Inborn SL. 1987. *J Infect Dis*. 156(3):442–48
14. Meschievitz CK, et al. 1984. *J Infect Dis*. 150(2):195–201
15. Rocha ALS, Pinheiro JR, Nakamura TC, da Silva JDS, Rocha BGS, et al. 2021. *Sci Rep*. 11(1):15960
16. Zhang N, Chen X, et al. 2021. *J Infect*. 83(2):207–16
17. Sommerstein R, Fux CA, Vuichard-Gysin D, Abbas M, Marschall J, et al. 2020. *Antimicrob Resist Infect Control*. 9(1):100
18. Moreno T, Gibbons W. 2022. *Geoscience Frontiers*. 13(6):101282
19. Tang JW, Bahnfleth WP, Bluyssen PM, Buonanno G, Jimenez JL, et al. 2021. *J Hospital Infec*. 110:89–96
20. Weinstein RA, et al. 2003. *Clin Infect Dis*. 37(8):1094–1101
21. Cannell JJ, Zasloff M, et al. *Virol J*. 5(1):29
22. Rosenbaum MJ, et al. 1971. *Am J Epidemiol*. 93(3):183–93
23. Reed SE. 1975. *Journal of Hygiene*. 75(2):249–58
24. Gwaltney JM, et al. 1978. *Trans Am Clin Climatol Assoc*. 89:194–200
25. MacMichael I. 1962. *The Common Cold*. Edinburgh: University of Edinburgh
26. Hassan SA, Sheikh FN, Jamal S, Ezeh JK, Akhtar A. 2020. *Cureus*
27. Gaitonde D, et al. 2019. *Am Fam Physician*. 100(12):751–58
28. Kindt PH, Chakraborty T, et al. 2022. *Commun ACM*. 65(1):56–67

29. Kerr W, Lagen J. 1934. *Exp Biol Med.* 31(6):713–15

30. Buckland FE, Bynoe ML, Tyrrell DAJ. 1965. *J Hygiene.* 63(3):327–43

31. Gwaltney J, Moskalski P, Hendley J. 1978. *Ann Intern Med.* 88(4):463

32. D'Alessio DJ, et al. 1984. *J Infect Dis.* 150(2):189–94

33. Fildes P, McIntosh J. 1920. *Br J Exp Pathol.* 1(3):159–74

34. Gwaltney JM. 1980. *Ann N Y Acad Sci.* 353(1):54–60

35. Song F, Parekh-Bhurke S, Hooper L, Loke YK, Ryder JJ, et al. 2009. *BMC Med Res Methodol.* 9(1):79

36. Begg CB, Berlin JA. 1988. *J R Stat Soc Ser A.* 151(3):419

37. D'Alessio DJ, et al. 1976. *J Infect Dis.* 133(1):28–36

38. Jennings LC, Dick EC. 1987. *Eur J Epidemiol.* 3(4):327–35

39. Hall CB, Douglas RG. 1981. *J Pediatr.* 99(1):100–103

40. *Influenza (Flu).* 2022. Centers for Disease Control and Prevention

41. Townsend J. 1924. *U.S Public Health Service.* 48:1–68

42. Hirsch A. 1883. *Handbook of Geographical and Historical Pathology.* New Sydenham Society

43. Hope-Simpson E. 1992. *The Transmission of Epidemic Influenza.* New York: Springer Science

44. Sisley R. 1891. *Epidemic Influenza: Notes on its Origin and Method of Spread.* London: Longman, Green and Co.

45. Creighton C. 2014. *A History of Epidemics in Britain: Volume 2, From the Extinction of Plague to the Present Time.* Cambridge University Press

46. Wilson EA. 1905. *BMJ.* 2(2323):77–80

47. Ommanney F. 2023. *Richard E. Byrd.* Encyclopedia Britannica

48. Ellsworth L. 1937. *Geogr J.* 89(3):193

49. Kerr W. 1936. *JAMA.* 107(5):323

50. Allen TR, Bradburne AF, Stott EJ, Goodwin CS, Tyrrell DAJ. 1973. *Epidemiol Infect.* 71(4):657–67

51. Bean B, Moore BM, Sterner B, Peterson LR, Gerding DN, Balfour HH. 1982. *J Infect Dis.* 146(1):47–51

52. Hedblom E. 1965. Polar Manual

Chapter 16 References

1. Reeves RR, Ladner ME, Hart RH, Burke RS. 2007. *Gen Hosp Psychiatry*. 29(3):275–77

2. von Wernsdorff M, Loef M, Tuschen-Caffier B, Schmidt S. 2021. *Sci Rep*. 11(1):3855

3. Schweiger A, Parducci A. 1981. *Pavlov J Biol Sci*. 16(3):140–43

4. Moseley JB, O'Malley K, Petersen NJ, Menke TJ, Brody BA, et al. 2002. *NEJM*. 347(2):81–88

5. Fielding JWL, Fagg SL, Jones BG, Ellis D, Hockey MS, et al. 1983. *World J Surg*. 7(3):390–99

6. Meador C. 1992. *Southern Med J*. 85(3):244–47

7. Blakeslee S. 1998. *Placebos Prove so Powerful Even Experts are Surprised; New Studies Explore the Brain's Triumph Over Reality*. New York Times

8. Agnihotri K. 2020. *Can Fam Physician*. 66(11):862–64

9. Unknown. 1919. *An Official Test*. Glendale Evening News. 1–4 pp.

10. Barry JM. 2009. *Nature*. 459(7245):324–25

11. Kerr W. 1936. *JAMA*. 107(5):323

12. Dochez AR, Shibley GS, Mills KC. 1930. *J Exp Med*. 52(5):701–16

13. Jackson G, Dowling H, Anderson T, Riff L, Saporta J. 1960. *Ann Intern Med*. 53(4):719

14. Cohen S, Doyle WJ, Turner RB, Alper CM, Skoner DP. 2003. *Psychosom Med*. 65(4):652–57

15. Cohen S, Alper CM, Doyle WJ, Treanor JJ, Turner RB. 2006. *Psychosomatic Med*. 68(6):809–15

16. Pagnini F, Cavalera C, Volpato E, Banfi P. 2020. *Complement Ther Med*. 50:102396

Chapter 17 References

1. Fischer V, O'Mara SM. 2022. *Prog Brain Res.* 274(1):1–30
2. Riggio RE, Riggio CR. 2022. In *Reference Module in Neuroscience and Biobehavioral Psychology.* Elsevier
3. Bauch CT, Galvani AP. 2013. *Science (1979).* 342(6154):47–49
4. Jones T. 2000. *Am Fam Physician.* 62(12):2649–53
5. Prochazkova E, Kret ME. 2017. *Neurosci Biobehav Rev.* 80:99–114
6. Acharya S, Shukla S. 2012. *J Nat Sci Biol Med.* 3(2):118
7. Sonnby–Borgström M. 2002. *Scand J Psychol.* 43(5):433–43
8. Kelly JR, Iannone NE, McCarty MK. 2016. *Br J Social Psych.* 55(1):182–91
9. Rosenthal SB, Twomey CR, Hartnett AT, Wu HS, Couzin ID. 2015. *Proc Natl Acad Sci.* 112(15):4690–95
10. Morreall J. 1993. *J Phil.* 90(7):359–66
11. Buchanan TW, Bagley SL, Stansfield RB, Preston SD. 2012. *Soc Neurosci.* 7(2):191–201
12. Norscia I, Zanoli A, Gamba M, Palagi E. 2020. *Front Psychol.* 11(442):1–8
13. Palagi E, Celeghin A, Tamietto M, Winkielman P, Norscia I. 2020. *Neurosci Biobehav Rev.* 111:149–65
14. Massen JJM, Dusch K, Eldakar OT, Gallup AC. 2014. *Physiol Behav.* 130:145–48
15. Franzen A, Mader S, Winter F. 2018. *J Exp Psychol Gen.* 147(12):1950–58
16. Gupta S, Mittal S. 2013. *Int J Appl Basic Med Res.* 3(1):11
17. Lobstein T, Jackson-Leach R, Powis J, Brinsden H, Gray M. 2023. World Obesity Atlas 2023. London
18. Kolata G. 2007. *Study Says Obesity Can Be Contagious.* New York Times
19. Huang H, Yan Z, Chen Y, Liu F. 2016. *Sci Rep.* 6(1):37961
20. Christakis NA, Fowler JH. 2007. *NEJM.* 357(4):370–79
21. Ponterio E, Gnessi L. 2015. *Viruses.* 7(7):3719–40
22. Cancelier ACL, V. Dhurandhar N, Peddibhotla S, Atkinson RL, Silva HCG, et al. 2021. *J Pediatr (Rio J).* 97(4):420–25
23. Na HN, Nam JH. 2011. *J Bacteriol Virol.* 41(2):65
24. Pasarica M, Dhurandhar N V. 2007. *Adv Food Nutr Res.* 52:61–102
25. McClintock M. 1971. *Nature.* 229(5282):244–45

26. Graham CA, McGrew WC. 1980. *Psychoneuroendocrinology.* 5(3):245–52

27. Quadagno DM, Shubeita HE, Deck J, Francoeur D. 1981. *Psychoneuroendocrinology.* 6(3):239–44

28. Ziomkiewicz A. 2006. *Human Nature.* 17(4):419–32

29. Russell MJ, Switz GM, Thompson K. 1980. *Pharmacol Biochem Behav.* 13(5):737–38

30. Cutler WB, Preti G, Krieger A, Huggins GR, Garcia CR, Lawley HJ. 1986. *Horm Behav.* 20(4):463–73

31. Knight C. 1991. *Blood Relations: Menstruation and the Origins of Culture.* London: Yale University Press

32. Benedetti F, Durando J, Vighetti S. 2014. *Pain.* 155(5):921–28

33. Hendriksen E. 2016. *Is Depression Contagious?* Scientific American

34. Parkinson B, Simons G. 2012. *Cogn Emot.* 26(3):462–79

35. Foulk T, Woolum A, Erez A. 2016. *J App Psychol.* 101(1):50–67

36. Schut C, Grossman S, Gieler U, Kupfer J, Yosipovitch G. 2015. *Front Human Neurosci.* 9(57):1–6

37. Geangu E, Benga O, Stahl D, Striano T. 2010. *Infant Behav Dev.* 33(3):279–88

38. Fowler JH, Christakis NA. 2008. *BMJ.* 337(dec04 2):a2338–a2338

39. Provine RR. 2005. *Behav Brain Sci.* 28(2):142–142

40. Wild B, Erb M, Eyb M, Bartels M, Grodd W. 2003. *Psychiatry Res Neuroimaging.* 123(1):17–36

41. Cacioppo JT, Fowler JH, Christakis NA. 2009. *J Pers Soc Psychol.* 97(6):977–91

42. Hu F, Shi X, Wang H, Nan N, Wang K, et al. 2021. *Front Public Health.* 9(691746):1–15

43. MacKrill K, Gamble GD, Bean DJ, Cundy T, Petrie KJ. 2019. *Clin Psychol Eur.* 1(1):1–12

44. MacKrill K, Gamble GD, Petrie KJ. 2020. *Clin Psychol Eur.* 2(2):1–14

45. Faasse K, Gamble G, Cundy T, Petrie KJ. 2012. *BMJ Open.* 2(4):e001607

46. Giri SP, Maurya AK. 2021. *Pers Individ Dif.* 180:110962

47. MacKrill K, Morrison Z, Petrie KJ. 2021. *J Psychosom Res.* 150:110630

48. Witthöft M, Rubin GJ. 2013. *J Psychosom Res.* 74(3):206–12

49. Bräscher A-K, Raymaekers K, Van den Bergh O, Witthöft M. 2017. *Environ Res.* 156:265–71

50. Verrender A, Loughran SP, Dalecki A, Freudenstein F, Croft RJ. 2018. *Environ Res.* 166:409–17

51. Domaradzki J. 2021. *Int J Environ Res Public Health.* 18(5):2396

52. Surette R. 2017. In *Oxford Research Encyclopedia of Criminology and Criminal Justice.* Oxford University Press

53. Viridiana Rios, Ferguson CJ. 2020. *Justice Quarterly.* 37(6):1012–39

54. Helfgott J. 2015. *Aggress Violent Behav.* 22:46–64

55. Guilbeault D, Becker J, Centola D. 2018. In *Complex Spreading Phenomena in Social Systems,* pp. 3–25. Springer

56. Pandey J. 2022. In *Nature and Dynamics of Social Influence,* pp. 203–14. Singapore: Springer Nature Singapore

57. Hawkes N. 2010. *BMJ.* 340(2):c789–c789

58. Wagner-Egger P, Bangerter A, Gilles I, Green E, Rigaud D, et al. 2011. *Public Understanding of Science.* 20(4):461–76

59. Bonneux L, Damme W V. 2010. *BMJ.* 340(jun09 3):c3065–c3065

60. Tarafder BK, Khan MAI, Islam MdT, Mahmud SA Al, Sarker MdHK, et al. 2016. *Psychiatry J.* 2016:1–5

61. Ayehu M, Endriyas M, Mekonnen E, Shiferaw M, Misganaw T. 2018. *Int J Ment Health Syst.* 12(1):31

62. 2000. *Am Fam Physician.* 62(12):2655–56

63. Sirois F. 1974. *Acta Psychiatr Scand Suppl.* 252:1–46

64. Waller JC. 2008. *Endeavour.* 32(3):117–21

65. Waller J. 2009. *Lancet.* 373(9664):624–25

66. Rankin P, Philip A. 1963. *Central African J Med.* 9(5):167–70

67. Olkinuora M. 1984. *Scand J Work Environ Health.* 10(6):501–4

68. Radovanovic Z. 1996. *Eur J Epidemiol.* 12(1):101–13

69. Nemery B, Fischler B, Boogaerts M, Lison D. 1999. *Lancet.* 354(9172):77

70. Gallay A. 2002. *Am J Epidemiol.* 155(2):140–47

Chapter 18 References

1. Moncrieff J, Cooper RE, Stockmann T, Amendola S, Hengartner MP, Horowitz MA. 2022. *Mol Psychiatry*. 28:3243–56
2. Cappuccio FP, Campbell NRC, He FJ, Jacobson MF, MacGregor GA, et al. 2022. *Curr Nutr Rep*. 11(2):172–84
3. Neculita CS, McKay R. 2020. *Transnatl Corp Rev*. 12(2):173–92
4. Riley D. 1988. In *Interstitial Lung Diseases in Children*. 1:31–40. Taylor and Francis
5. Ananda Rao A, Johncy S. 2022. *Cureus*. 14(1):1–10
6. Nawroth JC, van der Does AM, Ryan (Firth) A, Kanso E. 2020. *Phil Transactions Roy Soc*. 375(1792):20190160
7. Ball M, Hossain M, Padalia D. 2023. *Anatomy, Airway*
8. Kippelen P, Anderson SD, Hallstrand TS. 2018. *Immunol Allergy Clin North Am*. 38(2):165–82
9. D'Amato M, Molino A, Calabrese G, Cecchi L, Annesi-Maesano I, D'Amato G. 2018. *Clin Transl Allergy*. 8(1):20
10. Hanstock HG, Ainegren M, Stenfors N. 2020. *Front Sports Act Living*. 2(34):1–11
11. Bustamante-Marin XM, Ostrowski LE. 2017. *Cold Spring Harb Perspect Biol*. 9(4):a028241
12. Bayramoglu A, Erdogan K, Urhan O, Keskinoz EN, Acikel Elmas M, et al. 2022. *J Cosmet Dermatol*. 21(3):1086–92
13. Taherali F, Varum F, Basit AW. 2018. *Adv Drug Deliv Rev*. 124:16–33
14. Kuek LE, Lee RJ. 2020. *Am J Physiol Lung Cell Mol Physiol*. 319(4):L603–19
15. Naeem A, Rai SN, Pierre L. 2023. *Histology, Alveolar Macrophages*
16. Williams R, Rankin N, Smith T, Galler D, Seakins P. 1996. *Crit Care Med*. 24(11):1920–29
17. Wolkoff P. 2018. *Environ Int*. 121:1058–65
18. Cui X, Lai W, Zhao Y, Chen C. 2023. *Environ Sci Technol*. 57(21):7891–7901
19. Serman E, Thrastarson H, Franklin M, Teixeira J. 2022. *Geohealth*. 6(2):e2021GH000469
20. Callahan CW, Elansari AM, Fenton DL. 2019. In *Postharvest Technology of Perishable Horticultural Commodities*, pp. 271–310. Elsevier
21. Lowen AC, Steel J. 2014. *J Virol*. 88(14):7692–95

22. Shaman J, Pitzer V, Viboud C, Lipsitch M, Grenfell B. 2009. *PLoS Curr.* 1:RRN1138

23. Shaman J, Goldstein E, Lipsitch M. 2011. *Am J Epidemiol.* 173(2):127–35

24. Wood W, Marshall S, Fargey S. 2018. *Earth Syst. Sci. Data*

25. Shaman J, Kandula S, Yang W, Karspeck A. 2017. *PLoS Comput Biol.* 13(11):e1005844

26. Shaman J, Pitzer VE, Viboud C, Grenfell BT, Lipsitch M. 2010. *PLoS Biol.* 8(2):e1000316

27. Mäkinen TM, Juvonen R, Jokelainen J, Harju TH, Peitso A, et al. 2009. *Respir Med.* 103(3):456–62

28. Lidwell OM, Morgan RW, Williams REO. 1965. *J Hyg.* 63(3):427–39

29. Simpson R. 1958. *Proc R Soc Med.* 51(267):267–71

30. Green J, Dyer I. 2009. *Anaesth Intensive Care Med.* 10(1):45–47

31. Shoji M, Katayama K, Sano K. 2011. *Tohoku J Exp Med.* 224(4):251–56

32. Shimmei K, Nakamura T, Ng CFS, Hashizume M, Murakami Y, et al. 2020. *Sci Rep.* 10(1):7764

33. NASA. 2022. *NASA Finds Each State Has Its Own Climatic Threshold for Flu Outbreaks.* Jet Propulsion Laboratory

34. Tamerius JD, Shaman J, Alonso WJ, Bloom-Feshbach K, Uejio CK, et al. 2013. *PLoS Pathog.* 9(3):e1003194

35. Jaakkola K, Saukkoriipi A, Jokelainen J, Juvonen R, Kauppila J, et al. 2014. *Environmental Health.* 13(1):22

36. Ikäheimo T, Jaakkola K, Jokelainen J, Saukkoriipi A, Roivainen M, et al. 2016. *Viruses.* 8(9):244

37. Deyle ER, Maher MC, Hernandez RD, Basu S, Sugihara G. 2016. *Proc Natl Acad Sci.* 113(46):13081–86

38. Lipsitch M, Viboud C. 2009. *Proc Natl Acad Sci.* 106(10):3645–46

39. Tamerius J, Nelson MI, Zhou SZ, Viboud C, Miller MA, Alonso WJ. 2011. *Environ Health Perspect.* 119(4):439–45

40. Baskerville EB, Cobey S. 2017. *Proc Natl Acad Sci.* 114(12):e2270–71

41. Kudo E, Song E, Yockey LJ, Rakib T, Wong PW, et al. 2019. *Proc Natl Acad Sci.* 116(22):10905–10

42. Kashef Z. 2019. *Flu Virus' Best Friend: Low Humidity.* Yale News

43. Eccles R. 2002. *Rhinology.* 40(3):109–14

44. Thai PQ, Choisy M, Duong TN, Thiem VD, Yen NT, et al. 2015. *Epidemics.* 13:65–73

45. Suntronwong N, Vichaiwattana P, Klinfueng S, Korkong S, Thongmee T, et al. 2020. *PLoS One*. 15(9):e0239729

46. Yuan H, Kramer SC, Lau EHY, Cowling BJ, Yang W. 2021. *PLoS Comput Biol*. 17(6):e1009050

47. Chew F, Doraisingham S, Ling A, Kumarasinghe G, Lee B. 1998. *Epidemiol Infect*. 121(1):121–28

48. Chumkiew S, Jaroensutasinee K, Jaroensutasinee M. 2007. *Int J Med Health Sci*. 1(12):364–67

49. Mello WA de, Paiva TM de, Ishida MA, Benega MA, Santos MC dos, et al. 2009. *PLoS One*. 4(4):e5095

50. Ndiaye K, Mathiot C, Spiegel A, Sagna M, Dosseh A. 2000. *Am J Trop Med Hyg*. 62(5):639–43

51. Moura FEA, Perdigão ACB, Siqueira MM. 2009. *Am J Trop Med Hyg*. 81(1):180–83

52. Yang L, Wong CM, Lau EHY, Chan KP, Ou CQ, Peiris JSM. 2008. *PLoS One*. 3(1):e1399

53. Viboud C, Alonso WJ, Simonsen L. 2006. *PLoS Med*. 3(4):e89

54. Lee VJ, Yap J, Ong JBS, Chan K-P, Lin RTP, et al. 2009. *PLoS One*. 4(12):e8096

55. Lofgren E, Fefferman NH, Naumov YN, Gorski J, Naumova EN. 2007. *J Virol*. 81(11):5429–36

56. Chen S, Liu C, Lin G, Hänninen O, Dong H, Xiong K. 2021. *Environ Health Prev Med*. 26(1):109

57. Noti JD, Blachere FM, McMillen CM, Lindsley WG, Kashon ML, et al. 2013. *PLoS One*. 8(2):e57485

58. Moozhipurath RK, Kraft L. 2021. *Sci Rep*. 11(1):2757

59. Anastasiou OE, Hüsing A, Korth J, Theodoropoulos F, Taube C, et al. 2021. *Pathogens*. 10(2):187

60. Sagripanti J, Lytle CD. 2007. *Photochem Photobiol*. 83(5):1278–82

61. Schuit M, Gardner S, Wood S, Bower K, Williams G, et al. 2020. *J Infect Dis*. 221(3):372–78

62. Sagripanti J, Lytle CD. 2020. *Photochem Photobiol*. 96(4):731–37

63. Ishmatov A. 2017. *PeerJ Preprints*

64. Yang W, Elankumaran S, Marr LC. 2012. *PLoS One*. 7(10):e46789

65. Davey ML, Reid D. 1972. *J Epidemiol Community Health (1978)*. 26(1):28–32

66. Sisley R. 1891. *Epidemic Influenza: Notes on its Origin and Method of Spread*. London: Longman, Green and Co.

67. Farr W. 1885. *Vital Statistics; A Memorial Volume of Selections from the Reports and Writings of William Farr*. London: Sanitary Institute London

68. Eade P. 1894. *BMJ*. 1(1738):846–48

69. Townsend J. 1924. *U.S Public Health Service*. 48:1–68

70. van Loghem JJ. 1928. *J Hyg*. 28(1):33–54

71. Semple A. 1951. *Proc Roy Soc Med*. 44:794–96

72. Johnson C, Eccles R. 2005. *Fam Pract*. 22(6):608–13

73. Lowen AC, Mubareka S, Steel J, Palese P. 2007. *PLoS Pathog*. 3(10):e151

74. Jackson G, Dowling H, Spiesman I, Boand A. 1958. *AMA Arch Intern Med*. 101(2):267

75. Douglas RG, Lindgren KM, Couch RB. 1968. *NEJM*. 279(14):742–47

76. Foster H. 2014. *The Reason for the Season: Why Flu Strikes in Winter*. Harvard University

77. Ellsworth H. 1920. *Ecology*. 1(1):6–23

78. Antunes L, Silva SP, Marques J, Nunes B, Antunes S. 2017. *Int J Biometeorol*. 61(1):127–35

79. Murtas R, Russo AG. 2019. *BMC Public Health*. 19(1):1445

80. Grant SB, Mudd S, Goldman A. 1920. *J Exp Med*. 32(1):87–112

81. Gahwyler M. 1922. *Schweiz Med Wchnschr*. 52:648

82. Bonadonna P, Senna G, Zanon P, Cocco G, Dorizzi R, et al. 2001. *Am J Rhinol*. 15(5):297–301

83. Scarupa MD, Kaliner MA. 2009. *World Allergy Org J*. 2(3):20–25

84. Silvers W. 1991. *Ann Allergy*. 67(1):32–36

85. Mudd S, Goldman A, Grant SB. 1921. *J Exp Med*. 34(1):11–45

86. Schade H. 1919. *Z Gesamte Exp Med*. 7(1):275–374

87. Mudd S, Grant SB, Goldman A. 1921. *Ann Otol Rhinol Laryngol*. 30(1):1–73

88. Wakamura T, Tokura H. 2002. *J Therm Biol*. 27(5):439–47

89. Wever RA. 1979. *The Circadian System of Man*. New York, NY: Springer New York

90. Teramoto Y, Tokura H, Ioki I, Suho S, Inoshiri R, Masuda M. 1998. *J Therm Biol*. 23(1):15–21

91. Koskela HO. 2007. *Int J Circumpolar Health*. 66(2):91–100

92. Liener K, Leiacker R, Lidemann J, Rettinger G, Keck T. 2003. *Acta Otolaryngol*. 123(7):851–56

93. Cruz A, Naclerio R, Proud D, Togias A. 2006. *J Allergy Clin Immunol.* 117(6):1351–58
94. Giesbrecht G. 1995. *Aviat Space Environ Med.* 66:890–902
95. Eccles R, Wilkinson JE. 2015. *Rhinology.* 53(2):99–106
96. Anderson SD, Daviskas E. 2000. *J Allergy Clin Immunol.* 106(3):453–59
97. Anderson SD, Kippelen P. 2008. *J Allergy Clin Immunol.* 122(2):225–35
98. Larsson K, Tornling G, Gavhed D, Muller-Suur C, Palmberg L. 1998. *Eur Resp J.* 12(4):825–30
99. Cruz A, Togias A. 2008. *Curr Allergy Asthma Rep.* 8(2):111–17
100. Clary-Meinesz C, Cosson J, Huitorel P, Blaive B. 1992. *Biol Cell.* 76(3):335–38
101. Zhao K, Cowan A, Lee R, Goldstein N, Droguett K. 2022. *Adv Geriatr Med Res*
102. Bailey K. 2022. *Adv Geriatr Med Res.* 4(2):e220005
103. Michael Foster W. 2002. *Pulm Pharmacol Ther.* 15(3):277–82
104. Yoshihara S, Geppetti P, Hara M, Lindén A, Ricciardolo FLM, et al. 1996. *Eur J Pharmacol.* 296(3):291–96
105. Proud D, Naclerio RM, Gwaltney JM, Hendley JO. 1990. *J Infect Dis.* 161(1):120–23
106. Naclerio RM, Proud D, Lichtenstein LM, Kagey-Sobotka A, Hendley JO, et al. 1988. *J Infect Dis.* 157(1):133–42
107. Shibayama Y, Skoner D, Suehiro S, Konishi J-E, Fireman P, Kaplan AP. 1996. *Immunopharmacology.* 33(1–3):311–13
108. Groneberg D, Harrison S, Thai Dinh Q, Geppetti P, Fischer A. 2006. *Curr Drug Targets.* 7(8):1005–10
109. Doyle WJ, Skoner DP, Gentile D. 2005. *Curr Allergy Asthma Rep.* 5(3):173–81
110. Davis N. 1891. *JAMA.* 17(7):245
111. Sundblad B-M, Larsson B-M, Acevedo F, Ernstgård L, Johanson G, et al. 2004. *Scand J Work Environ Health.* 30(4):313–21
112. Holma B. 1989. *Environ Health Perspect.* 79:109–13
113. Grose EC, Gardner DE, Miller FJ. 1980. *Environ Res.* 22(2):377–85
114. Helleday R, Huberman D, Blomberg A, Stjernberg N, Sandstrom T. 1995. *Eur Resp J.* 8(10):1664–68
115. Kienast K, Riechelmann H, Knorst M, Schlegel J, Muller-Quernheim J, et al. 1994. *Clin Investig.* 72(3):

116. Su W, Wu X, Geng X, Zhao X, Liu Q, Liu T. 2019. *BMC Public Health.* 19(1):1319

117. Pimple P, Doshi G. 2021. *Intl J Pharm Sci Res.* 12(2):97–232

118. Horvath EP, doPico GA, Barbee RA, Dickie HA. 1978. *J Occup Med.* 20(2):103–10

119. Unknown. 1889. *Science (1979).* 14(350):260–62

120. Oakes JA, Wang RY. 2017. In *Critical Care Toxicology*, pp. 2213–23. Cham: Springer International Publishing

121. Vaughan V. 1887. *Public Health Pap Rep.* 13:123–78

122. Knapp P. 1892. *Boston Med Surg J.* 127(11):253–57

123. Bryson L. 1890. *Southern Med Rec.* 20(3):104–7

124. Canger R. *Manicomio Moderno*, pp. 135–50

125. Dresbach M. 1900. *J Exp Med.* 5(3):315–18

126. Anders HS. 1899. *Trans Am Climatol Assoc.* 15:286–303

127. Bartlett FW. 1883. *Buffalo Med Surg J.* 23(1):1–14

128. Fell GeoE. 1883. *Proc Am Soc Microscopists.* 5:69

129. Augustus H. 1890. *Nature.* 41(1056):271–271

130. Dallas E. 1865. *Once a Week.* 12(287):94–96

131. Hill L, Flack M. 1911. *Proc R Soc London.* 84(573):404–15

132. Barlow J. 1879. *J Anat Physiol.* 14(Pt 1):107-130.3

133. Allegra L, Moavero NE, Rampoldi C. 1991. *Am J Med.* 91(3):S67–71

134. Ali ST, Wu P, Cauchemez S, He D, Fang VJ, et al. 2018. *Eur Resp J.* 51(5):1800369

135. Wang X, Cai J, Liu X, Wang B, Yan L, et al. 2022. *Environ Sci Pollut Res.* 30(4):10426–43

Chapter 19 References

1. Vohra K, Vodonos A, Schwartz J, Marais EA, Sulprizio MP, Mickley LJ. 2021. *Environ Res.* 195:110754

2. Bray F, Ferlay J, Soerjomataram I, Siegel RL, Torre LA, Jemal A. 2018. *CA Cancer J Clin.* 68(6):394–424

3. Wang M, Aaron CP, Madrigano J, Hoffman EA, Angelini E, et al. 2019. *JAMA.* 322(6):546

4. White C. 2023. *Breathing Toxic Air in New York Is Equivalent to Smoking 6 Cigarettes a Day.* The Science Times

5. van der Zee SC, Fischer PH, Hoek G. 2016. *Environ Res.* 148:475–83

6. Millner J. 2015. *Breathing in Beijing's Air is the Equivalent to Smoking FORTY Cigarettes a Day: Smog Map of China Reveals Shocking Extent of Pollution.* Daily Mail

7. Acres T. 2017. *Air Quality in New Delhi Worse than Smoking 50 Cigarettes a Day.* Sky News

8. Zhang Y, Wang S, Feng Z, Song Y. 2022. *Front Public Health.* 2(10):1071229

9. Lawrence H, Hunter A, Murray R, Lim WS, McKeever T. 2019. *J Infect.* 79(5):401–6

10. Li X, Xu J, Wang W, Liang J-J, Deng Z-H, et al. 2021. *PeerJ.* 9:e11397

11. Bhat TA, Kalathil SG, Bogner PN, Miller A, Lehmann P V., et al. 2018. *J Immunol.* 200(8):2927–40

12. Horvath KM, Brighton LE, Herbst M, Noah TL, Jaspers I. 2012. *Clin Immunol.* 142(3):232–36

13. Donaldson K, MacNee W, Stone V. 2006. In *Encyclopedia of Respiratory Medicine*, pp. 104–10. Elsevier

14. Yang J, Fan G, Zhang L, Zhang T, Xu Y, et al. 2023. *Influenza Other Respir Viruses.* 17(7):

15. Pope C. 1996. *J Exposure Analysis Environ Epidemiol.* 6(1):23–24

16. Trinh TT, Trinh TT, Le TT, Nguyen TDH, Tu BM. 2019. *Environ Geochem Health.* 41(2):929–37

17. Stephens ER. 1965. *Weatherwise.* 18(4):172–75

18. Yin P-Y, Chang R-I, Day R-F, Lin Y-C, Hu C-Y. 2021. *Applied Sciences.* 12(1):71

19. Stanway D, Schmollinger C. 2022. *Reuters*

20. Yu W, Ye T, Zhang Y, Xu R, Lei Y, et al. 2023. *Lancet Planet Health.* 7(3):e209–18

21. Toczylowski K, Wietlicka-Piszcz M, Grabowska M, Sulik A. 2021. *Viruses.* 13(4):556

22. Xu T, Liu B, Zhang M, Song Y, Kang L, et al. 2021. *Tellus B Chem Phys Meteorol.* 73(1):1898906

23. Sarkar T, Das S, De A, Nandy P, Chattopadhyay S, et al. 2015. *Comput Biol Chem.* 59:8–15

24. Poovorawan Y. 2014. *Pathog Glob Health.* 108(4):169–70

25. Wu X, Nethery RC, Sabath MB, Braun D, Dominici F. 2020. *Sci Adv.* 6(45):1–6

26. Cheney V. 1928. *Am J Pub Health.* 18(1):15–20

27. Ely TC. 1918. *JAMA.* 71(17):1431

28. Wang T, Zhang Y, Zhang R, Mao Y, Yan J, et al. 2023. *Front Public Health.* 15(11):1145669

29. Kullmann T, Barta I, Antus B, Valyon M, Horvath I. 2008. *Eur Resp J.* 31(2):474–75

30. Rehman T, Welsh MJ. 2023. *Cells.* 12(8):1104

31. Cu Y, Saltzman WM. 2009. *Nat Mater.* 8(1):11–13

32. Clary-Meinesz C, Mouroux J, Cosson J, Huitorel P, Blaive B. 1998. *Eur Resp J.* 11(2):330–33

33. *Particle Pollution Exposure.* 2023. United States Environmental Protection Agency

34. Samet JM, Cheng P-W. 1994. *Environ Health Perspect.* 102(S2):89–103

35. Holma B. 1989. *Environ Health Perspect.* 79:109–13

36. Holma B, Lindegren M, Andersen JM. 1977. *Arch Environ Health Int J.* 32(5):216–26

37. Tony Eissa N, Huston D. 2003. *Therapeutic Targets in Airway Inflammation.* Boca Raton: CRC Press

38. Douglas RG. 1976. *Hosp Pract.* 11(12):43–50

39. Kirkpatrick GL. 1996. *Primary Care: Clinics in Office Practice.* 23(4):657–75

40. Turner RB, Hendley JO, Gwaltney JM. 1982. *J Infect Dis.* 145(6):849–53

41. Kreutzberger A, Sanyal A, Saminathan A. 2022. *Proc Natl Acad Sci.* 119(38):

42. Jacoby DB, Tamaoki J, Borson DB, Nadel JA. 1988. *J Appl Physiol.* 64(6):2653–58

43. Polosa R, Hasani A, Pavia D, Agnew JE, Lai CK, et al. 1992. *Thorax.* 47(11):952–56

44. Munkholm M, Mortensen J. 2014. *Clin Physiol Funct Imaging.* 34(3):171–77

45. Quraishi MS, Jones NS, Mason J. 1998. *Clin Otolaryngol Allied Sci.* 23(5):403–13

46. Naclerio RM, Proud D, Lichtenstein LM, Kagey-Sobotka A, Hendley JO, et al. 1988. *J Infect Dis.* 157(1):133–42

47. Vaughan J, Ngamtrakulpanit L, Pajewski TN, Turner R, Nguyen T-A, et al. 2003. *Eur Resp J.* 22(6):889–94

48. de Lima TM, Kazama CM, Koczulla AR, Hiemstra PS, Macchione M, et al. 2013. *Clinics.* 68(12):1488–94

49. Holma B. 1989. *Environ Health Perspect.* 79:109–13

50. Thangavel P, Park D, Lee Y-C. 2022. *Int J Environ Res Public Health.* 19(12):7511

51. Schlesinger RB. 1985. *Environ Health Perspect.* 63:25–38

52. Hussein T, Atashi N, Sogacheva L, Hakala S, Dada L, et al. 2020. *Atmosphere (Basel).* 11(1):79

53. Erupe ME, Benson DR, Li J, Young L-H, Verheggen B, et al. 2010. *J Geophys Res.* 115(D23):D23216

54. Tricker R, Tricker S. 1999. In *Environmental Requirements for Electromechanical and Electronic Equipment*, pp. 158–94. Elsevier

55. Kalbarczyk R, Kalbarczyk R, Kalbarczyk E, Ziemiańska M. 2019. *J Elem*

56. Lin W, Xu X, Ma Z, Zhao H, Liu X, Wang Y. 2012. *J Environ Sci.* 24(1):34–49

57. Khalaf EM, Mohammadi MJ, Sulistiyani S, Ramírez-Coronel AA, Kiani F, et al. 2022. *Rev Environ Health*

58. Reno AL, Brooks EG, Ameredes BT. 2015. *Environ Health Insights.* 9s1:EHI.S15671

59. Pan X. 2019. In *Encyclopedia of Environmental Health*, pp. 823–29. Elsevier

60. Riechelmann H, Maurer J, Hafner B, Mann WJ, Kienast K. 1995. *Laryngoscope.* 105(3):295–99

61. Chen T-M, Kuschner WG, Gokhale J, Shofer S. 2007. *Am J Med Sci.* 333(4):249–56

62. Zhou X, Gao Y, Wang D, Chen W, Zhang X. 2022. *Front Public Health.* 31(10):854922

63. Ravelli AC, Kreis IA. 1991. *Public Health Rev.* 19(1–4):93–101

64. Su W, Wu X, Geng X, Zhao X, Liu Q, Liu T. 2019. *BMC Public Health.* 19(1):1319

65. Scialla JJ, Anderson CAM. 2013. *Adv Chronic Kidney Dis.* 20(2):141–49

66. Remer T, Manz F. 1995. *J Am Diet Assoc.* 95(7):791–97

67. Vormann J, Goedecke T. 2006. *Swiss J Integrative Med.* 18(5):255–66

68. DiNicolantonio JJ, O'Keefe J. 2021. *Open Heart.* 8(2):e001730

69. Robey IF. 2012. *Nutr Metab (Lond).* 9(1):72

70. Carnauba R, Baptistella A, Paschoal V, Hübscher G. 2017. *Nutrients.* 9(6):538

71. Frassetto LA, Todd KM, Morris RC, Sebastian A. 1998. *Am J Clin Nutr.* 68(3):576–83

72. Osuna-Padilla IA, Leal-Escobar G, Garza-García CA, Rodríguez-Castellanos FE. 2019. *Nefrología.* 39(4):343–54

73. Naude D. 2022. *J Evid Based Integr Med.* 27:2515690X2211423

74. Sikter A. 2022. *Neuropsychopharmacol Hung.* 24(3):126–33

75. Lambert DC, Abramowitz MK. 2021. *Kidney360.* 2(11):1706–15

76. Pham AQT, Xu LHR, Moe OW. 2015. *F1000Res.* 4:1460

77. Østergaard HB, Demirhan I, Westerink J, Verhaar MC, Asselbergs FW, et al. 2022. *Eur J Clin Invest.* 52(9):e13814

78. Rodrigues M, de Castro Mendes F, Paciência I, Cavaleiro Rufo J, Silva D, et al. 2023. *Children.* 10(2):263

79. Fischer H, Widdicombe JH. 2006. *J Membrane Biol.* 211(3):139–50

80. Zajac M, Dreano E, Edwards A, Planelles G, Sermet-Gaudelus I. 2021. *Int J Mol Sci.* 22(7):3384

81. Kostikas K, Papatheodorou G, Ganas K, Psathakis K, Panagou P, Loukides S. 2002. *Am J Respir Crit Care Med.* 165(10):1364–70

82. Cho D-Y, Hajighasemi M, Hwang PH, Illek B, Fischer H. 2009. *Am J Rhinol Allergy.* 23(6):e10–13

83. Mousa HA-L. 2017. *J Evid Based Complementary Altern Med.* 22(1):166–74

84. Gawade A, Bale S. 2020. *Indian Jour Trad Knowledge.* 19(4):S158–63

85. Mammas I, Drysdale S, Theodoridou M, Greenough A, Spandidos D. 2020. *Exp Ther Med.* 20(6):1–1

86. Sokullu E, Soleymani Abyaneh H, Gauthier MA. 2019. *Pharmaceutics.* 11(5):211

87. van der Want JPH, Dijkstra J. 2006. *Arch Virol.* 151(8):1467–98

88. Wang Z, Walker GW, Muir DCG, Nagatani-Yoshida K. 2020. *Environ Sci Technol*. 54(5):2575–84

89. Borowy I. 2021. *University of Chicago Press Journals*. 26(3):411–24

90. Power AL, Tennant RK, Jones RT, Tang Y, Du J, et al. 2018. *Front Earth Sci (Lausanne)*. 6(131):1–18

91. Rajak S, Raza S, Tewari A, Sinha RA. 2022. *Dig Dis Sci*. 67(8):3497–3507

92. Naidu R, Biswas B, Willett IR, Cribb J, Kumar Singh B, et al. 2021. *Environ Int*. 156:106–16

93. European Union. 2022. *Chemicals Production and Consumption Statistics*. Eurostat

94. No Plastic in Nature: Assessing Plastic Ingestion From Nature to People. 2019. Newcastle

95. Rolle-Kampczyk U, Gebauer S, Haange S-B, Schubert K, Kern M, et al. 2020. *Sci Total Environ*. 15(748):142458

96. Lawton G. 2022. *How Our Environment is Making Us Sick – And What We Can Do About It*. New Scientist

97. *Influenza (Seasonal)*. 2023. World Health Organisartion

98. Brahney J, Hallerud M, Heim E, Hahnenberger M, Sukumaran S. 2020. *Science (1979)*. 368(6496):1257–60

99. Carrington D. 2022. *Microplastics Found Deep in Lungs of Living People for First Time*. The Guardian

100. Wang C, Wu W, Pang Z, Liu J, Qiu J, et al. 2023. *J Hazard Mater*. 446:130617

101. Johnstone K, Capra M, Newman B. 2007. Organophosphate Pesticide Exposure in Agricultural Workers. Newcastle

102. Sherpa Awasthi M. 2019. *Open Access J Environ Soil Sci*. 2(2):206–8

103. Antonini JM. 2014. In *Comprehensive Materials Processing*, pp. 49–70. Elsevier

104. van Coevorden AM. 2002. *Arch Dermatol*. 138(6):840–41

105. Wong A, Greene S, Robinson J. 2012. *Aust Fam Physician*. 41(3):141–43

106. Marcovitch H. 2006. *Black's Medical Dictionary*. Scarecrow Press. 41st ed.

107. Weidner C. 1989. *Pediatrics*. 84(6):1124–1124

108. Chen F, Ye Y, Jin B, Yi B, Wei Q, Liao L. 2019. *J Forensic Sci*. 64(3):941–45

109. Borzelleca JF, Skalsky HL. 1980. *J Environ Sci Health, Part B.* 15(6):843–66

110. Björkman L, Sandborgh-Englund G, Ekstrand J. 1997. *Toxicol Appl Pharmacol.* 144(1):156–62

111. Silva MJ, Reidy JA, Samandar E, Herbert AR, Needham LL, Calafat AM. 2005. *Arch Toxicol.* 79(11):647–52

112. Nigg HN, Wade SE. 1992. *Rev Environ Contam Toxicol.* 129:95–119

113. Drobitch RK, Svensson CK. 1992. *Clin Pharmacokinet.* 23(5):365–79

114. Hussain J, Cohen M, O'Malley CJ, Mantri N, Li Y, et al. 2023. *Int J Hyg Environ Health.* 248:114091

115. Kuan W-H, Chen Y-L, Liu C-L. 2022. *Int J Environ Res Public Health.* 19(7):4323

116. Sears ME, Kerr KJ, Bray RI. 2012. *J Environ Public Health.* 2012:1–10

117. Wagner U, Schlebusch H, van der Ven K. 1990. *Fresenius J Anal Chem.* 337(1):77–78

118. Melikian AA, Sun P, Prokopczyk B, El-Bayoumy K, Hoffmann D, et al. 1999. *Cancer Lett.* 146(2):127–34

119. Stachel B, Dougherty RC, Lahl U, Schlösser M, Zeschmar B. 1989. *Andrologia.* 21(3):282–91

120. Pichini S, Zuccaro P, Pacifici R. 1994. *Clin Pharmacokinet.* 26(5):356–73

121. Mehta R V., Sreenivasa MA, Mathew M, Girard AW, Taneja S, et al. 2020. *BMC Public Health.* 20(1):1877

122. Mekonen S, Ambelu A, Wondafrash M, Kolsteren P, Spanoghe P. 2021. *Sci Rep.* 11(1):22053

123. Genuis SJ, Lane K, Birkholz D. 2016. *Biomed Res Int.* 2016:1–10

124. Saieva C, Aprea C, Tumino R, Masala G, Salvini S, et al. 2004. *Sci Total Environ.* 332(1–3):71–80

125. Aijaz A, Vinaik R, Jeschke MG. 2022. *Methods Cell Biol Methods Cell Biol.* 168:191–219

126. Mo Y, Chen J, Humphrey DM, Fodah RA, Warawa JM, Hoyle GW. 2015. *Am J Physiol Lung Cell Mol Physiol.* 308(2):L168–78

127. Roslan N, Urgena K, Wahab M. 2023. *Asia Pac J Med Toxicol.* 12(1):33–37

128. Slager RE, Poole JA, LeVan TD, Sandler DP, Alavanja MCR, Hoppin JA. 2009. *Occup Environ Med.* 66(11):718–24

129. Rastogi S, Tripathi S, Ravishanker D. 2010. *Indian J Occup Environ Med.* 14(2):54

130. Robb EL, Baker MB. 2023. *Organophosphate Toxicity*

131. Geronimo J, Beevers H. 1964. *Plant Physiol.* 39(5):786–93

132. Hardwick K, Wood M, Woolhouse H. 1968. *New Phytologist.* 67(1):79–86

133. Patharkar OR, Walker JC. 2018. *J Exp Bot.* 69(4):733–40

134. *Why Do Trees Lose Their Leaves?* 2020. Forestry and Land Scotland

135. Nesse R. 2019. *Good Reasons for Bad Feelings: Insights from the Frontier of Evolutionary Psychiatry.* Penguin Books Limited

Appendix References

1. Davis D. 1906. *J Infect Dis*. 3(1):1–36
2. Kruse W. 1914. *Munch Med Wschr*. 61:1547
3. Foster G. 1916. *JAMA*. 66(16):1180
4. Dold VH. 1917. *Munch Med Wschr*. 5:143–44
5. Nuzum J, Pilot I, Bonar B, Stangl F. 1918. *JAMA*. 71(19):1562
6. Selter H. 1918. *Deutsche Med Wschr*. 44(34):932–33
7. Nicolle C, Lebailly C. 1918. *Compt Rend*. 167:607–10
8. Dujarric de la Rivière R. 1918. *Compt Rend*. 167:606–7
9. Rosenau M, Keegan W, Goldberger G. 1918. *Hygienic Laboratory*. 123:5–30
10. McCoy G, Richey D. 1918. *Hygienic Laboratory*. 123:42–51
11. Rosenau M, Keegan W, Richey D, McCoy G, Goldberger J, et al. 1919. *Hygienic Laboratory*. 123:54–90
12. Yamanouchi T, Sakakami K, Iwashima S. 1919. *Lancet*. 193(4997):971
13. Michelli F, Satta G. 1919. *J R Acad Med Turin*, pp. 115–36
14. Paraf J, Goubalt A. 1919. *Soc. méd. des hôp. de Paris*. 3(4):63
15. Schofield F, Cynn HC. 1919. *JAMA*. 72(14):981
16. Lister F, Taylor E. 1919. *Public South African Inst Med Res*. 12(9):9–23
17. Wahl HR, White GB, Lyall HW. 1919. *J Infect Dis*. 25(5):419–26
18. Sellards A, Sturm E. 1919. *Bull Johns Hopkins Hosp*. 30:331
19. Bloomfield A. 1920. *John's Hopkins Hospital Bulletin*. 31(349):1
20. Schmidt P. 1920. *Deutsch Med Wschr*. 46(43):1181–82
21. Cecil RL, Steffen GI. 1921. *J Infect Dis*. 28(3):201–25
22. Williams A, Nevin M, Gurley C, Mann A, Hussey H, Bittman F. 1921. *J Immunol*. 6(1):5–24
23. Robertson R, Groves R. 1924. *J Infect Dis*. 34(4):400–406
24. Walker J. 1929. *J Infect Dis*. 1929:254–56
25. Shibley G, Mills K, Dochez A. 1930. *JAMA*. 95(21):1553
26. Dochez AR, Mills KC, Kneeland Y. 1931. *Exp Biol Med*. 28(5):513–16
27. Dochez AR, Mills KC, Kneeland Y. 1931. *Exp Biol Med*. 29(1):64–66
28. Powell HM, Clowes GHA. 1931. *Exp Biol Med*. 29(3):332–35
29. Costa-Mandry O, Morales-Otero P, Suarez J. 1932. *Puerto Rico J Public Health Trop Med*. 8:205–19

30. Dochez AR, Mills KC, Kneeland Y. 1933. *Exp Biol Med*. 30(8):1017–22

31. Kerr W, Lagen J. 1934. *Exp Biol Med*. 31(6):713–15

32. Andrewes C, Smith W, Laidlaw P. 1935. *Br J Exp Pathol*. 16(6):566–82

33. Smorodintseff AA, Tushinsky MD, Drobyshevskaya AI, Korovin AA, Osetroff AI. 1937. *Am J Med Sci*. 194(2):159–70

34. Francis T, Magill TP. 1937. *Journal of Experimental Medicine*. 65(2):251–59

35. Burnet F, Lush D. 1938. *Br J Exp Pathol*. 19(1):17–29

36. Francis T. 1940. *Exp Biol Med*. 43(2):337–39

37. Topping NH, Atlas LT. 1947. *Science (1979)*. 106(2765):636–37

38. The Commission On Acute Respiratory Diseases. 1947. *J Clin Invest*. 26(5):957–73

39. Andrewes CH. 1949. *The Lancet*. 253(6541):71–75

40. Andrewes CH, Lovelock JE, Sommerville T. 1951. *Lancet*. 257(6645):25–27

41. Lovelock JE, Roden AT, Porterfield JS, Sommerville T, Andrewes CH. 1952. *Lancet*. 260(6736):657–60

42. Quilligan J, Minuse E, Francis T. 1954. *Journal of Laboratory and Clinical Medicine*. 43(1):43–47

43. Bell JA. 1957. *J Am Med Assoc*. 165(11):1366

44. Dowling H, Jackson G, Inouye T. 1957. *J Lab Clin Med*. 50(4):516–25

45. Jackson G, Dowling H, Spiesman I, Boand A. 1958. *AMA Arch Intern Med*. 101(2):267

46. Dowling H, Jackson G, Spiesman I, Inouye T. 1958. *Am J Epidemiol*. 68(1):59–65

47. Tyrrell D, Bynoe M. 1958. *The Lancet*. 272(7053):931–33

48. Jackson GG, Dowling HF. 1959. *Journal of Clinical Investigation*. 38(5):762–69

49. Tyrrell DAJ, Bynoe ML, Petersen KB, Sutton RNP, Pereira MS. 1959. *BMJ*. 2(5157):909–11

50. Jackson G, Dowling H, Mogabgab W. 1960. *Journal of Laboratory and Clinical Medicine*. 55(3):331–41

51. Tyrrell DAJ, Hitchcock G, Bynoe ML, Pereira HG, Andrewes CH. 1960. *The Lancet*. 275(7118):235–37

52. Kapikian AZ. 1961. *JAMA*. 178(6):537

53. Bynoe M. 1961. *The Lancet*. 277(7188):1194–96

54. Buckland FE, Bynoe ML, Rosen L, Tyrrell DAJ. 1961. *BMJ.* 1(5223):397–400

55. Taylor-Robinson D, Bynoe ML. 1963. *Epidemiol Infect.* 61(4):407–17

56. Taylor-Robinson D, Bynoe M. 1964. *Br Med J.* 1(5382):540–44

57. Cate TR, Couch RB, Johnson KM. 1964. *Journal of Clinical Investigation.* 43(1):56–67

58. Buckland FE, Bynoe ML, Tyrrell DAJ. 1965. *J Hygiene.* 63(3):327–43

59. Fleet W, Couch R, Thomas C, Vernon K. 1965. *Am J Epidemiol.* 82(2):185–96

60. Hoorn B, Bynoe ML, Chapple PJ, Tyrrell DAJ. 1966. *Arch Gesamte Virusforsch.* 18(2):226–30

61. Gordon D, Alford R, Cate T, Couch R. 1966. *Ann Intern Med.* 64(3):521

62. Bradburne AF, Bynoe ML, Tyrrell DA. 1967. *BMJ.* 3(5568):767–69

63. Douglas RG, Lindgren KM, Couch RB. 1968. *NEJM.* 279(14):742–47

64. Allen TR, Bradburne AF, Stott EJ, Goodwin CS, Tyrrell DAJ. 1973. *Epidemiol Infect.* 71(4):657–67

65. Gwaltney J, Moskalski P, Hendley J. 1978. *Ann Intern Med.* 88(4):463

66. D'Alessio DJ, Meschievitz CK, Peterson JA, Dick CR, Dick EC. 1984. *J Infect Dis.* 150(2):189–94

67. Bardin P, Sanderson G, Robinson B, Holgate S, Tyrrell D. 1996. *European Respiratory Journal.* 9(11):2250–55

68. Bischoff WE. 2010. *Infect Control Hosp Epidemiol.* 31(8):857–59

69. Killingley B, Enstone JE, Greatorex J, Gilbert AS, Lambkin-Williams R, et al. 2012. *J Infect Dis.* 205(1):35–43

70. Nguyen-Van-Tam JS, Killingley B, Enstone J, Hewitt M, Pantelic J, et al. 2020. *PLoS Pathog.* 16(7):e1008704

Made in United States
North Haven, CT
15 May 2024

52521367R00252